Solitary Sex

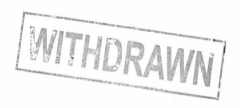

Solitary Sex

A Cultural History of Masturbation

Thomas W. Laqueur

ZONE BOOKS · NEW YORK

2003

© 2003 Thomas Walter Laqueur
Zone Books
40 White Street
New York, NY 10013

Printed in Canada.

Distributed by The MIT Press,
Cambridge, Massachusetts, and London, England

Library of Congress Cataloging-in-Publication Data

Laqueur, Thomas Walter
    Solitary sex : a cultural history of masturbation /
Thomas W. Laqueur.
        p. cm.
    Includes bibliographical references.
    ISBN 1-890951-32-3 (cloth) – ISBN 1-890951-33-1 (pbk.)
    1. Masturbation – History. 2. Masturbation in literature.
3. Sex – Religious aspects. I. Title.

HQ477.L36 2003
306.77′2–dc21

                                        2002028055

Contents

Acknowledgments

Books — or at least my books — are intimately connected to great blocks of life, to conversation, collaboration, and thinking with friends, teachers, colleagues, and students over decades. They are lodged in a history. Finishing is a pleasure: the task is done; the rest refreshing; the glances back to where one has been exhilarating; the offering of thanks a small gesture for great gifts. But the end is also melancholy: the book will not become better, friends have died, and the inevitable changes in one's community — however expected and necessary — speak of finitude and loss.

Lawrence Stone, my mentor and my model for intellectual seriousness and academic engagement, said in the late 1970s that someone really should find out why what he called the hysteria about masturbation appeared so dramatically in the eighteenth century at a time when, he thought, all signs pointed to great acceptance of sexual pleasure. I was past choosing a thesis topic by then and, in any case, he made clear that this was not the sort of problem a young person should take up. I cannot claim that his posing of the question began this book or that in an oedipal moment I set out to disprove his mistaken, if provocative, views on the subject. He was perhaps the greatest venture capitalist of the historical profession during the second half of the twentieth century, but this book is not, in any direct sense, the fruit of his investments in ideas. It is, however, a product of his investment in me. It is buoyed by his energy and his insistence that we engage with history at both the level of intimate life and social change. I wish that he had lived to see my account of a problem he pondered.

7

Except for a short and somewhat misguided few pages in my previous book — not so much wrong as too narrowly framed — this book really began when Roy Porter asked me in 1992 to address a conference at the Wellcome Institute on sexuality and Enlightenment medicine. I delivered on that occasion a paper on the pathophysiology of masturbatory death and disease, on why doctors suddenly came to think that there was an epidemic of solitary sex that was mortally dangerous to the many who succumbed to it. He liked my ideas — truth be told, there were few ideas he did not like — and offered all sorts of support and information. But mostly he was the genie of creativity whose scores of books buoyed up my own and many, many other people's work. He died a few weeks ago and I wish that he could have seen what had come of his invitation and encouragement.

To be truthful, this book did not literally take very long to *write* if one counts not thinking about and researching the topic or the years discussing short preliminary essays, but actually getting words on paper. I wrote the entire draft in one wonderfully happy year as the Berglund Senior Fellow at the National Humanities Center in Research in Triangle Park, North Carolina, whose librarians, staff, and administration — not to speak of my fellow fellows — made it an almost unimaginably agreeable place to work. When Robert Connor, the center's genial, tolerant, and wise director invited me, it was with the understanding that I would spend my time writing a book not on this subject but on memory and mortality. That book, *The Dead Among the Living*, will come soon, but for the time being I want to thank an institution that represents all that is right and good about American academic culture for making this one possible.

Several generations of graduate students, many now teaching around the country, have helped me. I am indebted to: Nasser Hussain for a dossier on the imagination; Lisa Cody for some preliminary prowling around in British libraries; Vanessa Schwartz for checking out some French nineteenth-century medical dissertations in Paris; Arianne Cherncok for a dossier on late-twentieth-century feminism; Kate Fullagar for material on American popular medicine; Catherine Gilhuly for her remarkable report on classical sources, Suzanne Jeblonsky for her reports on Tissot's letters, and Azzan Yadin for his research on the rabbis.

On specific issues well beyond my scholarly competence, I also owe debts to many learned friends. I could not have written about onanism and the Jewish tradition without the help of Daniel Boyarin, Brian Britt, Naomi Janowitz, Davie Biale, and Jack Levison; Herbert Schreier, MD, Chief of Psychiatry at Oakland Children's Hospital, answered many questions about masturbation and various neurological and psychological conditions; Guy Micco, MD, provided alternative diagnoses to some offered by the doctors I had read. I have acknowledged the generosity of particular scholars on particular points in the endnotes but I want especially to thank: Yaron Toren of St. Johns College, Oxford, for his translation and analysis of Gerson and more generally for helping me with medieval sources; Irv Schiener and Andrew Barshay for their help with Japan generally and Sabine Frühstück for letting me see the manuscript of her forthcoming book on Japanese sexology in the late nineteenth and early twentieth centuries; James Spohrer, the German bibliographer in the Berkeley library, for many years of being ready to resurrect the most obscure and incomplete of references into something findable; Cory Silverberg of Come As You Are in Toronto for information on sex toys; Robert Folkenflix of the Department of English at the University of California, Irvine for a constant stream of late-seventeenth-century literary references; Seth Koven of Villanova for various nineteenth-century tidbits; and Elizabeth Dungan for introducing me to the question of masturbation in contemporary art and for her comments on Chapter 6.

My daughter Hannah did research among her friends regarding the title and suggested that I think about the work of Vito Acconci. Herb and Marion Sandler, in addition to being such good company over the decades and offering help with marketing, about which they are expert, came to represent for me the demanding general reader who might be interested in my subject but not in every twist and turn of academic debate. I hope they find the end result readable. Lee Grossman helped me to become clear that I really wanted to write this book. Meighan Gale has

9

been all an author could ask for in seeing the manuscript into print; Ingrid Sterner was a copyeditor of preternatural precision who brought order to an entropic manuscript. I am also grateful to Amy Griffin and Heather MacDonald for their expert picture research.

Solitary Sex would have been finished at least six months sooner were it not for a generous and intellectually demanding community of friends. Jerry Seigel alone cost me many weeks with his acute criticisms; he has read and encouraged my work since I was in graduate school and I only wish that I could have met his queries more fully in this instance; Cathy Gallagher has been an intellectual soul mate for almost thirty years, from whom I have learned so much that to thank her only for her usual rigorous reading of this particular manuscript is far too small a gesture; Carol Clover, too, has been a longtime partner in various intellectual pursuits, and thanking her for specific references, for insisting on the seriousness of jokes, and for making me take the gender implications of my story more seriously does not quite capture my debt; Marty Jay offered many suggestions for expanding various points and saved me from various errors; Ramona Naddaff and Michel Feher as editors, but far more importantly as friends, have worked through the arguments and organization of this book at various stages of its conception and execution right down to the last minute. I could not have written it without them. Steve Greenblatt saved me from one really embarrassing mistake but, more importantly, has been there as a friend for almost three decades. James Vernon and Thomas Metcalf of my department, although interested in very different questions than those treated in this book, kept me to their high standards of clarity and relevance. Henry Abelove and Harry Oosterhuis, both of whom generously read the entire manuscript, made specific suggestions, and assured me that I was more or less right on the areas in the history of sexuality in which they are expert. My best friend since college, Alexander Nehemas, has seen me through a lot and certainly did his part to help this book along. He was on call for all matters Greek — he found the Venetian Greek late-eighteenth-century translation of Tissot's epochal book on onanism; he helped with ancient Greek words and with Plato and Aristotle. He read and commented on the entire manuscript, although not without some nudging. But what matters most is that he was almost always there to talk. Finally, the historian Carla Hesse has discussed the project with me at every stage. Her moral seriousness, clear analytic intelligence, and fearless, demanding criticism — not every wife is willing to engage a partner who is so quarrelsome in the face of truth — have made this a better work and me a better historian. I am full of love and gratitude to her for not giving up on this book and for the challenge she offers of living with a brilliant colleague.

Finally, the customary release of everyone from any liability for errors of fact and judgment: those that remain are not their fault.

Berkeley, CA
May 2002

CHAPTER ONE

The Beginning

Modern masturbation can be dated with a precision rare in cultural history. It was born in, or very close to, the same year as that wild and woolly and profoundly self-conscious exemplar of "our" kind of human, Jean-Jacques Rousseau. It arrived in the same decade as Daniel Defoe's first novels and the first stock-market crashes. (Readers will remember the repeated jokes — new at the time — in the first chapter of *Gulliver's Travels* that Swift began in 1719: "Mr. Bates, my master"; "my good master Bates.") It is a creature of the Enlightenment.

Modern masturbation is profane. It is not just something that putatively makes those who do it tired, crippled, mad, or blind but an act with serious ethical implications. It is that part of human sexual life where potentially unlimited pleasure meets social restraint; where habit and the promise of just-one-more-time struggle with the dictates of conscience and good sense; where fantasy silences, if only for a moment, the reality principle; and where the autonomous self escapes from the erotically barren here and now into a luxuriant world of its own creation. It hovers between abjection and fulfillment.

Sometime between 1708 and 1716 — "in or around 1712" — the then-anonymous author of a short tract with a long title not only named but actually invented a new disease and a new highly specific, thoroughly modern, and nearly universal engine for generating guilt, shame, and anxiety. Its title: *Onania; or, The Heinous Sin of Self Pollution, and all its Frightful Consequences, in both SEXES Considered, with Spiritual and Physical Advice to those who*

13

have already injured themselves by this abominable practice. And sea-
sonable Admonition to the Youth of the nation of Both SEXES....
There exists, the author warned, "so frequent and so crying an
offense" that the usual sources of moral corruption — "ill books,
bad companions, love stories, lascivious discourses, and other
Provocations to Lust and Wantoness [*sic*]" — will not alone account for it. Whatever its proximal causes, this sin is so widespread because those who engage in it do not know they are doing
something wrong, because what they are doing seems free from
the usual constraints of conscience and community, and because
it seems to have no ill consequences.

Ignorance thus accounts for a great deal. Through "wantonness," or just by being "idle and alone," or by the instruction of
intimates, the young learn to abuse themselves without learning
how wrong and dangerous it is. Secrecy is the reason for ignorance: "All other actions of uncleanness must have a witness, this
needs none." It promises its victims freedom from shame, guilt,
and the restraints of social convention: bashful boys who are too
delicate to approach a girl can satisfy themselves anyway; girls
can use it to "combat strong desires" and refuse disadvantageous
matches without "revealing their weakness to anyone." And,
finally, there is the supposed impunity of the act: no death penalty, as there would be for sodomy; no criminal or social sanctions,
as there would be for fornication or adultery; no punitive consequences of any sort. Or so masturbators, to their peril, might
think. There can be no other explanation for the existence of so
terrible, endemic, but largely unremarked-upon sin, for willful
self-pollution.

To be precise, the problem that had been so long ignored but
that would come to play such a large role in the modern Western
understanding of self and sexuality was this:

> That unnatural Practice by which persons of either sex may defile
> their own bodies, without the Assistance of others. Whilst yielding
> to filthy imagination, they endeavor to imitate and procure for
> themselves that Sensation, which God has ordered to attend the Car-
> nal Commerce of the two sexes for the Continuance of our Species.

The universe of potential perpetrators is capacious: "either sex," alone without the help of others. This offense — unlike sodomy, nocturnal pollution, and a host of others — was one that men and women were equally likely to commit and one for which they were equally morally liable. It was the most democratic and luxuriantly available of unnatural practices. Would-be sinners need only yield to "filthy imagination" in order to "imitate and procure for themselves" the sensations of orgasmic intercourse. This artful practice that had once signified so little would come to represent the psychic depths of boys and girls, men and women — as well as a danger to their relationships with their family, lovers, and the social order more generally — for the next three centuries.

The author — anonymous, but in fact, as we will discover soon, a surgeon of sorts who wrote soft-core medical pornography — invents the brilliant, almost entirely original, and wildly successful association of "willful self-abuse" with the Genesis story of Onan, who spilled his seed upon the ground rather than into the wife of his dead brother and was struck down. Onanism is born. The new sin, he suggests, has the same terrible consequences as the one in the Old Testament: death. Not the hand of God this time but a wounded nature will fell the sinner. In a sense, *Onania* and all that followed are one long effort to support Freud's later claim that it is easy to commit a crime but difficult to remove its traces; both secrecy and impunity are illusory.

Situating this text — and the years around 1712 — in the history of sexuality and selfhood is in some measure an exercise in the history of medicine. Our author says that he was initially of a mind to offer only religious remedies. But he showed his work to a pious physician, whom he told about the problem of people suffering from a secret sin and that no help was available to them. This putative encounter changed history. The pious physician — like the author, anonymous — "imparted to me [the narrator, who identifies himself as the author] two medicines of great efficiency." The one cures oozing and gleets (discharges) of all sorts, in men and women, that are not the result of venereal disease — *fluor albus* (a white vaginal flux), nocturnal effusions, seminal emissions upon urination or defecation; the other cures infertility and impotence, whether caused by venereal disease or not.

Ask for them by name, the publisher Mr. Varenne — a third voice — advises: the "Strengthening Tincture" and the "Prolific Powder." There were also tie-ins: the "Strengthening Tincture" works best with the "Decoction" and the "Injection," for example. Medicine seems to have hijacked morality. The author/narrator in fact distances himself from *Onania*'s therapeutic hucksterism by telling his readers that the physician — not he — started printing up editions of the tract at his own expense — two thousand at a go — and that he "has administered the Medicines with greatest benefit and success in the world" ever since.[1]

Remarkably, this shameless effort to invent a new disease and at the same time offer its cure at a steep price became the founding text for a medical tradition that would draw in the pillars of high-Enlightenment medicine and help create modern sexuality. Scores of dissertations, hundreds of articles, encyclopedia entries, didactic tracts, and many learned tomes would find their origins in 1712. Almost two hundred years later, when many had come to doubt that masturbation caused serious physical harm, a noted French doctor could still find almost a hundred conditions that were either signs or consequences of self-abuse.[2]

But the history of medicine tells only part of the story. Well before and well after 1712, the body was thought to suffer from bad behavior. Medicine had always been something of a moral guide, a kind of ethics of the flesh. That role increased dramatically in the eighteenth century as moral norms became, at least in progressive circles, rooted more in nature and taught in schools, the world of physicians and pedagogues, and less in divine authority and preached in church, the province of priests or pastors. In this context, it is not surprising that cultural anxieties were translated into disease: diseases of civilization, for example, caused by a variety of bad things — too much luxury, too much mental activity and not enough exercise, too much sympathy or too much novel reading, which stirs up the body and its nerves, or diseases that followed upon too much sexual activity. But excessive venery, to take the last example, had been recognized as a medical problem since Antiquity. The fundamental question, therefore, is not why sometime around 1712 masturbation came to be regarded as a medical problem or why around 1920 it stopped being thought to cause disease. More puzzling is why solitary sex in particular became so troubling a moral problem at precisely the time when sexual pleasure itself was enjoying ever more secular approval. The problem is in explaining an ethical transformation of considerable magnitude and staying power; masturbatory diseases were but one of its putative manifestations.

In fact, masturbation continued to be a morally fraught, much-thought-about arena of human sexuality — indeed a critical component of what came to be understood as "sexuality" — long after it stopped being regarded as a cause of real physical harm. It remains so today, even though its most virulent opponents no longer claim that it causes blindness, madness, or other bodily ills. Moral passion and medical danger grew up together, the latter as an expression of the former. But when the threat of physical harm ceased to be persuasive, the anxiety about solitary sex — first voiced around 1712 — did not go away. To the contrary.

Queen Victoria's surgeon, Sir James Paget, for example, wrote in 1879 that the putative ill effects of the solitary vice were best regarded as a form of "sexual hypochondriasis" and that physicians should tell their patients — both adult and adolescent — that it was no more, or less, harmful than "sexual intercourse practiced with the same frequency." But he mixed this admission with regret: he was sorry that he could say nothing worse of "so nasty a practice; an uncleanliness, a filthiness forbidden by God [and] despised by men." Why, we must wonder, this hyperbole — "so nasty...forbidden by God...despised by men" — for a medically benign practice?[3] Freud and his circle debated passionately whether onanism caused organic harm and whether it was generally injurious — the Master tended to be old-fashioned on such matters — but all the founding fathers of psychoanalysis, and many of their successors, agreed that it was critically important in understanding the history of the self and its place in the social order. In 1995, the surgeon general of the United States, Jocelyn Elders, was fired, ostensibly because she answered a question,

17

put to her at a press conference, with a somewhat tentative yes: children should be taught about masturbation in the appropriate health or social-studies classes. As a culturally significant aspect of our sexuality, in other words, onanism has easily survived its tenure as a disease.

The more general problem is this: Why, in or around 1712 (at the dawn of the Enlightenment) does masturbation move from the distant moral horizon to the ethical foreground? For millennia, it had been dwarfed by other, seemingly far more important matters regarding the ethics of the body in general and the desiring body in particular: the purpose and regulation of sexual pleasure within marriage or the question of same-sex love, for example. For millennia, doctors, philosophers, rabbis, theologians, and preachers who expounded on sexual ethics had concentrated on men. But all this changed within decades. As sex with oneself became a topic for the most serious reflection, the young — boys and girls — and especially women were said to be its prototypical practitioners. Not just in Europe but wherever the issue of the modern desiring self arose, there too one came to find the problem and the novel attractions of what had been largely unspoken. Masturbation is the sexuality of modernity and of the bourgeoisie who created it. It is the first truly democratic sexuality. Why, for the first time, then, does the regulation of a form of sexual gratification said to be so dangerously attractive to boys and girls, men and women alike become so worrisome when before, insofar as it was discussed at all, it was largely regarded as a relatively marginal problem for adult men and especially monks?

Beginning in or around 1712, the trajectory forward of this new "trouble and agony of a wounded conscience," as *Onania* labels it, this "heinous sin ["crime" in later editions] of self pollution," is clear and sharp. Its rise to prominence constitutes one of the most spectacular episodes of intellectual upward mobility in literary annals: in just over fifty years, it moved from Grub Street to the *Encyclopédie*, the greatest compendium of learning produced by the high Enlightenment. Churchmen and cultural conservatives were not responsible; modern masturbation was born of a new secular moral world; it was that world's dark, other side.

The Enlightenment project of liberation — the coming into adult-hood of humanity — made the most secret, private, seemingly harmless, and most difficult to detect of sexual acts the center-piece of a program for policing the imagination, desire, and the self that modernity itself had unleashed.

The crucial moment in my history is around the late seven-teenth or early eighteenth century, when the sin whose history we are tracing came into its own. This is the age that invented the notion of morality as self-governance; it insisted that all humans shared a common moral capacity and the specific psychological capacities that we needed to exercise our freedom.[4] In these years, a profoundly individualist culture came into being: "It prizes autonomy; it gives an important place to self-exploration;... and its visions of the good life generally involve personal commit-ment." The formulation is the philosopher Charles Taylor's, and we can turn it to our purposes. The individual has broken free from a cultural world in relation to which we were not autono-mous, not self-exploring in quite the same way, and in which the good life was something to be found in an order of things and not within each of us. In the pre-modern world, broadly speaking, what is right and good is to be sought in a providential order, in the authority of religion, in the authority of the state, and more generally in one's relationship to a metaphysical reality beyond oneself. When Aristotle writes that the happy man ought to live pleasantly among friends and that "if he were a solitary, life would be hard for him," he expresses a truth about sociability and the good life that is underwritten by a reality beyond humans and their particular social arrangements. Nature gives us this as the human default mode. That is, in one form or another, the individ-ual's relation to the cosmos was given in the hierarchic, organic universe in which most people imagined themselves before the late seventeenth century. Imagining such a connection has been increasingly difficult in the West since the late seventeenth cen-tury. In this sense, the problem of the individual to society is dis-tinctly modern.[5]

There is, however, no single vision of this "modern self"; the whole idea is wildly contested. My point is simply that all the people I deal with in this book, the famous and the not famous, are engaged with what is essentially the same problem: How is the autonomous individual in a world without fixed poles going to negotiate the relationship between himself, or herself, and others? Or, put differently, they are engaged with creating the kind of inner discipline that makes individualism and liberty possible.

Why masturbation became so central to the history of the self in relation to the broader cultural history of the last two hundred years, to the history of gender, and to the history of individual guilt, anxiety, and autonomy — I leave for Chapters 5 and 6. Before giving an explanation, however, I have other stories to tell. I will begin, in the next chapter, by mapping the spread of masturbation as a culturally resonant sexual practice from its beginnings in the early eighteenth century to the present. This is the story of how, with awesome adaptability, *Onania* filled the available ecological niches across first a nation, then a continent, and finally the world, how the vice it proclaimed came to rank among the most spectacularly successful ever, anywhere. (I also reveal, for the first time, the name of the author of the long-anonymous tract that began it all.)

For the purposes of recounting how modern masturbation conquered the world of sexuality, I assume that it did, in fact, begin in or around 1712. But the act itself, of course, did not begin then nor did talk about it. Chapter 3 tells masturbation's prehistory, first from a medical perspective, and then, more extensively, from the perspective of sexuality and ethics: from the eponymous Old Testament Onan himself — probably not a masturbator at all — and later Jewish commentary on what he might have done wrong, through classical Antiquity and almost two millennia of Christian writing and preaching on the subject, to the eve of the Enlightenment. Compared with what came afterward, the story is relatively thin, relatively unfocused; not very much was said on the subject, and what was said quickly veered off in other directions. Equally important, it was almost entirely directed to adult men. This prehistory is about what did not happen. It is about the eclipse of an ethics of sex with oneself by serious thinking about other sexual practices through which a man's relationship to the

20

social and the divine order was monitored and regulated. Chapter 3 thus stands at the opposite pole from the rest of this book; if masturbation represented so much after the eighteenth century, it explains why it meant so little before. It makes the case that it is indeed the sexuality of modernity, the first democratic, equal-opportunity would-be vice.

The next question is, *What*, exactly, became so threatening about masturbation at the dawn of the Enlightenment? It was not that there was more of it. There may or may not have been but, in either case, neither we nor contemporaries would know. No one in the eighteenth century thought this was the problem. Nor was hostility to masturbation an aspect of hostility to sexual pleasure generally. Far from it. Seminal loss was not the new problem. It was a chestnut of ancient medicine, and it could not have been what so disturbed people about the masturbation of young boys and girls and especially of women, who produced in their orgasmic exercises nothing except fantasy and desire. The answer in brief is that three things seem to have been regarded as the core horrors of sex with oneself: it was secret in a world in which transparency was of a premium; it was prone to excess as no other kind of venery was, the crack cocaine of sexuality; and it had no bounds in reality, because it was the creature of the imagination.

By Chapter 5, we have been prepared for an explanation. I have already hinted that the history of masturbation is part of the history of how the morally autonomous modern subject was created and sustained. Specifically, an explanation of why it became so exigent depends on understanding why its core elements — imagination, excess, solitude, and privacy — became so problematic. Modern culture encourages individualism and self-determination and is threatened by solipsism and anomie; it asks that individuals always desire more than they have and imagine far more than is real and at the same time that they learn to moderate their desires and limit their imaginations themselves. The reality principle comes not from the next world, or even directly from this world, but from within ourselves. Masturbation is the sexuality of the self par excellence, the first great psychic battlefield for these struggles.

21

Chapter 6 takes the story up to the present. It begins with how an increasingly dense tradition that extended from the early eighteenth to the early twentieth century is transformed by sexology and psychology. Masturbation becomes a stage of development and abandoning it at the proper time a mark of maturity, mental health, and social conformity. Freud is the master of the new model, and he became the focus of debate on the left and the right.

Masturbation changed its valences again during the last forty or fifty years of the twentieth century. Beginning in the 1950s, picking up energy with the feminism of the 1960s and early 1970s, with the subsequent sex wars, and with the worldwide gay movement of the last quarter of the century, it would become an arena for sexual politics and for art across a wide spectrum of society. The disconnected, imaginative, individualist, resolutely ahistorical qualities of masturbation — no form of sexuality is more profligate with time or less linked to family and inheritance — that so disturbed eighteenth-century critics had, for a time in the Freudian story, subsisted as a kind of infantile sexuality that normal people transcend through the processes of civilization. Now it became a practice of individual autonomy and of sexual energy, an instrument of freedom, or, in the minds of some, a sign of abjection and despair. Self-pleasuring teeters between utopia and its opposite. Walt Whitman's most romantic reveries jostle with the bleakest visions of self-indulgence, egocentrism, and anomie.

The history of masturbation thus goes through three stages although the earlier ones are never left behind: Rousseau and Freud live on in us. But there is change. Beginning in the eighteenth century, solitary sex came to represent the relationship between the individual and the social world, a sort of crossroads where men and women, boys and girls could go terribly wrong, where they might, if not carefully watched and taught otherwise, choose the wrong kind of solitude, the wrong kind of pleasure, the wrong kind of imagination, the wrong kind of engagement with their inner selves. A false step led not so much to sin as to disease and decay; it was a secular waywardness. Then came the Freudian revolution. Now masturbation was less a crossroads where one might go astray than a stage that one had to pass through in an appropriate way. We

22

all have to struggle in the shoals of autoeroticism to emerge with a socially useful articulation of the ego with its sexual energies. Finally, masturbation becomes an experience of self-esteem or self-love, a form of personal autarky that allows each of us to form relationships with others without losing ourselves. What the philosophes had regarded as the surest road to ruin has become for some a road to self-realization, the nearest thing we have in our day to the Hellenistic care of the self but now available not only to the leisured gentleman, as it was in antiquity, but to everyone democratically. None of these developments is so clear or so straightforward, but complexity can wait. First I need to fill in the terrain, to show *how* an obscure vice became a sexual superstar over three centuries.

CHAPTER TWO

The Spread of Masturbation

from *Onania* to the Web

Onania, masturbation's primal text, was swept up in the burgeoning popular print culture of eighteenth-century England.[1] It was
carried along, in the first instance, by a seemingly limitless flood
of words that brought with it the news of a horrible new and debilitating vice along with much else. Without a booming commerce in books and medicines, and without the profit motive,
onanism, as we know it, would not exist.

The founding text itself tells the story a little differently. The
author's intentions were pure. His plan, he tells us, was to publish
his own warnings about the moral and physical dangers of the
"abominable practice" of "self pollution" accompanied by translations of various "eminent physicians'" prescriptions for cures to
the ills that it caused.[2] But this plan proved impractical. The ingre-
dients for the nostrums he was about to impart would have been
terribly costly, he says considerately, and the medicines were too
complex for patients to have them compounded discreetly. No one
would want to go to an apothecary and ask him to make up a complicated brew to cure the most embarrassing of ills. So, the author
continues, he had the medicines made up wholesale and generously transferred his rights over them to a "man of skill" — his
medical friend — who, in turn, had two thousand copies of *Onania*
printed at his own expense. This doctor supposedly offered the
cures for free at first. But that proved too expensive. All the
editions we have until the late eighteenth century, when *Onania*
ceased being tied into the quack-medicine market and became a
freestanding work of soft-core pornography, sold potions to cure

25

the ill effects of the solitary vice. They were not cheap: 12 shillings for the full treatment, enough money to buy almost 290 cups (dishes, actually) of coffee at a coffeehouse, more than two weeks' wages for a footman. Readers are advised to apply for the medicines, by name, at the various booksellers who published or sold *Onania*.

Except for the brief allusion to philanthropy at the beginning, this story in broad outline is not implausible. Giveaway or cheap books — pamphlets made from a single print sheet — to sell medicines were commonplace, and one such family of productions hawking an "anodyne necklace" for toothache, sugarplum drops for purging, and various purported remedies for gout, rheumatism, and venereal disease itself came to play a part as well in the diffusion of onanism.[3] Booksellers and printers were often the outlets for both print and potion. Thus a hack writer might well have produced the pamphlet and someone else made the medicine both in league with people in the book trade who organized the whole operation.

But in *Onania* as it has come down to us, the "frame tale" distinction between a moralist — a nonmedical author — and the inventor of the "Prolific Powder" or "Strengthening Tincture" who also provided advice had broken down. Readers are told they can consult *the author* by arrangement through the booksellers: "But then he expects his fee." And the publishers, printers, and booksellers expected, of course, to sell books.[4] There was thus a market for the book and a separate, though intimately connected, tie-in market for the medicine.

Advertisements for both, and for a *Supplement* that soon joined them, began to appear regularly in the London weeklies around 1716. In form, they were much like other ads, small boxes, similar to modern want ads, filled with copy: transcriptions of *Onania*'s elaborate title page; frequently updated reports on how many copies of various editions had been sold; the news that a new edition contained a curious letter from a lady on the use and abuse of the marriage bed. *Onania* jostled, cheek by jowl, with all the other stuff being hawked in the booming marketplace of popular print. One week the ad appeared just before an announcement for a book on the imminent destruction of the papacy and just after one for a dumb gentleman who was famous for knowing the names of everyone he met. *Onania*'s commercial success alone made it a *cause célèbre*: "I was desirous to see a book which had so long made such a noise in the world" and been so successful "as to require so many editions in so short a time," wrote a critic in 1724 as he launched into a vicious attack born, no doubt, of envy. Wherever papers like the metropolitan *Saturday Post* circulated there too went the newly discovered horror. (My example above came from the November 22, 1718, issue, picked at random.) And its fame radiated from provincial centers as well. In fact, the foundational text of solitary sex, proclaiming the dangers of that "filthy Commerce with oneself" daily practiced by young and old, men and women, single and married, was one of the first books to be extensively advertised in the nascent country press.[5]

Quickly *Onania*'s success became part of its ongoing story. The author of one reprinted letter (January 25, 1723 — genuine or not we do not know) confesses that he first encountered the book — and the word "onanism" — through an advertisement for the sixth edition in the *London Journal*, which he had read in a public house. "I asked a friend what it meant, who explained it to me, which so terrified me, that I vowed never would do the like any more." He bought the book, as did tens of thousands of others. In that sense, modern masturbation and the sales of the book that brought it to the world's attention owe their success to the hype of Europe's first mass media and to the public spaces in which it circulated. By one estimate, London had 2,000 coffeehouses in 1700. There is a precise list for a more limited area in 1739: 551 coffeehouses within the Bills of Morality, the parishes of the London conurbation for which statistics on death had been gathered since the sixteenth century. These not only made available the newspapers that advertised *Onania*, among many other books, but also sold the quack medicines that *Onania* made its readers feel they needed. In the absence of postboxes, mail orders could be addressed to, and packages picked up from, these hubs of information and commerce. Most provincial cities of any size also had coffeehouses by 1700.[6] A broad commercial infrastructure for the spread of the new vice was well in place.

Onania and its *Supplement* also made their way in the world through an extended print family that looked out for its own. For a start, each part extolled the virtues of the other. In its end matter, an undated edition of the *Supplement*, for example, offers for sale a new edition of *Onania* that, it proclaims, is "to be read by all sorts of People of both Sexes of what Age, Degree, Profession or Condition soever, Guilty or Not Guilty of the Sin declaimed against." Everyone, in short, needs this book. A carnivalesque hucksterism beckons the potential customer with breathless hyperbole: "Strange effects of that Practice in Women hardly ever till now taken notice of."

From these self-referential testimonials a network branches out. The "strange effects" being shouted about to attract readers refers to the case of two nuns, each discovered to have an enlarged clitoris. The pope authorized some cardinals to investigate whether these women had changed sex, as some would have had it. Their translated "report" is excerpted from one of those mildly salacious popular medical works that were a staple of Grub Street and a reservoir of stories for *Onania* and the *Supplement*. It found that there had been no miracle; the facts described did not "exceed the bounds of nature"; the nuns had taken on their appearance through "the uncommon Exercise of the clitoris which, as it is used to frequent imitations, thrusts out and enlarges its dimensions not unlike the human penis." Only "imitations" suggests masturbation in this standard bit of anticlerical pornography, but *Onania* could make gold out of the dross of its literary neighbors.[7] The trope is a commonplace of eighteenth-century pornography and of female masturbation in its pantheon of titillation. "Near these forts is the metropolis, called CLTRS," much delighted in by the Queens of Merryland, announces the narrator of a "traveler's guide" to the distant shores that are a woman's body. Their "chief palace, or rather pleasure seat," it was at first small until "the pleasure some of the Queens have found in it, has occasioned their extending its bounds considerably."[8] This, of course, is the nuns' story in one of its many guises.

Onania also made itself known through established channels of popular literature. The men and women who sold or published it were all major players in the early-eighteenth-century publishing world who collectively controlled great swaths of print and publicity. Thus, for example, Thomas Crouch advertised his *Wonderful Prodigies of Judgment and Mercy Discovered in Near Three Hundred Memorable Histories* and a "Volatile Aromatik Snuff" that was said to be restorative in the back of one edition of *Onania* that he co-published. Paul Varenne — he had a varied list with an emphasis on books in Latin and French, including a translation of the *Book of Common Prayer* — published (with Crouch) in 1718 a book on venereal disease that said nothing about masturbation but carried a prominent advertisement for the fourth edition of which he owned a share.[9]

The same consortium that printed and sold *Onania* and its *Supplement* had a few years earlier, in 1708, launched John Marten's treatise on venereal diseases, in which the word "masturbation" in its modern spelling first appeared in English. The mention is brief but to the point: a list of what might cause gleets, impotence, and infertility includes the vice "too liberal using of *Friction* with the hand when schoolboys." "Women using Titillations in themselves" could end up with the same debilities. A year later the group published another of Marten's works, a manifestly "scandalous book — *Gonosologium novum; or, A new system of all the secret infirmities and diseases natural, accidental, and venereal in men and women*" — that had the honor of being the first such work indicted for pornography in Queen's Bench once the authorities got serious and removed such cases from the Guildhall. The indictment failed.[10]

And it had little impact. Future editions of *Onania* profited from the same voyeuristic, sensationalist stuff that had been published in *Gonosologium novum*. Here Marten introduces a long section on the parts of generation in women with the observation that "every man's passion is inflamed by the sight of them, so every man is desirous of their being treated upon." He particularly draws attention to the clitoris, as both a verb and a noun, "which signifies lasciviously to grope the privities," and suggests masturbation to "allay the fury" of women's desire. Of course, he adds a mild hint of rebuke against this alternative but in the next breath

29

counters with fulsome descriptions of how "for both sexes the pleasures of love are quick and excessive."[11] John Marten is also a link between the invention of modern masturbation and whole other worlds of soft-core-porn medical works; large parts of his books are compilations from Nicolas Venette's immensely popular *The Mysteries of Conjugal Love Reveal'd*, translated into English in 1703, and from *Rare Verities; or, The Cabinet of Venus Unlocked* that had brought the best of expensively printed Italian erotica to a general English audience in 1658. The publishers of *Onania*, in short, launched the new vice into a market eager and prepared to embrace and nourish it — a market that they themselves had helped to develop.

Their new book, like many of its literary confreres, was something of a magpie that lived from what it could gather round about. *Onania*, like an epistolary novel, added more and more putative letters about the sexual initiations and adventures of boys and girls followed by their inevitable comeuppance. It even transformed attacks into more copy. Despite the promise of "no more addition to this BOOK, howsoever, it may be reprinted," the fifteenth edition, and sixth of the *Supplement*, justified new material on the grounds of countering falsehoods circulated by that "scurrilous libel, 'Onania Examined and Detected'" and other, now lost interlocutors.[12] The still-anonymous author denies he is "a pretending, whining, cantering preacher" who has produced "the most lascivious Rhapsody" known to man. He is no preacher at all, he protests. And as for the accusation that all this fuss about onanism is really an implicit license for fornication and "whoredom," he denies it. Graciously responding to the charge that he had elevated masturbation into the "most superlative Kind of Uncleanness" so as to sell more quack medicines for the diseases it supposedly caused, he admits that he has perhaps given short shrift to adultery, sodomy, bestiality, and incest. But, he rejoins, there is little new to say on these subjects, whereas self-pollution "has never been touched upon yet by any able pen, at least not yet." And as for the allegation that he said masturbation is harmless if done simply to be rid of semen, our author replies that the biggest part of the sin is "an impure imagination" and that in fact one could not commit it "free of mental impurity." Scrupulously hygienic masturbation is not possible. (This dispute was sparked by a harebrained account, which does seem to suggest what its critics claimed, of the relief practiced by the husband of a thirteen-year-old bride whose father would not allow her to have intercourse.) Until the late 1720s, this is the literary neighborhood of *Onania*: solidly Grub Street.

And it is the literary sniping of the gutter that allows us to discover finally, after almost more than three hundred years of anonymity, who actually wrote the primal text of modern masturbation. In 1727, a longish tract appeared, under the pseudonym "Mathew Rothos," called *A Whip for the Quack; or Some remarks on M——n's Supplement to his "Onania."*[13] It was produced by the same publishers who gave the public "Philo-Castitatis'" attack on *Onania* in 1723 and 1724 and who, like *Onania*'s and its *Supplement*'s publishers, straddled the gap between high-minded religious and pedagogical works and scurrilous semipornography.[14]

Rothos' excuse for writing is that M——n had not responded to the earlier critique — *Onania Examined* — and that he had been asked to enter the fray as the ignored tract's champion. Perhaps this literary gambit reflects public debate; perhaps people were upset that someone was claiming for masturbation the status of worst possible sexual vice and thereby shoving aside old standbys; perhaps the repeated graphic stories of self-seduction by the private vice were genuinely offensive. Equally likely is the hope of squeezing a bit more profit out of the masturbation business.

For whatever reason, the literary marketplace thrived on nasty point and counterpoint. What ought one to expect, Rothos asks with a rhetorical flourish, from a quack with his "ill natured, rambling falsehoods, misrepresentations, self contradictory Billingsgate language," from someone who produced "a multiplicity of sham letters as if they were so many credentials and testimonials," from someone who "flattered and complimented himself," paraded "worthlessness for merit, impertinent harangues for demonstrative argument," and wrote so "full of Billingsgate and Grub Street dialect" because he hoped to attract an audience to whom such language would seem natural.

31

M——n stands accused — not without some justification — "of carefully cultivating and blowing the Fire of Lust in Youth by all incitements Words are capable of" and then offering a secret and expensive medicine to cure the disease allegedly caused by the activity to which he had provoked his young readers in the first place. That fornication led to venereal disease, the cornerstone of quackery, is old news. That solitary, private sex caused disease was an amazing invention. Worse, M——n was said to be a hypocrite who probably practiced himself what he would deny to others: while claiming that the solitary vice was the "most superlative kind of uncleanness" (highly dubious), he "profited by it"; he "feigned dislike" and "pretend[ed] an aversion" to masturbation, which he assumed everyone — boys and girls, men and women — did, because he and his family did. We are really down in the dirt here.

The identity M——n can have offered only the thinnest of disguises in 1727, because the author of *Gonosologium novum* and other medical soft-core pornography was well known to be John Marten, the surgeon and quack prosecuted for obscenity in 1708. Not only do his earlier works and *Onania* share the same publishers but also a similar language and style. Seldom has a cultural innovation of such magnitude had such humble beginnings. But even if John Marten did not write *Onania*, the little contretemps between the pseudonymous "Mathew Rothos," as the representative of one publishing consortium, and *Onania* and its *Supplement*, as representatives of another, can stand as a synecdoche for the energy of commercial print culture that gave life and energy to the new private vice.[15]

Onania had legs, as they say in publishing. Even after two of its publishers died, it kept going. But its monopoly on masturbation was short-lived; others moved in to make the private vice ever more public and profitable. Next in the field, in the mid-1720s, was the most successful of London's quack-medicine establishments, led by the famous Mrs. Garroway, scion of the well-known coffeehouse family. From a secure base in "Dr. Chamberlayne's Anodyne Necklace for Children's Teeth" and a subsidiary line that included gout cures, purging sugarplums, ague plasters, saffron drops, and ophthalmic tobacco that the firm made, sold, and advertised lavishly, she branched out into the self-pollution business. The whole array — her new cure for the newly discovered masturbatory disease and the old standbys — could be had in London or the provinces, retail and wholesale, in person and by mail. Hundreds of pamphlets, each slightly different from the others, as well as weekly notices in newspapers, spread the fame of this wide-ranging pharmacopoeia and of onanism. In short, others rushed into the niche that *Onania* had pioneered.[16]

Toothache continued to be Garroway's biggest market, but masturbation offered enormous opportunities. She linked up with Henry Parker, also a child of commerce, and together they ventured forward in this new phase of the business. (Parker was probably the son of the well-known anti-Whig printer of almanacs and purveyor of medicines.) We learn this prehistory from the advertisements in the front or back matter of twenty-four- to thirty-page cheaply printed tracts variously titled *Eronania; or, The Misusing of the Marriage Bed by Er and Onan* and *The Crime of Onan (together with that of his brother Er); or, The Heinous Vice of Self Defilement* that first appeared in 1724 and continued for some years. Like *Onania*'s, their purpose was, first of all, to make people aware that what they had been doing was not only terribly wrong but also terribly dangerous and then, once customers knew that they needed help, to offer a costly restorative. In a world in which low-grade infections, bad diet, excessive drink, and the stresses of life must have made many people feel unaccountably tired, lethargic, headachy, and generally out of sorts, it did not take much to convince them that maybe masturbation contributed to their malaise and that some potion might pep them up.[17]

There is no specific reference in these tracts to *Onania*, although parts are clearly plagiarized: the definition of the crime — to "imitate with themselves that carnal pleasure" — is stolen almost word for word from its predecessor.[18] Like *Onania*, they treat masturbation as a newly exposed corruption and not as the old enemy concupiscence in all its many familiar forms, natural and unnatural: a great many treatises have been written on "the several branches and Sins of Impurity but very few (if any) really

33

SERIOUS ones upon this ... the most COMMON of all." Moreover, the new vice offered "more and stronger inducements to
it than ... any other" and was especially threatening because one
might be tempted to believe that one could get away with it:
"IT in particular" seems to escape attention. All people — and the
"authors" specifically include men and women — are in greater
danger of succumbing to solitary sex than to any other kind because "the fuel and treacherous enticements to it always accompany us, wherever we go." (This, too, is a reworking of a phrase
in *Onania*.) As in *Onania*, the words that matter are all about interiority: "SECRECY," "WITHIN OURSELVES," "Persons USING
THEMSELVES Separately and Alone." And, as in *Onania*, moral
warnings are interspersed with tales of horrible illness, death, or
redemption.

But *Eronania* and *The Crime of Onan* are altogether shabbier,
more plebeian productions, hopeless shambles of capital letters,
bits and pieces from the anodyne-necklace empire's other publications, and lists of contents that bear little relation to what follows. Both were given away free, although the medicines they
advertised were decidedly not: a purge by clyster cost a staggering 7 shillings, 6 pence, and 1 guinea when combined with "a
great specific remedy." Both were clearly also playing to the
salacious interests of readers, who are promised details of "those
wicked Clubs and Societies of Women Haters and others who
meet to defile themselves" (the so-called molly clubs and other
such venues of a new sodomitic subculture), "of the Crime in
Ministers and Clergymen and travelers and others absent from
their wives" of "SELF EMASCULATION." Nothing so juicy ever
materialized. And both are from the slummier end of Grub Street,
where they remained.

Not so *Onania*. Its tenth edition — "above fifteen thousand of
its former editions have been sold" — traveled to the American
colonies in 1724 to be printed by a respectable publisher. The
year before, the aged Puritan divine Cotton Mather had offered
an attack on the newly discovered vice for the first time in his life,
although he had, it seems, long been worried about it. How he
came to the subject we do not know.[19]

34

And then, in 1728, *Onania* began in earnest its ascent into elevated secular company. Just over two decades after its initial notice in a humble tract, the new sin and its neologism made their way into the first of the great eighteenth-century encyclopedias. "Onania" and "onanism" had become nouns worthy of the definition of so intellectually ambitious a work as Ephraim Chambers's *Cyclopaedia*. ("Onanism," which in its French form became the title of an eighteenth-century best-seller, seems to have come from the title of a now-lost tract attacking the third edition of *Onania* that we learn about only from its future editions. Thus the first extant appearance of "onanism" is coterminous with the first extant appearance of *Onania*.) In any case, both are neologisms, Chambers tells us, "terms which some late empirics have framed, to denote the crime of self pollution, mentioned in Scripture to have been practiced by Onan and punished in him by death." The entry's author is skeptical of the biblical origins of the Onan/masturbation link, as well he might be. In the entry "Self Pollutions," we read "that Onan, and, as some critics also think, Er, were severely punished for polluting themselves by spilling their seed onto the ground, whence the crime has been denominated by some empirics, Onania. See ONANIA." A contemporary learned source thus acknowledges the originality of the anonymous progenitor of modern masturbation and identifies him — rightly — as a quack doctor while at the same time treating his creation as worthy of attention.[20]

The whole idea of *self*-pollution is presented as novel. "Pollution" or "pollutio" standing alone, we are told, in the voice of detached rationality that British Protestantism adopts when discussing other religions, means "profaning a sacred place," something that seems to worry superstitious Indians, Jews — who think they are polluted by the menses of women and by touching dead bodies — and Romanists, who need to consecrate a church anew if it is "polluted by effusion of blood or of seed." "Self-pollution" seems to absorb this history of superstition and take on new meaning: "pollution" or "*self*-pollution" is "also used for the abusing or defiling of one's own body by means of lascivious frictions and titillations, raised by Art, to produce emission. See

'Emission.'" "Raised by Art" is crucial here. It is the first suggestion we have of what would become a tradition of worry about
masturbation as the work of fiction — of the imagination — under-
mining the place of the individual in society. Securely in the first,
1728, edition of the first major English encyclopedia, "Onania"
and its allied words and ideas appeared again and again in the
more than twenty eighteenth-century English editions that followed, not to speak of foreign translations. It was launched in
intellectual high society.[21]

Then, in 1743, *Onania* crossed the Channel and made it into
Johann Heinrich Zedler's *Universal Lexicon*, the second of the three
great eighteenth-century encyclopedias. Its opening paragraphs
constitute, more or less word for word, the entry "Selbst-befleckung, Onanie" (self-pollution, onanism) in volume 36 of this sixty-
four-volume compendium of old and new scientific learning.
Barely thirty years from first being brought to the world's attention as a serious problem, masturbation had found a place in the
cultural center of German-speaking Europe. Zedler may have
excerpted his text from Carl Albert Carus's 1736 translation of the
ninth English edition that would itself go through at least five German editions before 1800. How Carus came to *Onania* we do not
know. Nor has anyone done a sufficiently careful bibliographical
study to make clear the relationship among *Onania*, Carus's text
in its various editions, and a work that may have been the first
book on our subject originally written in, as opposed to translated
into, German. That honor probably belongs to *Persuasive and lively
warnings against all the sins of uncleanness and secret lewdness* by
the Halle pietist Georg Sarganeck, whose several editions had
made something of a splash in the learned newspapers of major
German cities. It shared a lot with *Onania*, including the literary
framing device — a friendly doctor helps the moralist, who is
actually the narrator — and the offer of recovery from masturbation's ill effects. But in whatever forms *Onania* bounced around
the increasingly vibrant world of German print, by 1740 translations had spawned oft-reprinted literary hangers-on tied to the
quack-medicine market, more pious but still money-generating
upmarket books like Sarganeck's, and, within a few more years, an

entry in a major encyclopedia of the age. Not bad for an upstart that, as in England, straddled popular commercial culture and learned culture, religious and secular morality.[22]

Next came France. How — or when — *Onania* got there is not clear. There seems to have been no full French translation in the eighteenth century, and by the time a French-language derivative was published, in Leipzig in 1775, *Onania* had already been well enshrined in the best of circles.[23] We do know that the celebrated Enlightenment physician Samuel Auguste David Tissot, who would finally bring respectability to the exposure of onanism in 1759, had the first edition of Chambers's *Cyclopaedia* in his Lausanne library and the 1752 edition (the seventeenth), of *Onania* as well.[24] Perhaps interest in the subject was generated by the entry "manustrapratio" in the second volume of Robert James's famous *Medicinal Dictionary* that Denis Diderot, the philosophe and intellectual entrepreneur, helped to translate. Perhaps it inspired him to commission the masturbation article in the encyclopedia he was organizing. Perhaps a man as fascinated by vision as Diderot had been drawn to James's account of a boy who, as a result of this "preposterous entertainment," this "preposterous way of venery," that is, masturbation, had come to write in a smaller and smaller script until he ended up nearly blind. The diagnosis: amaurosis, impairment of vision without manifest fault of the eye.[25]

But this is speculation. We know that the eminent physician Jean Jacques Menuret de Chambaud, author of the long article "Manstrupration or Manustupration" — among others — in Diderot's epoch defining *Encyclopédie*, credited *Onania* with making masturbation a question worthy of serious attention even as he criticized it for being a hopeless muddle. By 1765, little more than fifty years after an anonymous empiric claimed to be the first to alert the world to a secret, unnamed, and too-little-noticed vice, his work had made it into the last and the greatest of the eighteenth-century encyclopedias. *Onania* from Grub Street had reached the pinnacle of the high Enlightenment.[26]

The main authority for the *Encyclopédie* article, however, was not the lowly *Onania* but a far more learned, respectable work by one of the eighteenth century's most famous, influential, and prolific physicians: Tissot's *L'Onanisme; ou, Dissertation physique sur les malades produites par la masturbation*, published in a 1760 French edition that was one-third longer than the original Latin one of 1759. Tissot was not generous to the earlier work from which he stole both title and story line. It "is a real chaos…one of the most unconnected productions that has appeared for a long time." There is no similarity between the two books, he insists. Do not, he cautions, be misled by the "affinity of title"; anyone who reads both will be clear on their differences. But he protests too much; *Onania* had arrived.[27]

Tissot's introduction suggests how extensively the work of the anonymous English empiric had penetrated high culture. Since the publication of this work — he is referring to the interval between publication of the original Latin and the French translation — he had been told by an indisputable authority that some facts in *Onania* were not true, that the work had been accused — falsely — of obscenity, and that a German edition had been suppressed for lack of an imperial privilege.[28] For all these reasons, he considered omitting all mention of *Onania*. On the other hand, some criticisms pertained only to the German edition; there might be "imaginary facts," but in general what *Onania* says is "all too true." But the deciding factor for including a discussion of the earlier work was a letter he had received from a distinguished physician named Johann Rudolph Stehelin, that informed him of a case reported by Friedrich Hoffman at Halle. (Hoffmann was famous for his views that an ether-like fluid was transmitted by the nerves to the muscles and thereby kept them in a state of semi-contraction. Versions of this view were widespread and explain why the dissipation of this ethereal energy through masturbation would be thought to produce slack jaws, limp hands, and other signs of the secret vice.) One of Hoffmann's patients, Stehelin wrote, apparently suffered from masturbatory disease. By taking the remedies of *Onania*'s author, he was cured and, indeed, subsequently had children. In short, *Onania* got around in the best medical circles as well as among its clients. One patient in Switzerland, we know, picked up a copy in Frankfurt.[29]

But Tissot's *L'Onanisme* succeeded on an altogether different scale; it was an instant literary sensation throughout Europe. Unlike *Onania*, it did not sell medicine; it was not tied to quack products and offered very little immediate help beyond advising readers never to begin masturbating or to give it up if they had already succumbed. Its prescriptions for cure were anodyne, commonsensical, and cheap: healthy living, good company, some strengthening potions perhaps. *L'Onanisme* (in the rest of the book, I will call it by its English title, *Onanism*) thus thrived independently of the sort of quack-medicine market that had sustained *Onania*. For whatever reasons — more about this later — it almost immediately captured the public imagination.

There is no complete, systematic bibliography. But we know about scores of eighteenth-century editions: in London, and Bristol, and Bath, and Dublin; in Tissot's native Lausanne, in Bern, and in Geneva; in Frankfurt, Leipzig, Augsburg, Hamburg, and Eisenach; in Utrecht and Amsterdam and Louvain; in Madrid, Philadelphia, Vienna, and Venice (at least one each in Italian and in Greek).[30] (This list does not include excerpts or plagiarisms.) In sheer number of editions alone, *Onanism* ranks high among eighteenth-century best-sellers. There were at least 35 editions in French, 61 in all languages, not including 6 editions and 4 translations of the shorter Latin version; by comparison, there were 137 eighteenth-century editions of Rousseau's most popular novel, *La Nouvelle Héloïse*. In short, this first "serious" book on masturbation was a genuine best-seller and continued to be widely reprinted and quoted in the nineteenth century in ever more languages. (There were 5 editions in Russian, for example, by 1855.[31])

Tissot was already well known, well connected, and widely respected when *Onanism* was published. He had studied with some of the leading lights of eighteenth-century medicine and was the editor and translator of one of its real luminaries — Albrecht von Haller. His 1754 book on smallpox had been an international success and the acknowledged basis for the *Encyclopédie* article on inoculation. The year *Onanism* appeared, he was elected to the Royal Society, and the next year, with the publication of *Advice on the Health of the People*, his name became a household word; the medical philosophy in which onanism was embedded swept

Europe. When one of her servants was ill, Mrs. Thrale — Dr. Johnson's friend — called to her son, "Fetch me Buchan's *Domestick Medicine* . . . , or rather . . . fetch me Tissot, 'tis the better book." "'Tis so," he replied wittily, and went for *Advice*. It existed in more than 130 eighteenth-century editions in at least fourteen languages, including two in Telugu. John Wesley introduced an abridgment of *Advice* and sold it "at Methodist Preaching Houses in Town and Country" with the endorsement that Tissot was a person of "strong understanding, extensive knowledge, and deep experience." What is said to be the first scientific medical tract in Yiddish relied heavily on the German and Hebrew translations.[32] And through his other writings as well, Tissot was on the night tables of Europe. James Boswell spent the better part of Sunday, June 25, 1769, in bed reading *On the Health of Literary Persons*, which, he said, "gave him some curious thoughts." And well it might, since this book portrays the diseases caused by prolonged mental activity and those caused by masturbation — about which Boswell felt immense guilt and repulsion — in much the same light.[33]

Thus Tissot, with his impeccable credentials, huge reputation, and a widespread correspondence that included both the intellectual greats and the crowned heads of Europe, definitively launched masturbation into the mainstream of Western culture. He claimed that his brief was limited, that he was not interested in self-pollution as a "crime," as a moral disorder, or as a "sin," to use the old-fashioned language of religion that he and his colleagues generally eschewed. The problem, as he saw it, was not, in the first instance, one of ethics. His subject was corporeal pathology; the disorders that masturbation occasioned — the diseases that it brought on — would be of concern.

But this is a bit disingenuous. Tissot avows that he is only doing what a doctor is supposed to do: "Quod medicorum es Promittunt medici," only what relates to medicine is permitted the doctor, he protests, quoting Horace. In fact, he knows he is part of a major imperialist enterprise in which science is claiming the authority that had for so long belonged to religion. The body suffers — so argued Enlightenment medicine — when social practices violate the natural order; medicine was a — arguably *the* — foundational moral science because it alone had the expertise to determine whether such a violation had taken place. If norms were to be grounded not in divine revelation but in an understanding of what nature demanded, and if violations of such norms were made evident through pathology, then doctors were both guides to what was right and diagnosticians of what was wrong. Johann Georg Zimmermann — the eminent German physician, *belletrist*, and good friend of Tissot's — represents this version of medico-morality beautifully. On the one hand, he writes a tract in which the stern voice of the physician warns of masturbation in young girls and announces, "No one can fill some of the holes in the moralist's knowledge and warnings like the doctor." On the other, he was best known to the European and American literary public for his book on solitude, a meditation on the importance of self-reflection in a socially ever more demanding civilization. For a man like Zimmermann, who explored "the secret recesses of the human heart" (the phrase is from Tissot's memoir), at the limits of solitude stood the solitary vice.[34] Morality spoke through medicine.

Masturbation moved easily from medico-moral literature to all manner of other writing. It quickly came to represent for the great thinkers of the Enlightenment a derangement of sociability that might well be hideously destructive to the body but that was terrible even if it had no organic effects. Voltaire, for example, takes up the subject with characteristic gusto. He, like Tissot and others, gives credit to the English doctor who wrote *Onanism* — he means *Onania* — for starting it all. Nowhere, he points out, does the Bible say that Onan masturbated as opposed to using some other method to avoid conception. He recognizes the enormous success of the English tract, "one counts around eighty editions" — where Voltaire gets this figure is not clear — with the proviso that this "prodigious number" is not but the "common trick of booksellers to lure readers." And then he sketches in some of the history we have just surveyed. The famous doctor from Lausanne who wrote *Onanism*, S.A.D. Tissot, is given credit for bringing clarity and method to the jumble of the English Grub Street tradition. Tissot's views seemed to interest Voltaire not so much because he was interested specifically in the medical dangers of masturbation as because they offered ammunition for his anticlericalism. Clerical celibacy, unnatural abstinence, led to unnatural pleasures; the one encouraged the other; monks, priests, and nuns masturbated. And, Voltaire says in the sarcastic tone he reserves for attacks on the Church, the claim that the eternal God was born of a tribe of prostitutes and thieves, from whose genealogy Onan opted out by spilling his seed on the ground, is ridiculous, but no more mysterious than much else that the savants of the Church would try to put over on unsuspecting believers. (Readers who want to hear immediately the whole lurid story of Onan's family might want to skip ahead to pp. 112–15.) When, however, Voltaire is pressed to characterize the sin of Onan, known by his day as masturbation, he says only that it is the result of "perverted self-love" — what Havelock Ellis and Freud would think of as narcissism. But the point for now is that Voltaire, like most of those who helped invent modern masturbation, cared about autoerotic sexuality because it was at odds with social and moral life as it ought to be lived.[35]

Jean-Jacques Rousseau understood this explicitly. When Tissot sent him a copy of *Onanism* on July 8, 1762, it was in the spirit of a fellow worker in the vineyards of a great moral cause for which his distinguished countryman had already done so much. What would become the most influential Enlightenment work on education, *Emile*, had appeared two months earlier, in May 1762; Tissot must have read it immediately and recognized that he and its famous author shared a great deal. He asked for, and was quickly granted, an audience. Afterward Tissot offers his compliments: "The moments I spent with you are among the most interesting of my life." And he allies his own book, which he sent along, with Rousseau's masterpieces: "*Onanism* will show you that finally there is a doctor who sees all the dangers of the odious practice which you have so sharply attacked and had the courage to make known." The allusion is to the moral foreboding about masturbation that haunts the sexual awakening of Emile, Rousseau's eponymous protagonist, and, by extension, that of all adolescents. "If he [an educator's pupil] were to know one time the dangerous supplement" as a way of satisfying his sexual instincts, "he is lost," declares Rousseau unequivocally. Not only would "he carry the doleful [*triste*] effects of this habit, the most disastrous to which a young man can subjugate himself, to the grave," but by the very act he would be lost to his teacher. Medicine is part of the story; heart and body, to be sure, are enervated. But even more troubling is the fact that through masturbation Emile would become hopelessly enslaved to himself. Better to fall in love with an inappropriate woman; from such a fate, Rousseau is sure, he might be saved. But to be rescued from himself as the engine of sexual desire and satisfaction would be altogether another matter. Complex as Rousseau's feelings were about the role of society in making us who we are, society still offered grounds for redemption; pure interiority was harder, perhaps impossible, to reach. And pure interiority, driven by the possibility of endless, self-generated sexual pleasure was the most extreme case.[36]

Masturbation and the creation of the self are major themes in Rousseau and ones to which we will return. But for now, while the project is still to describe how a new guilt made its way in the world, the point is that masturbation as a morally serious question had escaped the bounds of popular as well as learned medicine, pedagogy, anticlerical polemics, and the learned encyclopedias to figure powerfully in a literary best-seller. Over 30,000 copies of *Emile* in the original French were in print at the end of 1762; nearly 200,000 at the end of the century. And this does not count translations. Two of the most prominent German educators of the eighteenth century said that in *Emile* Rousseau had "taught thinkers how to think."[37] The vice that had scarcely spoken its name in 1700 was proclaimed to millions of readers and listeners as holding the gravest possible threat to an individual's moral integrity less than a hundred years later.

Rousseau thanked Tissot on July 22, 1762, for sending him *Onanism*. He must have read the book very soon after he received it — clearly the subject was near to his heart — and he responded appreciatively. In his thank-you note, he says that although he did not read very much anymore — and especially not medical books — he could not put this one down once he had started. He only

43

regretted that he had not come upon it earlier so that he could have used its authority and learning to strengthen what he himself had had to say on the subject.[38]

How Rousseau originally came to the problem we do not know. The famous account of his relationship to his own masturbation and its place in the making of his sexuality comes in the *Confessions* and is the reflection of an older man on his younger self.[39] But the general point is clear enough: by the 1760s, one of the most read and influential of Enlightenment doctors and the greatest, most original of the philosophes, had made common cause against a vice that had emerged from almost complete obscurity barely fifty years earlier. Tissot continued to be quoted extensively on the subject by learned and popular writers for at least another century and a half. And Rousseau's autobiographical reflections resonated, at least in educated circles, as the definitive formulation of the new vice.

"Have I not often told you that I was another Rousseau," wrote John Ruskin, the Victorian sage, to Mrs. Cowper, asking her to use this information to convince the family of Rose La Touche, whose daughter he was courting, that his marriage to his former wife Effie had been annulled not because he could not get an erection but because he could not get one with her in particular. The irony of confessing that he had been a masturbator to prove that he could be a lover — the common assumption would have been the opposite — was lost on him. All he wanted to get across was that his masturbatory days were over. He had already been saved from sin, he tells Mrs. Cowper. Those days were past, "indeed past as the night,"[40] although they still bore testimony to his potency under the right circumstances.

Along the two intertwining and ever broadening streams that Tissot and Rousseau represent — medicine on the one hand, moral philosophy and pedagogy on the other — masturbation would make its way forward. Each stream, in turn, had its tributaries, low-life and more respectable, which ran their separate intertwining ways through essentially the same territory. First, a brief account of the course of the now-no-longer-so-new vice in popular medicine.

The spirit of the John Marten who created the illness and was

44

the first to sell a cure lived on for at least two centuries. In the late eighteenth century, Dr. Solomon's Balm of Gilead, for example, exploited the medico-moral market first opened up by *Onania* and the Anodyne-Necklace empire with spectacular success. The "doctor" had been a shoe-polish salesman in Newcastle before he bought his M.D. from Aberdeen — not the famous university but a late-eighteenth-century diploma mill. He began selling the balm as a general restorative, but by the early nineteenth century his nostrum had become more targeted. A hundred thousand copies of his company's *Guide to Good Health* offered pharmaceutical respite to the masturbator. (The guilt would have to take care of itself.) Like *Onania*, Solomon's *Guide* was ever growing; the fifty-second edition had 283 pages, the sixty-fourth, sometime around 1814, had 312, including nine pages with the names of agents in Britain and the United States from whom one could buy both book and balm. In good years, the firm spent a stupendous £5,000 — one hundred times a solid artisan's annual wage — on advertising, which announced that a certain "delusive habit" is "the most destructive thing that can be practiced." As before, but on a far larger scale, anxiety about masturbation — and perhaps information about the deed itself — came before the public through a marketplace of print and products that was large and always on the lookout for new customers.

Goss and Company's *Hygeiana* (at least a score of editions by 1830) used the authority of Tissot to claim that girls suffer the ill effects of masturbation as much as, or more than, boys, and they too therefore were in need of the firm's medicines. In a blatant bit of self-promotion, James Hodson, another late-eighteenth-century fake doctor, announced that he had "the most extensive practice, in a particular line, of any one of the professions in this kingdom," that all sorts of "so-called physicians" sought to steal his prose and product, and, finally, that his Persian Restorative Drops would cure those "who have been unfortunately allured in the practice of a certain secret vice." For Hodson, as earlier for the Anodyne-Necklace crowd, coffeehouses, with their ever-circulating clientele, offered the venue for both sales and correspondence — requests for advice, offers of testimonials, and mail orders could be dropped there. And once again a buoyant market spread the word; edition after edition, variant upon variant mixed up *Onanism* with good advice and helpful products for a price.[41] Tissot's book itself had a continuous publication in all European and many non-European languages right up to the twentieth century and no doubt encouraged sales of the various medicines offered in newspaper ads.

By the middle of the nineteenth century, devices of all sorts had joined the potions and pills of the anti-masturbation marketplace. Driven by anxiety and guilt, there was a seemingly inexhaustible demand for something, anything, that would stop the depredations of the supposedly secret vice. Capitalism and technology rose to the challenge: a steady stream of appliances — erection alarms, penis cases, sleeping mitts, bed cradles to keep the sheets off the genitals, hobbles to keep girls from spreading their legs — earned at least twenty patents in the United States alone.[42] And parents were urged by many a guidebook to exercise the utmost vigilance even without the help of technology. Right up to the Great War, in short, an extensive commercial medical network profited from the disease and the guilt born in or around 1712.

Popular medicine of many sorts, as well as health-related public policy debates, which held out no immediate prospects for gain, also kept masturbation before the public throughout the nineteenth and early twentieth centuries. They spoke in the service of a wide variety of often mutually incompatible causes, but out of this cacophony one clear message emerged: masturbation was the universal negation of, the most disastrous alternative to, everything good that one might affirm about the sexual body and the root of everything bad, corrupting, and antisocial to which it might fall prey. More than a half million copies of a book on sexual perversions by the nineteenth-century phrenologist O.S. Fowler, for example, let it be known that masturbation was "man's sin of sins, vice of vices" which had caused "incomparably more sexual dilapidation, paralysis, and disease as well as demoralization than all other sexual vices combined." Fowler was not suspicious of sexual pleasure per se. Others were. J.H. Kellogg, the American health reformer and founder of the cereal dynasty, circulated through his network the news that masturbation was the worst possible instance of the generally unfortunate human propensity to want sex. He could scarcely contain his repulsion: the "moloch of the species," "a crime doubly abominable" than the "heinous sin" of illicit commerce between the sexes. Sylvester Graham, the eponymous creator of the cracker that would ensure his fame, was of similar mind.[43]

The eighteenth-century tradition that mixed medicine with moral pedagogy also grew cancerously; word of the solitary vice's peculiarly insidious threat metastasized everywhere. *Scouting for Boys*, to take one of many later examples, brought elite jeremiads of an earlier age squarely into the early twentieth century and into the front parlors of a class well below those who might have read the earlier authors. If this "beastliness" becomes a habit, Chief Scout Lord Baden-Powell intoned, it "quickly destroys both health and spirits"; its hapless practitioners are liable to end "in a lunatic asylum." In the forward to a much-circulated pamphlet, the chief scout of the Boy Scouts of America warned that he had "seen boys as young as twelve years, or slightly more, in insane asylums from excesses of this kind. The cure is almost hopeless." Slightly older boys were not spared. Members of the Royal Navy, each given Arthur Trewby's *Healthy Boyhood*, learned that meddling improperly with the private parts would cause the brain to suffer. Anyone with a shred of manliness would resist.[44]

Girls got it even worse. The author of one of the books for boys, introduced this time by the chairman of the Social Hygiene Committee of the American Federation of Women's Clubs, warned them, in their very own pamphlet, that they faced a complete collapse of their nervous systems, which could send them, like boys, to an asylum but also "to an early grave." The full weight of the well-meaning U.S. Department of Labor Children's Bureau echoed these views in a pamphlet that advised mothers lest their children be "wrecked for life."[45] In short, *Onania*'s reach became ever greater and ever more connected with the great questions of the day and with almost every organization concerned about human welfare and morality.

Masturbation also figured prominently in the medico-moral

debate about birth control. For almost all Roman Catholic commentators over the millennia "the sin of Onan" had meant coitus interruptus. (I tell the story of theological interpretations of Onan later, and readers anxious to get it now might skip to pp. 125–35.) In more technical Catholic medico-moral discussions of the nineteenth century, the neologism "onanism" was defined as a new version of the old "peccatum Onan" and consisted, as it always had, in this: "when the man after beginning copulation, withdraws before semination and spills the semen outside its proper vessel so as to impede conception."[46] By extension, in the nineteenth century the sin came to include the use of any form of birth control. But now the traditional sin could be made to seem worse than ever by taking on board the visceral wickedness associated with the notorious new one: masturbation. Thus the redundant "marital" was added to "onanism" to create the hybrid "marital onanism" and make the old-fashioned kind appear even more wicked.

Doctors were generally not interested in sinfulness. But quite aside from whether onanism was wrong, what it did *not* produce occasionally brought it into the arena of medicine and public policy. In population-conscious France, for example, serious people called for a national self-pollution police — surprise inspections of the young at school to make sure that they kept their bodies fit for the state.[47] Such tactics would either keep them from masturbating in the first place for fear of detection and public humiliation or, at the very least, stop the damage before it could go too far. From an entirely different political and moral perspective, Anthony Comstock's campaign in the United States against birth control was rooted in his deep guilt about and hostility to masturbation, which sexual intercourse for pleasure alone seemed to approximate.

The story was not so different on the other side. Proponents of birth control, whatever their motivations — an interest in improving the lot of the poor by helping them limit their families, a worry about overpopulation, belief in freedom from procreation for all sorts of cultural reasons — ended up using the same antimasturbatory rhetoric as those who thought that all non-reproductive sex was morally wrong. Opponents as well as proponents

48

of sexual pleasure for its own sake thought alike about solitary pleasures.[48] In fact, masturbation was the bottom line of the full range of *reductio ad absurdum* arguments. On one side was the claim that birth control was dangerous because it was just another form of masturbation. The internal organs of a woman who masturbates are identical to those of married women who use birth control, said Dr. Elizabeth Blackwell, the best-known woman doctor of the late nineteenth century. She had already addressed the profound dangers of masturbation for women and was now arguing against devices that blocked the entrance to the womb. Her general point is that tender love is a physiological necessity, because it allows the mind to supply the body with the extra nervous energy it needs for sex; masturbation demands the energy without the love impulse or physical exchange, and birth control is, she makes clear, just another version of the same thing.[49]

The other side turns the tables. Physiology proved, it was said, that the reproductive instinct — the desire for sexual intercourse — was "superior to all others in universality and violence" (the words are those of the eighteenth-century German anatomist and anthropologist Johann Friedrich Blumenbach, but they might as well have been spoken by Thomas Malthus). From this follows a call not for abstinence but for sexual intercourse freed from the danger of conception; the failure to provide a socially and personally safe outlet in the good old heterosexual fashion for the unstoppable instinct would lead inevitably to its finding gratification in "a mischievous manner." Birth control prevented conception, but it also prevented masturbation. "Having recognized that sex-starvation is as serious as food-starvation," neo-Malthusians argued that the moral restraint Malthus himself had advocated — celibacy or late marriage — could, and should not be relied upon to stop sexual intercourse. It was immoral and unworthy of the age of progress to allow the disastrous consequences of a lack of sexual constraint — Malthus's so-called positive checks of famine, death, and extreme poverty kept population in line with food supply — to prevail. And relief through the "mischievous manner," that is, through "the unnatural habit of Onanism or Solitary gratification," was no solution at all. It was "an anti-social and demoralizing habit"; it did not give "quietus to the mind" of those who resorted to it; but, worse, it impaired its victims' "bodily powers as well as mental and not infrequently le[d] to insanity." Onanism always had "bad consequences." By contrast, a temperate and natural gratification "of the reproductive instincts," with no fear of unwanted pregnancy, was "attended with good — besides the mere attendant pleasures." Birth control, in short, prevented masturbation. Everyone, of whatever view, thought that masturbation was the enemy, and that almost anything bad followed from it.[50]

Supporting the sales of cures for masturbatory diseases and the public-policy debates about masturbation — that is, the gigantic medico-moral apparatus through which the solitary vice came to the consciousness of the laity — was the high medical tradition of professional journals, doctoral theses, encyclopedias, and books. There were hundreds of articles in the learned press about this or that new ailment that could be attributed to masturbation; all the major scientific reference works had one or more entries on the subject; specialist textbooks in urology, gynecology, psychiatry, neurology, and sexology supplied popular authors with more than enough material in this charged area. Their wisdom echoed in lay reference works and many other places as well. Nineteenth-century readers could hardly avoid the topic. A public-minded citizen of Ontario, Canada, for example, might pick up the report of a provincial hospital to find the warning that "every man in society who knows anything of the evil under consideration," that is, masturbation, and who remains silent or refuses to take public action to remove or mitigate the danger should be regarded as a criminal.[51] Silence itself was a sign of deviance. Those worried about women in sweatshops might see the problem refracted in the well-known medical observation that thigh friction from operating a sewing machine could be masturbatory. Likewise riding a bicycle, that dangerous conveyance of modernity and freedom. Masturbation, in short, could focus anxiety about almost anything.[52]

In the early twentieth century, when the swell of specific diseases attributable to it began to ebb, masturbation's more general medico-moral dangers flooded into new areas. Sex hygiene became part of eugenics, and eugenics became an instrument of national security and of a perceived international struggle of race against race. And in the middle of it was onanism. Masturbation was of primary concern, for example, to the reformers and modernizers who brought sex education and eugenics to Japan. It was, so said the founding director of Japan's first medical school for women in 1908, "the most terrible ailment related to the sexual instincts"; their only true purpose was to produce healthy children and therefore self abuse had fatal consequences not only for every individual's reproductive capacity but for society at large. The private vice had become a major question of public policy wherever science was mobilized in the competition between states.[53] Nothing will bring back the procreative powers once they are destroyed by "disobeying natural laws," warns a Western guide to sexual hygiene. Self-abuse destroys unwary boys physically by ruining their muscles and nerves and morally through the imagination. Our author suggests, in this age of individualism, that mothers might help by keeping watch but "the boy must realize that salvation rests with himself."[54]

The old paradigm also died hard. Germs, not self-abuse, had taken the blame for consumption and spinal tuberculosis by 1900. But reflex physiology and research into the biochemistry of metabolism offered new pathways by which masturbation could account for heart murmurs, optical cramps, and a wide variety of neurological and psychological debilities. Modern biological science did not give up on the sexual vice of modernity until well into the twentieth century, and even then it maintained a foothold through the social sciences. A major thinker like G. Stanley Hall—the professor of psychology who more than anyone developed the modern idea of adolescence and who, as president of Clark University, where Freud was invited for his first lectures in the United States—still found an audience for his claim that "masturbation is the most perfect vice and sin," "one of the very saddest of all the aspects of human weakness and sin as well as the cause of a host of nervous and cardio-vascular symptoms." Almost every great evil—social and individual—was, in his view, caused by, or mirrored in, its perversity. And his is only the most famous of the high tide of nineteenth-century criticism that swept — as we shall see in Chapter 6 — into the twentieth century. The medical tradition that began with *Onania*, that was consolidated by Tissot, and that flourished in the later eighteenth and the nineteenth century did not end until the 1920s, if then.

But medicine, high and low, is only one of the two streams through which *Onania* made its way into the world. Neither crass commercialism, nor medico-moral public-policy questions, nor the research tradition in masturbatory diseases would alone account for the spread of the new vice from its early-eighteenth-century Grub Street origins. Widely distributed tracts like Dr. Solomon's and Goss's and Hodson's had no intellectual ambitions, but they shared with Rousseau's *Emile* the view that self-abuse posed a peculiar moral danger from which, somehow, its medical dangers seemed to arise. Exploring here the reasons for the public's receptivity to the moral worries of philosophers, learned physicians, or quack doctors would take us beyond the present story of how the new vice spread from London ever outward. (The impatient can skip ahead to Chapters 4 and 5.) But the moral problem of masturbation follows its own channels, ones that widen and multiply well after masturbatory diseases and debilities are things of the past.

Low and more cultivated literature alike agreed that the fundamental problem with masturbation — or pleasure, depending on what one reads — was its autarkic existence. It was the avatar of a seemingly impossible land of sexual plenty and unlimited freedom; no need of anyone or anything, it taunted, because everything required — the desire and its satisfaction — was securely lodged within the individual. "The criminal carries forever about him the instruments and the incentives of his own guilt." "We wantonly, or without occasion, subject ourselves to lascivious desires; it is the imagination... and not nature that importunes them." (The last phrase is an almost exact translation of what the *Encyclopédie* had to say on the subject some forty years before; words circulated.) The usual way of preventing vice — avoiding temptation — was useless against a practice generated entirely from within. And conversely, masturbation was thought to be rampant because this uniquely attractive and available sin had — so to speak — no natural predators. Because it was generally practiced alone and in secret — or among like-minded miscreants — it was understood as almost uniquely free from the social opprobrium or fear of punishment that constrained the proliferation of other vices. (The secrecy of the vice it was exposing had been one of *Onania*'s big self-justifications for going public with so scandalous a subject.) Women, for example, who would not dare risk their reputations on extramarital satisfaction might think that they could satisfy themselves risk free. "What can hinder the odious propensity from taking frequent effect?"[55]

Something had to break into this circle of solipsism, and it was to be a new pedagogy. Schools and teachers would expose the secret vice; once public, its evils could be reckoned with. We might have suspected as much. In the first place, there were more schools, for both boys and girls, than ever before. The problem of adolescent sexuality, always just beyond the supervision of adults, was thus especially acute. Moreover, the education of the young was regarded as critical to the eighteenth-century project of creating a new sort of self-determining, self-governing, morally autonomous person. Pedagogy, in short, was at the heart of the Enlightenment.

The wide dissemination of *Emile* and its many interlocutors had already carried the anxiety about masturbation far from its starting point, and a whole new educational literature carried it farther. The prominent and widely published English headmaster of Tunbridge School Vicesimus Knox, for example, wrote in 1783 that teachers could not be too terrifying in their anti-masturbatory jeremiads; paint its consequences, he advised, "in colors as frightful as the imagination can conceive." This, like almost all eighteenth-century jeremiads against masturbation, came from the pen of a progressive. Knox and his family were driven from the Brighton theater by a reactionary mob when their presence there was discovered because he had preached against the counterrevolutionary French war in 1793; he favored Catholic emancipation. Masturbation, once again, is the sin of the moderns.

53

Nowhere did *Onanism* find a bigger audience than in Germany, where the pedagogues engaged with building a new civic culture from the ground up became deeply worried about the secret new vice. Johann Georg Zimmermann, the great friend of Tissot, of Goethe, and of almost everyone else in the intellectual elite, wrote an article in the leading progressive journal of his day — the same one in which Kant published his famous essay on what is Enlightenment — in which he solemnly declared that girls masturbated as much, and with as much danger to themselves, as boys. Dr. Samuel Gottlieb Vogel — famous for his educational writings and for introducing the word "paranoia" into medical practice — listed the dangers to each sex separately but argued that they were far greater for girls.[56] And one of the best known internationally of the German educators, C.G. Salzmann, produced more than three hundred pages on the topic by accumulating story after story of fallen youth, one more alarming than the next. His influence was wide. One of the founding mothers of feminism, Mary Wollstonecraft translated — adapted would be more accurate — his main work. She herself takes up the subject elsewhere in a context not altogether different from that of her German colleague: what is learned in school, she argues, has real social consequences. Specifically, "the little respect paid to chastity in the male world is ... the grand source of many of the physical and moral evils that torment mankind." In school, boys learn vices — "nasty indecent tricks" — which "render the body weak, whilst they effectually prevent the acquisition of any delicacy of mind." "[S]elfish gratifications," which "very early pollute the mind," she concludes, "render private vices [the standard term for masturbation] a public pest."[57] Whether Salzmann was behind the English feminist's views or not, he was a big name in pedagogical circles, and his 341-page *On the Secret Sin of Youth* was a major intervention.[58]

The narrator in this book suggests that he writes very near to the originary moment of a new sin, even before its name is generally known. In an early episode — the book is in the form of letters mostly from hapless suffering masturbators with the author/narrator's commentary — a young boy reports that he kept hearing the word "onanism" (*Onanie*) but that he did not know what it meant. He thought, in fact, that it referred to bestiality, but then why did the speaker use this "incomprehensible word" instead of a good German one? *Onanie* was a new word in German and, Salzmann acknowledges, the more descriptive term would be "self-pollution." (*selbst-befleckung*). It is also probably true, as this and other letter writers report, that teachers and parents were not fully committed to acknowledging that masturbation was the primal sin. Or they may well not have known about it. Thus Salzmann justifies his evangelizing for the new vice. One ought not to speak of sin, even a newly exigent one, lightly.[59]

There is also a sense in which masturbation here, and more generally, was always waiting to be discovered; it always needed to be condemned and guarded against not by external constraints — ineffective against a secret vice — but through guilt, which each generation had to be taught anew. It seemed by its very nature to be perpetually on the increase and thus constantly in need of censure. As with tobacco, to which it was compared, there was always more and more of it to meet an endless, self-referential desire; unlike tobacco, however, masturbation involved no exchange, no regulating economy. Of all sins, Salzmann argued, this one seems on first reflection to be the least wrong, the least prevalent, the least dangerous, which explains why for millennia it had been scarcely noticed at all. Every inquiry, beginning with *Onania*, remarks on how shockingly misguided this analysis is and how, in consequence, the vice is rampant. "I asked 94 of my pupils," reports one schoolmaster who wrote to Salzmann, and forty-nine admitted masturbating; he said he had "no reason to assume that all of the remaining forty-five are innocent."[60]

He thinks them all guilty because no vice is more attractive or easier to accomplish. It can be carried on without anyone's help. "The opportunity to embrace it is always there." It is not subject to public censure because "it is incredibly easy to keep secret." And it is subject to none of the quotidian obstacles to action in the real world. The laws of resistance and inertia do not seem to apply in relations to oneself. "At least" — here Salzmann perhaps echoes Rousseau's *Confessions*, which had been published in German two years before his book[61] — "in liaisons between the sexes there are restraints. There are always interruptions [*Unterbrechungen*] of various sorts ... one needs time and space ... one has to make arrangements not to be caught and to keep one's good name; it takes efforts." And also, because masturbation is solitary, it has the potential to enslave a soul with a nearly unbreakable habit before the victim is even aware of its dangers. The book is full of confessions of just how hard boys tried to give up onanism only to lapse again. The self seems haunted by the power to addict itself to a drug-like practice whose effects are every bit as deadly as those of any narcotic. Like heroin or some other horribly seductive drug that ensnares those who try it even once, masturbation makes addicts of the innocent.

Most eighteenth-century writers speak of social corruption — schools, bad companions, nursemaids, or servants that start children on their paths to perdition — but Salzmann is, as Freud would be, clear that masturbation comes essentially from within and that only guilt could redeem the young and transform the easy sexuality of the self into the far more demanding sexuality of society. In other words, the very structure of this vice — its limitless potential, its unknown extent, its secrecy — demanded excesses of censure. Precisely because masturbation was so covert, so insidious, so occult in origin, teachers had to attack it with nuclear intensity.

"I was not led astray by others," writes one thirteen-year-old boy who discovered self-pollution all on his own. His letter to Salzmann continues: "I had never heard it spoken of; I did not even know the difference between the sexes." For years, he says, "I did it without any sense of it being bad." It seemed as free from guilt as tickling, no more meaningful than being stroked under the chin by one of his friends. He says he simply enjoyed himself — every two weeks, maybe more often, he cannot remember — and felt so innocent that he would have told his parents if they had asked. Extreme naïveté perhaps, but paradigmatic of the danger of the pure sexuality of the self. Before Freud offered a model of sexual ontogenesis in which masturbation was ubiquitous but not, within limits, a calamity, the war against it was never ending and unsparing.[62] As if by parthenogenesis, this vice seemed self-generative from within the bodies of even the youngest children.

Rousseau's call for vigilance in *Emile* became ever more terrifyingly precise, and with each warning, of course, the vice became more known and feared. "It is immediately after birth" that the danger is greatest, just when the development is at its most rapid, wrote the major French medical encyclopedia of the early nineteenth century, published by what was probably the most important firm in France, the same house that had commissioned the *Encyclopédie*. "If by some unfortunate accident" or through "foreign contact the child [boys are the reference here but not everywhere] discovers a sensation located in the genital organs," the site where "the forces of life are concentrated," then all is lost. "The subject is carried away by a deceitful pleasure and abandons himself with a furor to a vice which will soon be his perdition, or draw upon him ills that are more terrible than death." "All is lost," the entry concludes, a phrase contemporary readers might have remembered from *Emile*. "Foreign contact" is an allusion to the much-lamented practice of nurses' tickling the penises of infant boys to keep them quiet. This worry itself is new, a creation, I suspect, of the discovery of masturbation. In the early seventeenth century, Louis XIII's doctor had no qualms about telling the world how the future king was calmed by his nanny's playing with his penis and indeed offered no criticism of the boy's unabashed masturbation, even though he was not happy with much else in the sexual culture of the court. Two generations earlier, the physician and anatomist Fallopius had encouraged parents to rub a son's penis repeatedly, bringing it again and again to erection. This would enlarge it and help ensure his future wife the pleasure necessary for conception.[63] Much had changed.

By the last third of the eighteenth century, after Tissot and Rousseau, the once-novel "trouble and agony of a wounded conscience" announced by *Onania* were everywhere. Masturbation had taken on a moral significance that would have seemed unimaginable a century earlier. And it continued to make its way along the high and low roads of late-eighteenth-century culture and then nineteenth-century culture. No less a figure than

Immanuel Kant, who thought more deeply about what it meant to be an ethically self-determining subject than any other modern philosopher, took up the subject with an extraordinary mixture of hyperbole and hard reason. Before we look more closely at his arguments, a glance over the linguistic field will tell us a great deal about his stakes in the matter. *Selbstschändung*, "self-abuse," is out there with *Selbstbewusstsein*, "moral self-consciousness," *Selbstschätzung*, "self-esteem," and *Selbsterkenntnis*, "moral self-knowledge." It is considered alongside *Selbstmord*, "self-murder," that is, suicide, and is followed by a discussion of *Selbstbetäubung*, "self-stupefaction through immoderate drink or food." Masturbation is abuse of the self whose moral foundations Kant is trying to create. Its evilness arises not from its being one more instance of concupiscence but from its being an attack on the whole enterprise of putting morality on a new footing.

Sexuality within marriage, a central concern in Christian moral theology, was, Kant argued, relatively unproblematic. This is surprising on its face. Sexual inclination is only tenuously "love" and more plausibly "the strongest possible sensuous pleasure in an object." So-called sexual love has almost nothing in common with moral love or love of benevolence but, to the contrary, is a manifestation of "the appetitive power in its highest degree, passion." And, most important for Kant, sexual pleasure is unashamedly "pleasure from the use of another person," the use of another as a means to self-gratification rather than as an end. Still, it could be assimilated into a modern rational ethics. Men and women of reason — both sexes are equal contracting agents here — could essentially agree to use each other in return for other things. They could enter into a marriage contract through which they "reciprocally obligate each other" and thereby bring sexual pleasure "into close union with [moral love] under the limiting conditions of practical reason."

Passion, in other words, is managed by civil society, by a whole repertoire of duties that militate against the selfish use of another — or oneself — merely for one's own pleasure. Kant says nothing about concupiscence, impurity, or chastity, which had dominated earlier discussions of sexual union. Nonreproductive intercourse

— sexual pleasure outside the natural purpose of sexual love — may be a hard but not intractable case. It is only superficially unnatural. But masturbation — about which moral theology had been largely silent — was another matter. It is, for Kant, a species of moral insanity, deeply "unnatural," an abrogation of all that it was to be an ethical subject; to masturbate was to embrace naked animality.[64]

The question he poses is this: Given that one can contract, through marriage, with another person to use him or her for one's own sexual pleasure, can one make a similar contract with oneself? Or, more generally, does one have a duty not to use one-self as an object, specifically not to use oneself as an object for one's own pleasure? Kant's answer is an emphatic, exaggerated yes. No violation strikes more deeply at the core of ethical being: it is called "defilement" (*Schändung*) and "not merely a debase-ment [*Abwürdigung*] of one's humanity in one's own person." The instinct to self-pleasure is called carnal lust; the vice is called impurity; and the virtue "with regard to this sensuous instinct" is called chastity. Chastity, in other words, is no longer primarily a virtue with respect to others but is "to be set forth now as the duty of a person toward himself."

The case is transparent; there is no possible ambiguity. It is clear to "everyone, immediately," that carnal self-defilement is "contrary to morality in the highest degree." The mere thought of it stirs up such an aversion that "we consider it indecent even to call it by its proper name." This is not the case, Kant reminds us, with self-murder, which we are all prepared "to lay before the world's eyes in all its heinousness." Of course, talking about sexual pleasure — even married love — requires some delicacy "in order to throw a veil around it." But masturbation is the wrong that dare not speak its name. Medieval theologians had spoken similarly of sodomy, of which some thought masturbation was a subspecies. But no secular thinker had gone quite this far.

It was, Kant said, worse than suicide. It violated a higher law of reason: self-murder breaks only the law of individual preserva-tion, whereas masturbation mocks the greater law of preservation of the species. But more important, the very impulse to do it was unnatural. Lust is called unnatural, he explains, if man is aroused to it, not by its real object, but by his imagination of this object, and so in a way contrary to the purpose of the desire, since he himself creates its object. For in this way the imagination brings forth an appetite contrary to nature's purpose ... [or to the contract of mutual pleasure that is marriage].

Freud might say that one uses the self as a fetish, that sexual self-love is a perversion.

At the end of the day, the general context for the question of carnal pleasure remains for Kant, as it had for Aquinas, one of nonreproductive sexuality, but he arrives at an answer by a highly significant detour. He is not primarily upset about misdirecting or misusing an existing sexual appetite. The problem is not concupiscence; normal sexual drives can be civilly regulated within marriage. Masturbation represents the abandonment of both reason and society. It is not so much a cause of insanity, as the doctors would have it, as its sign: *prima facie*, self-pollution is an act of moral madness.

I have given so much attention to Kant because of his prominence in the history of thinking about the morally autonomous modern self. It was Kant who defined "enlightenment" as throwing off the shackles of tutelage, of moral childhood, and becoming a self-determining adult whose actions would be governed by reason. Within this great project, masturbation mattered. But his interest in the subject was by no means unusual for his generation. In 1786, the *Berliner Monatsschrift*, which had published his "What Is Enlightenment" two years earlier, invited submissions on the prize topic "How children and young people can be spared the physically and spiritually devastating vices of unchastity in general and onanism in particular, or, insofar as they are already infected by these vices, how they can be healed." An "aristocratic friend of humanity" donated a generous prize of 60 Dutch ducats — about a year's salary for a fully employed laborer — and the most prominent education reformer of his day, Joachim Heinrich Campe, was appointed judge. After surveying a sizable pool of submissions, Campe chose four that he published, in whole or in part, in his massive project for a general review of German education that was meant to reshape the pedagogy of the new civil society. Prize essays of the sort generated by essay contests generally appeared, and were debated, simultaneously in learned journals, various periodicals, and newspapers; thus the reading public could not escape learning about the horrors of the solitary vice.[65]

With Kant, Campe, and their colleagues the solitary vice reached a new level of ethical centrality. But it had already established itself all over the Western world; at the end of the eighteenth century, no sexual act was so protean a signifier. The new vice and modernity went forward together everywhere except where one might have expected: the Church. This bastion of moral education was, remarkably, not part of the story until much later. It was reluctant to suggest vices that the young might not have thought of, and in any case, this one was not terribly interesting from a traditional perspective. As late as 1844, a priest who was also a doctor chided his colleagues for not taking masturbation seriously enough, but he based his arguments on his secular, not his clerical, calling, that is, on the many horror stories he had gathered from the annals of medicine and physiology about men and women, boys and girls dead from onanism. These, he said, could teach moral theology about dangers that it ignored.[66]

If not as extensively present in moral theology and pastoral practice as some would have liked, masturbation was everywhere else by 1800, richly elaborated and available for all manner of cultural work. It was there as metaphor, for example, as a way of linking eighteenth-century associations of a suspect interiority — a mental life unconstrained by external reality — with madness and dissimulation. Byron's views on Keats's poetry come to mind: "a Bedlam vision," "signifying nothing," "a sort of mental masturbation — frigging his Imagination," "Self-Polluter of the human mind." "The *onanism* of Poetry" sums it up; Keats had pushed the Romantic fascination with endless desire and plays of the imagination over the abyss. Wordsworth accused his verse of "outrageous stimulation." It is a set of images that stuck. Walt Whitman's celebration of masturbation in "Song of Myself" is, claims a prominent modern critic, the "genuine scandal" of his poetry.[67]

There is, of course, a certain irony in all this. Literature in general, and the emotional intensity of Romanticism in particular, seem to have actually caused people to masturbate. Or so they said. Moralists were not making up the danger. Vissarion Belinsky, the founder of Russian realism, one of the towering critics of his age, and a man who examined his own private life relentlessly, confessed to the anarchist Mikhail Bakunin that reading Byron and Schiller had driven him to masturbation when he first encountered them as a nineteen-year-old student.[68]

Whether some literature — or a certain way of living — was "masturbatory" or caused masturbation, the new vice had become an adjective and would live on as such through the nineteenth and into the twentieth and twenty-first centuries: always pejorative, always pointing to an excess of imagination, to a lack of seriousness, to a retreat from reason and from proper, polite behavior. Richard Wagner used the term with great virtuosity, blending the figurative and the literal seamlessly. Quick to blame the moral, mental, and physical failings of former friends on masturbation, he also singled out Jewish art as masturbatory in the same terms that Byron used to attack Keats: "Fundamentally separated from life...[a world] in which art only plays with itself." Wagner was not original in this. The connection between Jews and onanism goes back at least to Abbé Grégoire, a major player in French revolutionary cultural politics and an advocate of Jewish emancipation, who identified *unassimilated* Jews as masturbators in a tract arguing that only when they were secularized and assimilated would they be ready for citizenship — and for a decent sex life, too, one supposes. And late-nineteenth-century cultural anti-Semites would take up Wagner's themes: Jews (Felix Mendelssohn was their prime example) made art that referred only to itself and was not grounded in a national project; Jews were degenerate because they masturbated, and they masturbated because they were degenerate. Wagner, for example, knew full well that the young Jewish poet Theodor Apel's blindness was caused by a riding accident but nevertheless ascribed it to onanism.[69]

If the vice that was almost unheard of in secular circles less than a century earlier had become ripe for metaphor by the late eighteenth century, it had also become — and would continue to be — the stuff of political scandal great and small. Among the charges brought against Marie-Antoinette in 1793 by the radical revolutionaries was that she had taught her son, the nine-year-old dauphin, to masturbate. Hébert told the tribunal that the king's son, a boy already suffering ill health, had been surprised in an act of self-abuse "fatal for his condition." When pressed on where he had learned the "criminal ruse" — once again the emphasis is on dissimulation, on the trickery and fantasy inherent in the act — the boy replied that "he owed his familiarity with the criminal habit to his mother and his aunt."[70] Of treason she was probably guilty; perhaps, given the great array of kinky sex available in aristocratic circles, she had had a liaison with her intimate friend the duchess de Polignac and others; but of this she was surely innocent. The juxtaposition of treason with masturbation, however, makes the revolutionary's point with exquisite precision. In the minds of the queen's enemies, there could be no more perfect sexual parallel for her political crimes, for the rottenness of the old regime, and for the corruption that emanated from the foreign queen than the secret, hidden, polluting, and paradigmatically dishonest act of onanism through which she sought to corrupt her son.

At the other end of the social spectrum and a century later, masturbation was among the charges brought by one branch of Theosophists against another in early-twentieth-century California: C.W. Leadbeater, a teacher of one faction — subsequently defended by the founder, Annie Besant — had supposedly taught boys to masturbate as a way of preventing worse offenses. No offense could be worse. The American branch wanted to distance itself from such perversion.[71] (In 1991, the comedian Pee-Wee Herman or, more accurately his creator, Paul Reubens, was arrested, and his career ruined, for masturbating in an adult movie theater. Nothing, it appears, is more scandalous.)

Anything so delicate and secret could easily become, or at least be imagined as, the basis for blackmail. Having sold quack medicines to terrified young men — so a major nineteenth-century British paper reported — companies would charge them more and more for successive doses and threaten exposure of those who did not comply.[72] And why not? Charles Dickens's shifty-eyed, pimply, sallow-complexioned, untrustworthy Uriah Heep is probably the most famous and easily recognized culprit in Victorian fiction, but there are many, many others. (There are also other, and literarily more interesting, uses of masturbation in Dickens: his play on Swift's old joke in *Oliver Twist* — "Charley Bates, Master Charles Bates, Master Bates" — and the long account of Pip's hiding his "wicked secret," his "secret burden down the leg of his trousers" in *Great Expectations*.)[73] He was building on a century-long tradition that believed that the masturbator was an easily recognizable type. "Pale, desiccated limbs, hollow chest, powerless, sunken head . . . dead white face . . . eyelids falling powerlessly over his dying fading eyes." Pictures in widely circulated popular medical books put faces to words like these (figure 2.1). And worse. The poor once-handsome eighteen-year-old whom the dramatist Heinrich von Kleist saw and wrote about to his fiancée was near death from "unnatural sin," "his entire life nothing but a single, crippling swoon." A recent survey of German literary allusions to masturbation in the eighteenth, nineteenth, and twentieth centuries can scarcely contain its many references, and several monographs offer still more. The masturbator had become a figure of public scorn, derision, pity, fear; little wonder the young would go to great lengths to escape detection.[74]

The medical and the moral clearly overlap in descriptions like these, but physicians interested in an ethics based in nature condemned masturbation even if they had no interest in its putative organic pathologies. One of the first woman physicians in the Anglo-American world, Dr. Elizabeth Blackwell, for example, brought the full weight of modern medicine to bear on the proposition that masturbation was one of two vices from which "all other forms of unnatural vice springs" and much domestic violence besides. This was standard stuff in the purity crusades of which her book was a part, but it had little if anything to do with masturbatory disease. Blackwell, in fact, mobilized the vice for a specific political argument: masturbation was at the heart of a feminist analysis of the double standard that figured in a major legislative campaign. Men and women had the same natural sexual passions, she claimed. There were, therefore, absolutely no

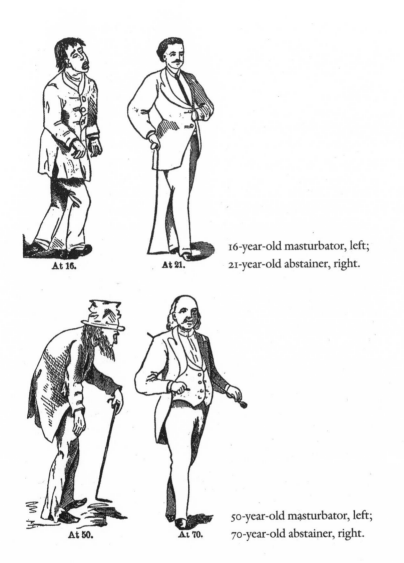

16-year-old masturbator, left;
21-year-old abstainer, right.

50-year-old masturbator, left;
70-year-old abstainer, right.

Figure 2.1. Faces of the masturbator, from Emery C. Abbey,
The Sexual System and Its Derangements (Buffalo, NY, 1875).

grounds for maintaining that men needed the release offered by prostitutes, a putative fact advanced by supporters of the Contagious Diseases Act, which, its opponents maintained, was trying to move late-nineteenth-century Britain toward a "French" system of state-licensed prostitution. Masturbation was dangerous, for both sexes, because it sharpened the sexual instincts — by exercising them prematurely — and because it decreased self-control, the basis of civilized humanity. Masturbation easily became obsessive, it was the most difficult form of sexuality to bring under the sway of reason, and hence it offered a model for unbridled sexuality generally.[75] It was the primal impurity, and that was enough; tuberculosis or madness had nothing to do with it.

By the turn of the new century, the organic dangers of self-abuse slowly, very slowly, had come to be regarded as the fears of another age, as the superstition or folk beliefs of the ignorant. But this was by no means the end of the story. It left what was really important about modern masturbation: the secret that stood at the heart of Western sexuality. Now largely stripped of its medical problems, it entered twentieth-century self-consciously modernist thought in three distinct but interconnected ways.

First, an enormous range of popular and professional work in anthropology, animal behavior, sexology, psychiatry, zoology, and other fields discovered not only that masturbation was nearly universal among the young — this had long been feared and known — but that it was practiced by all peoples everywhere, under an enormous range of circumstances, and by just about every animal one cared to observe as well. Horses and Welsh ponies, bears and ferrets, dogs, cats, apes, skunks, and deer all did it. So did the Balinese, Egyptians, Hottentots, Indians, Tamils, Kaffirs, Basuto, Chinese, and Japanese, not to speak of students, male and female, in the best schools as well as the reformatories of Europe. Techniques might vary; there were gender and racial differences. While all women, in whatever culture studied, seemed to masturbate, the use of artificial instruments seemed restricted in Europe and elsewhere to those "professionally devoted to some form of pleasure." But such nuances should not detract from the overwhelming fact that everyone did it. How the avalanche of data was interpreted varied. The evidence from humans could suggest the truth of degeneration theory — a favorite late-nineteenth-century view that saw in masturbation and prostitution, for example, signs of evolution gone wrong — or of the hypothesis that the premature development of sexual sensibility, before reproduction was possible, made some other form of release both natural and necessary, the view of the Nobel Prize winner Elie Metchnikoff. The German sexologist and physician Iwan Bloch, like Freud, goes back to Nietzsche, who suggested that the work of a learned man — that is, of civilization itself — depended on finding an appropriate outlet for basic and deep impulses. Some interpretations dealt with the zoological data; others did not. But taken together, the vast amount of new material on masturbation, widely available to the European and American reading public, greatly expanded the problem. It put the lie to the suggestion that masturbation was a perversion of young children and adolescents, something that could be prevented if only one had the correct pedagogy, or avoided bad servants, or kept children away from evil friends. It was, in a deep sense, natural and universal.[76]

The second major highway through which masturbation entered the twentieth century built on this mass of material and gave it a crucial psychological significance. In 1899, Havelock Ellis invented the term "autoeroticism," which laid claim to the whole empire of sexual emotion "generated in the absence of an external stimulus, proceeding directly or indirectly, from another person." Or creature. The new territory was immense. "Autoeroticism" described not only "those transformations of repressed sexual activity" that might result in various morbid conditions but everything that we would regard as the product of sublimation: "the normal manifestation of art and poetry, and indeed, more or less the color of life itself." In short, everything about sex that is in the mind — a great deal, as thinkers on the subject since Antiquity have known — was to be included under the new rubric. Indeed, every effort to achieve sexual satisfaction that came from within was included whether it was mindful or not.[77]

Masturbation, of course, constituted only one, somewhat arbitrarily delimited province of this vast realm, but, as Ellis pointed out, its significance could not be appreciated unless one regards it as "a sub-division of a great group of natural facts." At one extreme of this group is animal masturbation, which need not concern us here, although Ellis documents extensively the existence of self-stimulation in a variety of beasts. His point is that the propensity to generate sexual pleasure on one's own is grounded in nature; the beasts do it. But it is also a product of culture. Autoeroticism is greatly enhanced by that very faculty which makes us human, so that at the other extreme of this "great group of natural facts" are all those aspects of human experience where the imagination, sexuality, and art commingle. Masturbation becomes, in Ellis's formulation, the paradigmatic form of sex in the mind, the only sexual act, as the Italian novelist Alberto Moravia put it, that has an impact on culture precisely because it comes entirely out of fantasy.[78]

Masturbation, whose threat had long been regarded as its lack of articulation with the restraints of both society and morality, was now defined as a subspecies of a universal kind of pure sexuality, one freed from the constraints of body and society, time, place, and obligation and available for all manner of psychic work. Its moral valence now depended on how one viewed such matters. We could trace various positions through the twentieth century. On one side, for example, D.H. Lawrence, who famously despised the "sex-in-the-head middle classes" — hence the charm of Lady Chatterley's gamekeeper — clearly thought masturbation a poor substitute for the real, vital union of bodies. Those who complain that young men and young women are having sexual intercourse are really bewailing "the fact that they didn't go separately and masturbate." Sex has to go somewhere, and in "our glorious civilization, it goes to masturbation," that is, to the dead sex of the mind. The mass of popular literature and popular amusements, he suggests, seems to exist to fuel this secret in which the body remains, "in a sense, a corpse."[79] I might add that it is not just the cerebral quality of masturbation that so offended Lawrence; for him, as for eighteenth-century critics, it was its shameful privacy, more "private than excrementation."

On the other hand, Gore Vidal and André Gide — to take two

cases from the other side — are more sympathetic to Ellis's formulation: solitary sex is intimately bound up with the power to imagine and to create and, as Vidal wickedly notes, to have sex with someone else. *Onania*'s legacy expands still more. "Few lovers," Vidal suspects, "are willing to admit in the sexual act that to create or maintain excitement they may need some mental image as erotic supplement to the body in attendance." Rousseau's "dangerous supplement" has become domesticated and socially useful. Of course, we cannot take Vidal quite straight. That said, there is something to the idea that in order to make the solitary act meaningful for the adolescent — and why not for anyone? — "the theater of his mind early becomes a Dionysian festival." One consequence is that if someone does this well, then sex with another might become a boring disappointment, a standard eighteenth-century worry. But the other side of this prototypical occasion for fantasy is that it becomes the nursery of the imagination for a greater good.[80]

On the very first page of his autobiography — almost the first thing he says about himself — Gide describes parallel masturbation, himself a young boy with the son of a servant under the table at dinner, a scene suffused with guilt, sociability, and narcissistic autonomy. This memory is meant to be a prism for the making and the refraction of the self, and it is elaborated when masturbation once again becomes a trope for creativity. The "only possible explanation," Gide tells Roger Martin du Gard, for his "particular natural disposition" — by which he means his need and capacity to be emptied by multiple successive orgasms, which, in turn, he regards as central to his whole structure of desire, loss, production, enjoyment, taboo, and literature — is his early development of onanistic skills. There was less sin, he thought, if there was not complete orgasm; shock waves repeated, "often for a whole night long, without ever allowing himself to commit the 'full sin.'" As in Rousseau's *Confessions*, still resonant two centuries later in the more explicit language of our times, masturbation as a process of self-making was very much in evidence.

The third, and most important, way in which masturbation became a twentieth-century topic was through Sigmund Freud in whose work it became the great arena for human psychogenesis. Freud, of course, was not the only one of his contemporaries to make the subject central. We have already discussed Ellis, and there were many others. The pioneer sexologist Richard von Krafft-Ebing, for example, cared little about the corporeal effects of onanism but thought that "nothing contaminates like masturbation," in the sense that nothing is more likely to lead to the development of a "perverse feeling for the other sex," to an actual perversion of desire as distinct from merely engaging in a homosexual, perverted act. In other words, the failure to transcend infantile masturbation was the royal road to a very real distortion of the whole personality.[81] The American psychologist, G. Stanley Hall thought that more or less every unpleasant feature of adolescence, from excessive interest in theater to drug addiction, could be blamed on masturbation. But it was Freud who made it explicitly the secret of sex.

The great intellectual leap that made this possible was Freud's insight that the human sexual drive was not "naturally" directed toward reproduction or even toward a so-called opposite sex. Civilization had to struggle mightily to make out of the body and its desires the sort of useful, reproductive creatures — male and female — that it needed to sustain itself. And more generally, the struggle to sublimate the disorganized sexual energies of infancy into the organized sexuality of adulthood became the model for how desire itself had to be managed and directed if we humans were to attain higher goals: not only families, but art, music, literature, and all that culture stood for. In the beginning, there was the autoeroticism of the polymorphously perverse infant. On these insights and their multiple interpretations, the empire of masturbation, begun on Grub Street, expanded beyond the wildest nightmares of its eighteenth-century founders.

Few topics are discussed as extensively in Freud's work as masturbation and none is more deeply imbricated with his most foundational views. His thinking about it may well be the link between his early view that neurosis was rooted in actual trauma — the so-called seduction theory — and the view in which it is the result of the arrested erotic evolution of the self and its attendant guilt. By 1905, he could view Dora's claim to have been seduced as a phantasmic screen for unsuccessfully transcended infantile autoeroticism.[82] The struggle with masturbation became the psychic trauma he had looked for earlier in damage from actual sexual advances of an adult toward a child.

From this shift in Freud's thinking was born the notion that masturbation was the foundational form of sexual expression, perfectly natural and appropriate at an early stage of development but necessary to give up in the process of becoming a properly functioning adult. It was the site of the great struggles through which sexuality was channeled by civilization; and conversely, failure to manage it became the prototype for all other sorts of failure. "The insight has dawned on me," wrote Freud to his friend Wilhelm Fliess in late 1897, on the eve of *The Interpretation of Dreams*, "that masturbation is the one major habit," the "primary addiction," and, like addictions to alcohol, tobacco, or morphine, it served directly, or indirectly, as "a substitute for a lack of sexual satisfaction." In his analysis of Dostoyevsky, for example, he writes that masturbation gave way to compulsive gambling, emphasizing the common use of the word "play" at the gaming tables and with the genitals in the nursery.[83] It is in fact difficult to find major discussions in which autoeroticism does not figure. At one time or another, Freud traced anxiety neurosis, obsession, narcissism, hysterical vomiting, repressed memories of infantile sexuality, and, arguably, guilt itself to the psyche's confrontation with its primal source of sexual satisfaction. If masturbation was the enemy of adult sexuality, it was also its harbinger. Infantile masturbation proclaims the fact that the genitals are, as Freud says, "destined to great things in the future." Indeed, the entire organization of the human as a sexual being is negotiated through autoeroticism: "The future primacy over sexual activity exercised by this erotogenic zone was established by early infantile masturbation."[84]

What had been an ethically suspect and medically pernicious practice became with Freud an arena for normative psychogenesis. It was something one had to go through, to get beyond in a precise and orderly way. Masturbation constituted essential practice for the real thing: "preformative of the modes of erotic satisfaction that will be proper to the adult," as Freud's disciple Marie Bonaparte put it.[85] And for girls the process was especially treacherous, because their early rehearsals were for the wrong show. In becoming adult, they had to give up not only masturbation but also the kind of orgasm procured by their infantile efforts. Giving it up meant, in this account, giving up clitoral for vaginal sexuality, fantasies of active masculinity for the reality of passive femininity. The vice of *Onania* had attained a major role in the most influential psychological theory of the twentieth century, and the masturbation of girls and women in particular, entirely ignored for thousands of years, had a special place within it.

Freud, his colleagues, and their successors bridged a gap between a two-hundred-year-long history of condemnation and a new history of the role autoerotic sexuality plays in making us who we are and are not. No subject was, for them, more fraught. When members of the Vienna psychoanalytic circle met to discuss *Onanie* for three evenings in 1910, they had such disagreements that they dared not publish their proceedings. Two years later, they held nine further meetings, and Freud could barely salvage a fragile consensus; he concludes his report with the observation that "the subject of masturbation is quite inexhaustible." Precisely two hundred years after the "trouble and agony of a wounded conscience" emerged from Grub Street, it stood as "representative of the conflict...between instinct and repression," as Freud's colleague Wilhelm Stekel put it: sexuality with a decidedly modern twist and enormous potential for self-fashioning.[86]

Within psychoanalysis after the first generation, masturbation continued to have great theoretical import, whether this was always recognized or not. "Autoeroticism in Freudian theory is the prototype of human sexuality," the distinguished analyst Joyce McDougall opined, "an oft overlooked fact." It was significant both for relatively orthodox theorists and for later feminist writers like Luce Irigaray, who uses an argument against the Master's male-centered construal of female autoeroticism — the little girl will not "masturbate 'herself'" but rather a penis equivalent" — as a way of reconceptualizing and distinguishing the category "woman." Indeed, it is woman's particular relationship to autoerotic pleasure that defines femininity, or at least a direct, unmediated, constant feminine access to the self and to feeling: "As for Woman, she touches herself in and of herself without any need for mediation." She "touches herself all the time ... no one can forbid her to do so, for her genitals are formed of two lips in continuous contact."[87] Masturbation is still the model but not for the normative adult feminine sexuality that Freud imagined.

The influence of psychoanalysis quickly radiated far beyond the discipline. Freud's account of sexual development had enormous influence on what was taught about sex in works ranging from pediatric to moral-theology textbooks. In its new and less hostile register, masturbation played an even bigger part in discussions of growing up and becoming a person than it had during the Enlightenment and the nineteenth century. It was "neither a sickness nor a sin," as a leading German handbook of the 1920s put it, but still worthy of seemingly endless attention.[88] Once the clouds of organic harm had dispersed, the underlying ethical and psychological questions about solitary sex emerged with ever greater clarity. Now that it was "well demonstrated" "that masturbation does not interfere with physical health," as a prominent early American analyst concluded, great new psychological vistas opened up. It was — so enlightened opinion taught — to be regarded as something natural when practiced by the young, a stage of sexual development that they would outgrow. And conversely, "when practiced by any adult," it was the mark of arrested development. Not so much wicked, and certainly not physically threatening, it was now a symptom of abjection, a sign of failure, a font of guilt, and a token of inadequacy. Practiced without fantasy, it was said to relieve only a "physical chemical tension"; practiced with fantasy, it was at best an incomplete emotional outlet, never offering the "spiritual value" that sex was meant to offer a "socialized adult." Adolescence, in particular, became the crux, a fraught time between "natural" infantile autoeroticism and its sad holdover into maturity, the period when masturbation went from being a sign of "budding sexuality" full of promise to being an indication that its practitioner was unable to have a proper love object and, more generally, to make peace with the demands of society.[89] One's relation to masturbation tracked precisely one's willingness to go with the flow of the civilizing process.

This broadly Freudian interpretation opened still more avenues of sexual politics. Continuing to masturbate after childhood, or actively embracing it as an affirmative good, came to be regarded as a rebellion against the whole complex of norms and expectations implicit in the early-twentieth-century synthesis. One might date this new development from the Kinsey reports, which burst on the American and international scenes in the late 1940s and early 1950s. They reinforced in a broader and seemingly more scientific context what had been known for some time: that the so-called perversion of masturbation was in fact remarkably commonplace. It was most common not, as some late-nineteenth-century observers might have predicted, among the most ignorant. To the contrary, the more educated people were, especially women, the more likely they were to masturbate or to have masturbated, or at least to report doing so. Moreover, it did not, in general, detract from the pleasures of the marriage bed, as eighteenth-century critics had feared. Masturbation and sexual satisfaction from heterosexual intercourse seemed to go together.

Kinsey's data do not in themselves make a case one way or another for autoeroticism. But, like his more disputed data on homosexuality, they show that what might have been regarded as a suspect and even perverted practice was part of a complex gradient of sexual activities that seemed to run seamlessly from the most normative to the most perverse. Taken together and in all their popularized formats, the massive Rockefeller Foundation–supported studies by the Institute for Sexual Research received more publicity nationally and internationally than any previous studies of sexuality. Through them, masturbation appeared more normal than it ever had before.

Alternatively, one might date the post-Freudian era of masturbation from 1966, the year William Masters and Virginia Johnson published *Human Sexual Response*, the first of their widely reprinted and translated works. The point of this book and what followed it was not, of course, to rehabilitate masturbation. But especially for women it had this effect. First, it put the lie to the

74

Freudian claim that clitoral sexuality, and with it masturbation, were left behind by adult women. Based on interviews and extensive observation of female masturbation, Masters and Johnson concluded that "most women continue active manipulation of the clitoral shaft or mons area during their entire orgasmic experience." This meant that in heterosexual intercourse, mere penetration and thrusting simply would not do. But more generally, it suggested that, at least from a physiological perspective, masturbation represented the real truth of a woman's sexuality. The human female, they announced, "is not content with one orgasmic experience during episodes of clitoral automanipulation." Freed from "psychosocial distraction," concentrating "only on their own sexual demands, without the psychic distractions of a coital partner," they can have orgasms up to the limits of sexual exhaustion. Masters and Johnson do not advocate such freedom from "distractions"; their aim is to help women in heterosexual relationships achieve satisfaction by incorporating masturbation into their lovemaking. But the message was clear enough: self-manipulation was the gold standard of pleasure. And it was a message that resonated in many communities. The radical separatist feminist Jill Johnson, writing in *Lesbian Nation*, for example, quotes the pair approvingly to argue that the outer third of the vagina is an orgasmic platform, that Freud is right in holding vaginal orgasm to be more mature, but that this speaks not for the penis but for a dildo or a banana used alone or by another.[90]

‖ From these foundations, masturbation was embraced first by the women's movement and then by various parts of the male gay movement as a practice in the service of freedom, autonomy, and rebellion against the status quo‖ Of late, its domain within the spectrum of sexual politics has widened still further. Far from signaling abjection, it came to represent, for the first time, the affirmation of something positive and different. Sex with oneself came to stand for autonomy, even autarky. It was not reprehensible or frightening but liberating, benign, and attractive.

The key feminist text in this, the last section of our story of how the vice of Grub Street became culturally central in the modern West — and by now elsewhere — is *Our Bodies, Ourselves*, published in 1971 as an expansion of a somewhat earlier mimeographed book-let produced by the Boston Women's Health Book Collective called "Women and Their Bodies." It has been enormously successful. Still in print as of 2002, over four million copies have been sold in at least sixteen languages. (Italian in 1974, Japanese and Danish in 1975, Spanish in 1977, German in 1980 and Dutch in 1981, for example. In 1973, there was already an English Braille edition.)[91]

The discussion of masturbation begins with the confession and then rejection of a two-century-old guilt that had been given a new — so it was argued — anti-feminist inflection by Freud. A woman reports that, as a girl, she was sure that her father's infection and threatened leg amputation had been the result of her guilty pleasure and that he would die if she did not stop. *Our Bodies, Ourselves* continues with a more general critique of the Freudian story I have just sketched — the abandonment of clitoral masturbation and with it clitoral sexuality as part of the process of becoming a woman — and proceeds to affirmative arguments for autoeroticism: it is not a substitute for sex with a man or with another woman; "it's different from, not inferior to, sex for two."[92] One could not ask for a more explicit rejection of traditional Freudian thought on the subject. In a book on the emotional problems of single women, Dr. Laura Hutton, a clinician at the Tavistock Clinic, put the contrary view unequivocally: masturbation was the equivalent of going to a prostitute except that "no other human being has been made use of for purely self-centered ends." There is always something lacking in this "more or less unconscious self-love" even if the inferiority of the practice is not recognized for what it is: "a regression to the infantile stage of auto-eroticism."[93]

The "sensuous pleasure from one's own body," which Dr. Hutton so confidently condemns, is given a radically different twist in *Our Bodies, Ourselves*. Self-love is precisely the place to start, an essential path to a woman's self-knowledge, from which all else springs. Masturbation "is the first, easiest and most convenient way to experiment with your body," women are advised; it is about pure pleasure and hence about unencumbered autonomy. Masturbation, to put it differently, temporarily suspends the reality principle. Then come instructions on how to do it, followed by a valedictory meditation on the value of fantasy. And here too the eighteenth-century account and Freud's reworking of it are given a rebellious reinterpretation. Far from being a flight from reality — the danger it was in Rousseau — or a form of infantile regression, it is said to tell "us something about the reality we are in," to tell us about "accepting our feelings and then trying to understand them."[94]

By the 1970s, a whole new literature devoted to rewriting the Freudian story, the prototype of the modern patriarchal narrative, had grown up in the arena of feminist struggle. Anne Koedt's "Myth of the Vaginal Orgasm" in 1970 was the first to make the link with women's liberation explicit — to translate the sentiments of medical self-help into a more political register — but her message very quickly found resonance in a range of popular, less explicitly polemical works.[95] Betty Dodson's *Liberating Masturbation: A Meditation on Self Love*, for example, straightforwardly makes the case that autoeroticism is not only a politically but also a personally liberating act. Her book, too, was enormously successful; appearing first in 1974, it went through six subsequent editions, the latest in 1996. (Her other books, *Selflove and Orgasm* and *Sex for One: The Joy of Selfloving*, are variations on the same theme, as are numerous audio- and video-tape cassettes.) Dodson's claims go well beyond those of the Boston Women's Health Book Collective: from masturbation as an extension of the critique of the vaginal orgasm in the service of more satisfying heterosexuality to masturbation as a claim to autonomy. Whereas *Our Bodies, Ourselves* is predicated on a fundamentally social, if not heterosexual, world, one in which we need others for our own pleasure, Dodson's book assumes no such telos: "Masturbation is our primary sexual life. It is our sexual base. Everything we do beyond that is simply how we choose to socialize our sex life." Her views also go well beyond those of Masters and Johnson, who advocated clitoral stimulation so that women might attain their full orgasmic potential with their male lovers, not for its own sake.

By the late 1970s, writing about masturbation — both as an attack on the Freudian normative and, more positively, as a way to attain self-knowledge and autonomy — had reached new levels. Less clinical, less overtly political, the solitary vice of the imagination and of fantasy that had so terrified Rousseau had been transformed into a virtue: self-pleasuring was the path to self-knowledge, self-discovery, and spiritual well-being. Commerce spreads the word, as it had *Onania*'s: sex shops provided all that was needed in the way of tools and stimulation — dildos, vibrators, and much more, as well as how-to-do-it books, could be ordered by mail or bought in person. Of course, not everything was for the purposes of masturbation, but much was, and the market was strong. The West Coast store Good Vibrations opened in 1977 and was followed in the next decade by many more. In its first year, this leading non-chain sex shop had sales of $15,000; by 1995, its sales had reached $5,472,166, and by 2000, over $8 million. It sold 134,000 vibrators that year and if we assume it had, at most, a 10 percent share of the market, this figure suggests total U.S. sales of more than a million vibrators. Certainly, Doc Johnson, the world's largest sex-toy manufacturer — a major supplier of vibrators — has done fabulously well. Between 1990 and 2000, it went from an $8-million-a-year business to over $45 million a year; the firm claims that its sales doubled from 1999 to 2001. (These are wholesale figures in an industry with a 150–200 percent markup, so retail sales are in the $100 million range; there are three other major — more than 100 employees — manufacturers in the United States and probably a dozen in Europe.) There is also a specialty market that caters to customers with an attitude. A very flashy Web site, for example, offers a full line of 100-percent silicon dildos in the shape of religious figures: a Jesus dildo, a Virgin Mary dildo, a Buddha dildo allow customers to masturbate in ways that are offensive to almost everyone. Then, of course, there is the rest of the world. Europe's top dealer in erotic paraphernalia — Beate Ushe — for example, had almost three hundred shops in 2000 and a mail order business besides generating over $150 million in sales, up from $100 million in 1998. We cannot say how much of this was for masturbation-related products — porn, vibrators, dildos, for example — but they are prominently displayed in her shops. (The firm was founded by Beate Rotermund, a war

widow who began by selling birth control information from a bicycle and went on to become the world's most successful merchant of erotica.)[96] In other words, the solitary vice has become
the basis for a healthy and growing economy in self-pleasure, and
this is not even counting the gigantic pornography industry, probably the only part of the Web that is making money, which exists
to promote sexual fantasy and masturbation.[97]

Betty Dodson's and Lonnie Barbach's — Barbach is a psychologist whose *For Yourself* and *Women Discover Orgasm* are very much
the genre we have been discussing — books seem to have sold
mostly through specialized outlets, but best-selling authors like
Nancy Friday, publishing with major houses, brought masturbation as a form of commitment to an inner life and to pleasure for
its own sake to a broad public that did not frequent sex shops.
Self-love had been rehabilitated; solipsism had lost its sting; a
new version of the old Hellenistic care of the self was born. Take
a hot bubble bath, surround yourself with candles and mirrors,
relax, allow your imagination full rein; Barbach had suggested
that women tell themselves, "I love you."[98] Autonomous.

Friday's appeal was broader and her message less focused. She
made a fortune selling women's masturbatory fantasies, packaged
as sexual coming-of-age stories, or tales of self-discovery, or
paeans of liberation, to a wide world that apparently could not
get enough of them. Masturbation, with its moral valences reversed, had entered the mainstream of commercial culture. Her
My Secret Garden: Women's Sexual Fantasies was published in 1973
and proclaimed a new pride in the secrecy — and the fantasy —
that had once made solitary sex so suspect. It hit a nerve. The
twenty-fifth edition came out in 1998. *Forbidden Flowers*, with the
subtitle *More Women's Sexual Fantasies*, came out two years later,
and other spin-offs followed. Rebellion against the Freudian or
neo-Freudian model gave the epistolary genre that Friday borrowed from the eighteenth century a new twist: her letters reported not the death, debility, or shame but the life, health, and
honor that were to be had from self-pleasuring. To be accurate,
her correspondents often did report shame and guilt but only to
exult in triumph over emotions so atavistic and unnecessary for

79

engaging in so harmless an act. "From shame to pride" might be the lesson one should draw. French, Polish, Chinese, German, Dutch, Portuguese, and Spanish translations hailed masturbation as the safest, most pleasurable path to self-discovery and fulfillment, not as the "abominable" practice that had for two centuries been regarded as destructive of both mind and body and for most of another century — after Freud — as a guilty deviation from normal psychogenesis.[99]

All of this, in turn, created a counterattack. Sex-positive feminism, as it has come to be called, and the explicitly if perhaps falsely liberationist rhetoric of the 1960s and 1970s spawned an opposition. There was, for example, the antipornography, and arguably antisex, campaign associated with Catharine MacKinnon and Andrea Dworkin in which male masturbation in any case figured prominently as a fantasy-driven rehearsal for real sexual aggression. Not an outlet for sexual energies that might have gone more dangerously elsewhere — Stekel's view back in the 1920s — but a preview of worse to come. Ideas incorporated acts: "Pornography is masturbation material," MacKinnon asserts. "It is used as sex. It therefore is sex." (Where the truth lies in this matter is difficult to say but the South African Government recently sided with Stekel: "Join the Arm Struggle [the word play is on "Armed Struggle," that is, the battle against Apartheid] and stop raping our mothers, wives, sisters and children," urged an official campaign. "Masturbate, Don't rape.")[100]

For two decades, men were largely untouched by all this. The Freudian story of how a boy became a man certainly demanded that he give up masturbation but not that he give up the organ he had found so pleasurable earlier. There was no political exigency equivalent to that surrounding the question of the clitoral orgasm to motivate a liberatory pro-masturbation movement. For men far more than for women, masturbation continued to carry the freight of two millennia of jokes and two centuries of guilt. It was a silly thing to do; real men who could get girls did not need to do it. "Wanker" and "jerk-off" were bywords for the abject man or boy whose masturbation represented a more generalized ineffectiveness.

Norman Mailer infamously made this case in an interview with Paul Krassner of the *Realist*, which he reprinted several times in the early 1970s: "Masturbation is bad . . . in relation to everything — orgasm, heterosexuality, to style, to stance, to be able to fight the good fight." It is, quite simply, incompatible with masculinity: "Anybody who spends his adolescence masturbating generally enters his young adulthood with no sense of being a man." There is, of course, a feminist response, most forcefully Kate Millett's, to Mailer's view that seemed to suggest that even rape was better than doing it to oneself. More on this in Chapter 6; for the present, the point is simply that masturbation had entered deeply into the sexual politics of the 1960s and their aftermath and that for men it was still off bounds.[101]

There were some hints of change before AIDS. In the 1960s, Alan Dugan's poem "For Masturbation" had already made of his subject a declaration of independence (Dugan won the National Book Award for Poetry in 2001):

I have allowed myself
This corner and I am God . . .
I will do as I will.

But two things happened. First, with the spread of epidemic disease and the demise of bathhouses, masturbation became a new option for gay men. For a time, it was written about as second-best, a retreat from the revolutionary limits of the old venues. By the late 1990s, however, it had achieved a new autonomy, a new status as a genuine alternative to heterosexual norms. Jack-off clubs in scores of the world's cities were not only alternative bathhouses but places where men could masturbate side by side: community, as it had for the gentlemen of antiquity, began with autonomy. The secret vice had found among gay men at least, a public recognition, one that acknowledged, as eighteenth-century critics had done implicitly, that the private vice was not so private. It was social in the "wrong way."[102]

But one man's wrong way is another man's virtue. Masturbation, through its links to the gay movement — and perhaps through a sort of cultural fallout from the women's movement — came openly to represent alternative sexuality and sexual self-expression more generally. There are now clinics to teach men masturbation, as there had once been similar women's workshops; various kinds of spirituality have their masturbatory component, although, as one journalist observed, Tantric jacking off bears little resemblance to the more common variety. Masturbation is also decidedly queer. "To have so powerful a form of *sexuality* run so fully athwart the precious and embattled sexual *identities* whose meanings we always insist we know is only part of the revelatory power of the Muse of masturbation," writes the critic Eve Sedgwick.[103]

And this brief survey of the present does not touch masturbation in popular culture — television (the infamous Seinfeld episode, for example), film — in 2000, teenage humiliation through the discovery of real or impugned masturbation figured prominently in *American Pie* and *Something about Mary* — video, pop music; or on the Web, in tens of thousands of profitable pornography sites; or in sex shops (Good Vibrations sponsors National Masturbation Month, announced in posters all over certain neighborhoods). No sexual practice over the past three hundred years has signified quite so much, in quite so many places, to quite such a range of people. No sexuality, no putative vice was ever more democratic. Women and children, long ignored as subjects in sexual ethics, have become in modern masturbation sexual beings whose development might be stunted or furthered, degraded or refined. The "trouble and agony of a wounded conscience" announced to the world around 1712 is now everywhere. Or, in any case, talk about it is everywhere. But this does not mean that it was nowhere before; and that is the subject of the next chapter.

82

CHAPTER THREE

Masturbation Before *Onania*

I have taken it for granted so far that my history begins in the early eighteenth century: "in or around 1712." And if what I claim about solitary sex and the relationship of the individual to society in the modern world is right, then it does. But masturbation, by its own name and many others, has been around as far back as we have records and probably well beyond: rabbis may not have articulated the concept, but theologians certainly spoke of it; writers and painters depicted it; doctors even discussed it on rare occasion. Ordinary people seemed to have both done it themselves and joked about others' doing it.

This chapter circles back; it is about masturbation before it became a big deal, the prehistory of its modern significance. It holds an inverting mirror in front of my thesis: by showing why sex with oneself meant so little before the Enlightenment, I want to suggest why it came to mean so much after. There may be more detail here than some readers will find necessary to convince them of the modernity of modern masturbation; skip to Chapter 4 to get back to the story of sex with oneself from the eighteenth century on.

Masturbation and Medicine Before 1712
I begin with medicine because the story is relatively simple and uncontroversial. The editors of the most exhaustive of the nineteenth-century medical encyclopedias allotted more than twenty-six pages and a long bibliography to the article "Onanisme." No problem more deserves the attention of philosophers and doctors,

the author announces, which is presumably why he got so much space; masturbation is a question of social hygiene that touches on individual mental health; it represents a conjuncture of public and private interest. But this awareness, we learn, is new; it fell to the moderns to recognize the importance of the topic. The ancients, by contrast, "viewed onanism with the most serene indifference," and insofar as anyone in the classical world discussed the matter, it was the satiric and erotic poets. From doctors we hear nothing. Hippocrates, to be sure, addressed the danger of unbridled vene-real pleasure, but he was talking about newlyweds; Galen offered a few comments on continence; of medieval doctors one need say little: "They contemplated hardly any of the elements of the question except that of excess," which is, of course, only a very small part of the problem. Only in the eighteenth century, the article continues, did onanism become important. A "book enti-tled *Onania* [which the article authoritatively claims was written by a doctor named Bekker] had enormous repercussions."[1] Indeed it did.

We could quibble with a few details. Tissot first identified Bekker as the author, but this is not plausible. The name appears only once in the most complete bibliography of pre-1800 litera-ture that we have and it belongs to a Dutch clergyman, Balthasar Bekker, who died in 1698 and whose only extant work in English is an attack on superstitious belief in witches, ghosts, and evil spirits. This is not our man.[2] And, in any case, we now know who wrote *Onania*. Also, the occasional medical man did think about masturbation as part of his differential diagnosis before the early eighteenth century. An obscure London surgeon, writing in his private notebook in the 1650s, thought that his patient's scrotal fistula might be the result of nocturnal emissions and of his "sometimes a forcing of his seed to flow."[3] But no one knew about him. Basically, the learned author of the nineteenth-century arti-cle got it right and finds support in the most recent and thorough research on onanism as a disease: masturbation as a medical prob-lem dates from the early eighteenth century.[4]

Onania, of course, made precisely this claim. It cited no more ancient an authority than "Dr. Bayard" (Edward Baynard [1641-

1719?], that would be) in support of the view that there were "afflictions which may, and often do fall upon those who are or have been guilty of the sinful Practice of SELF POLLUTION."[5] This was a slender reed. Baynard was a reasonably well-known doctor who divided his time between Bath and London. He was most famous for an oft-reprinted long poem on health — "How to procure preserve and restore it" — and for an equally popular and long-lived book on cold bathing. But he had very little to say about self-abuse — one reference in one paragraph among the 450 pages of his book on the virtues of icy water — and that from 1706, two years before the putative first edition of *Onania*. It says only that "weakness of the penis and lost erections" may be due to "ill cured Gonorrhea and gleets [discharges]" and "sometimes by that cursed School wickedness of masturbation by which many a young gentleman has been for ever undone." He says he knows of twenty cases of such weakness that have been cured by the water treatment: "wound up their watch, and set their pendulum in Status quo." In addition to citing Baynard, *Onania* claims as a recent predecessor one Ettmüller, "a famous physician" who condemned masturbation as medically dangerous. Michael Ettmüller was in fact a Leipzig-trained physician — his dissertation was published in 1663 — who produced a multivolume compilation of medical and chemical learning in Latin during the 1670s. In 1699, a long abridgment was published in English, and there among its more than six hundred pages is indeed a two-word reference to our subject. There are three causes for involuntary emission of genital liquor, Ettmüller writes: too much of it, its being too sharp, and its "tenuity and wateriness." The remote cause of the third of these is excessive venery, especially in one's youth, and "manual violence." That is it. Nothing about women or girls and no further elaboration.[6] The quack doctor and medical pornographer John Marten, who wrote *Onania*, made much of his originality, and from the perspective of medicine he is right.

The learned Tissot, on the other hand, worked hard to give onanism, and his contributions to its study, a long pedigree. Like most scientific writers, he took pride in his footnotes, in standing triumphantly on the accumulated wisdom and observation of his great medical forebears, on the shoulders of giants. But the data simply were not there. His failure in creating a scholarly ancestry suggests, in fact, just how sharp the rupture was between the eighteenth century and the classical medical world.

He begins his genealogy at the beginning, with a case of Hippocrates's that illustrated the dangers of excessive venereal pleasure. The patient suffered from *tabes dorsalis* — literally, "consumption of the back," a wasting away of the spine, from whose marrow semen derives — which is characterized by a generalized cachexia that signals the approach of death. Symptoms include impotence, shortness of breath, heaviness of head, ringing of the ears; the body is racked by fever. In the nineteenth century, thanks to the worldwide success of *Onanism*, this cluster of symptoms and signs would indeed point to *tabes dorsalis* as a disease of masturbation. "Voy phthsie dorsale." So ends the article "Masturbation" in an authoritative French medical dictionary of the early nineteenth century. Wasting away through self-abuse was vividly rendered for the laity in widely circulated pictures, museum exhibits, and seemingly endless prose; doctors could read about it in journals and in at least six published M.D. dissertations.[7]

But in the Hippocratic corpus itself, this putatively foundational case has nothing to do with solitary vice. Tissot scrupulously quotes the Father of Medicine, who describes a disease that is said to strike "young married people, and those of lascivious disposition." The language of the Greek original makes it very clear that "lascivious disposition" refers specifically to those fond of sexual intercourse (*philolagnous*); nothing about an addiction to masturbation.

Other of Tissot's efforts to muster the ancients are even less to the point. He offers, for example, Pliny's mention of two "Roman knights" — Titus Helerius and Cornelius Gallus — who died "while with women." Again, the connection with masturbation is at best tenuous: they weren't alone; they weren't masturbating. And even as a warning against excessive venery and the stress of orgasm, their cases are unimpressive. The unfortunate knights come near the end of a long list of people who died in peculiar or unusual circumstances — none, therefore, a good candidate to

86

be exemplary of anything — which Pliny insists can be explained naturally and need not be regarded as miracles: the logician Diodorus died of shame when he could not immediately solve a problem he had been set; Sulla's doctor died in the course of drinking a draft of mead while sucking an egg after coming back from the bathhouse; and then the two knights who died more prosaically during heterosexual intercourse. In short, people die in the course of ordinary life, and we need not look for extraordinary causes.

Tissot gestures toward Galen, the most influential of ancient physicians, with two citations: one that refers to excessive seminal secretion leading to disorders of the brain and the other to a man dying while engaged in the conjugal act with his wife. Again, not quite on point; neither patient courted trouble through self-stimulation. And Tissot seems almost halfhearted in his efforts.

In fact, ancient doctors were almost entirely silent on the subject of masturbation, which is all the more striking because they offered extensive advice on what would, after 1712, come to be seen as some of the symptoms of self-abuse: "gonorrhea" — the leaking of seminal fluids in sleep or while awake — lassitude from venereal excess. They offered many of the same dietary cures — cooling foods, exercise — that Tissot would suggest for masturbatory disease; clearly, the new disorder took much from its classical predecessors. And they recognized the same causes. They thought that sexual excess was dangerous and that seminal loss was especially so. But in none of their pronouncements on these subjects did masturbation figure. On the practice itself and on its consequences the doctors of Antiquity had little or nothing to say.

This would be puzzling if we were to understand the dramatic rise to prominence of masturbation as a question in the history of medicine, because so much of the pathophysiology — to use an anachronistic term — of the eighteenth- and nineteenth-century pseudo disease, as well as treatments for it, was borrowed from Antiquity. But medicine in the ancient world, as in the eighteenth century, was about much more than fluids, illness, and death. The important point is that before the Enlightenment masturbation, unlike other kinds of sexuality, had almost no role to play in the

87

more general ethics of the body that doctors claimed as their domain. They were largely silent on the topic because it was not particularly exigent in thinking about how a reasonable man should live his life. In a world in which the upper-class male had available almost unimaginable possibilities for excessive behavior — slaves and prostitutes of both sexes, endless rich food, almost no external curbs on anger or violence — masturbation was off the lower end of the scale.[8]

Concern about any aspect of the sexuality of children and of what we would call adolescents, so central to writers from John Marten through Tissot and Rousseau to a host of nineteenth-century doctors and on to Freud and Hall, was almost nonexistent among ancient physicians. To be sure, they thought it might be unhealthy for a girl to remain long unmarried once she had reached puberty. (Boys were presumed to be able to find outlets elsewhere.) This issue, in turn, was part of a larger discussion of whether prolonged virginity was compatible with health, of when unmarried girls might begin to suffer from a lack of sex, and whether widows would become ill from the retention of seed after a lifetime of regular release. The major gynecological text of the early empire spends much time on these questions, and Galen takes them up in his discussion of hysteria and the greensickness. But the medical problem raised by the sexuality of women was usually not losing too much fluid or energy but, rather, not losing enough. Too little menstrual or seminal flow, excessive cold and wetness, were the most common signs that all was not right with the female body.[9]

Scrambling around, we can come up with what might be construed as a whisper or two about adolescents explicitly, but it would be a stretch. There is one reference in Aristotle — in a discussion of puberty in both boys and girls — where he mentions, as an aside, that "those who try by friction to provoke emission of seed" are apt to experience pain as well as pleasure. But doing it "by friction" (from the Greek *tribesthai* "to rub oneself") does *not* seem terribly dangerous, nor is Aristotle's censure, if that is what it is, terribly explicit. In a passage a bit further, Aristotle says that for girls, and for boys, "engaging in sex" when they are young will make them more likely to do so when they get older; that is, the passages may thereby become dilated, fluxes may ensue, former indulgences will thus create a longing for repetition, and the boys and girls might end up as adults lacking in self-control. This hints at the dangerous habit-forming qualities of masturbation that would so exercise eighteenth- and nineteenth-century doctors, but only because we read the passage with hindsight. There is no suggestion that the gerund *aphrodiasiazomenai*, usually translated as "giving way to wantonness" but more modestly something like "having sex," has anything to do with autoeroticism. Certainly no one in Antiquity thought so, and even learned eighteenth-century doctors looking for classical authority did not make the connection.[10]

Adult men mattered. And in regard to them, ancient physicians were deeply engaged with the finest nuances of both orgasm and seminal loss or retention as part of a larger medico-ethics of food, sex, pleasure, and desire. Doctors offered precise advice regarding risks and benefits of this or that circumstance under which semen, the most highly concocted and precious of fluids, might be lost. They also had much to say about ejaculation, because needs and pleasures of the body were understood to represent a corporeal economy of fungible fluids whose correct balance was essential to health, happiness, and fecundity. Age mattered. The dangers of ejaculation were greater for the young than for the old, greater in the throes of passion than in routine intercourse with one's wife. The advantages of rapid versus prolonged orgasm had to be considered; it was a small seizure, like epilepsy, and could lead to trouble if care was not taken. Doctors cautioned that prudence in the husbandry of semen was even more important than husbandry of other vital forces and that the threats of venereal excess to a decent, healthy use of the body were greater than other kinds of overindulgence. There were also the distracting aspects of sexual desire that also had to be considered and the advantages and disadvantages of various ways of mitigating it — diet, massage, and intercourse of different sorts, for example.

Venery, in short, put enormous strains on the corporeal economy and moral well-being of its votaries because of its potential for excess that was dangerous both medically and morally. But in all of this, there is almost no mention of masturbation and none that condemns it as a specific, dangerous form of sexual indulgence in general or of losing semen in particular. Nothing in the entire corpus of ancient medicine, Greek or Latin, or in the medieval and Renaissance tradition that derived from it, gives warning of what was to come after *Onania*.[11] Missing is the ethical problem of sexual modernity — the relationship of desire not to external temptations but to inner circumstances — which would allow eighteenth-century doctors to translate a two-millennium-old tradition into a wholly novel idiom.

There are two notorious breaches of silence on the subject of masturbation in the classical tradition, but neither suggests continuity with its modern history; indeed, they suggest the opposite. Both come from Galen, the Prince of Physicians, who unproblematically subsumed masturbation under the more general medico-ethical question of what is to be done with excess sperm. He offers a surprising answer from the perspective of the post-1712 era: it is to be eliminated as calmly and expeditiously as possible. Masturbation offers one possible, relatively safe and un-engaging way to achieve this end. Absent is any sense of moral fervor or indeed of interest in masturbation as an ethically sensitive form of sexual outlet. Nowhere is there a hint of purely physical harm; quite to the contrary. Galen's suggestions of masturbatory therapy would have a remarkable longevity — from the second to the twentieth century — but of them Tissot takes no note.

The first of his cases is all about men. Diogenes the Cynic, Galen tells us some four centuries after the event, was the most continent and temperate of men. But even he "engaged in sexual pleasures." He did it not because he took particular delight in them but because he shared with all humans the need to evacuate the surplus bodily fluids that inevitably built up in the course of life. Sexual desire in this model was understood basically as a question of burning and itching, of irritation, caused by highly wrought corporeal excess that demanded release. One day, the story goes, Diogenes made an appointment with a prostitute "so that she could come to him." Presumably, he did not opt for "marital pleasure" because it was psychologically or socially more complex and such complexity was inappropriate for men of his class, at least with wives. In any case, the point of the story is the Cynic's matter-of-fact way of dealing with the problem. The prostitute was late for the date, and he calmly applied "his hand to his genitals [and] rubbed himself off." Then, when she finally showed up, he sent her away untouched. His hand, he told her, had "sung the *hymenaion* [wedding song] first." Galen comments:

> And it is distinctly clear that moderate men come to intercourse not on account of pleasure, but because they want to heal their disturbance, even if it were without pleasure.[12]

A hundred years after Galen, Diogenes Laertius approvingly recounts the same story of the Cynic's public masturbation, but with a philosophical twist. Breakfast is not absurd, and therefore it is not absurd to have breakfast in public. The Greek Diogenes had said, while "using his hand continuously in public," that he wished he could satisfy his hunger as easily by rubbing his belly. Masturbating in public, when done in the right frame of mind, is in short like breakfasting in the agora. And "many other sayings are attributed to him."[13] In Stoic thinking, masturbation — like marital sexual intercourse — was to be practiced only according to nature; and sex with oneself was more easily confined to these bounds than sex with another. It was more likely to be moderate, which is, of course, precisely the opposite of the claims made by all but a tiny number of commentators after 1712.

Divorced entirely from its ancient medical and philosophical contexts, Diogenes's story enjoyed remarkable longevity. "That practice of Diogenes" was the euphemism Thomas Cogan, author of one of the best-selling health guides in Shakespeare's England, used for masturbation, which, along with fornication, buggery, and incest, he grouped as a class of unlawful ways to get rid of surplus semen. In case readers missed the allusion, he added both the phrase "*genitalia contrectando semen ejicere* [touching the genitals to ejaculate semen]" and the standard Protestant caveat that doing this was one of the bad consequences of popish celibacy. More than two millennia after masturbating in the agora, Diogenes pops up in Bernard Mandeville's argument for why one ought to let the market regulate sexual exchanges — as well as other desires. (His alternative was making sex free — creating an unlimited supply — by holding women in common, something Diogenes had not recommended!) Even philosophers could not make sexual wants go away, argued Mandeville, and although the Cynic did practice "manual venery" in public, he clearly thought that actually lying with a woman was preferable to lying with her in the mind.[14]

Of course, generations of Christian thinkers denied the possibility in postlapsarian man of the sort of moderation in the face of sexual desire that Galen recommended and Diogenes was said to have practiced. Such brutally physical treatment as a solution was out of the question for medieval and Renaissance doctors. But masturbation had no more moral resonance for them than it had for physicians of the ancient world. It occupied an obscure corner of the far more general problem of regulating sexual pleasure within a framework that sanctioned it within marriage and only for the purposes of procreation. Insofar as it was discussed at all, "manual venery" raised a specific casuistic question, not one with broad cultural resonance: Was one ever justified in deliberately inducing orgasm, inside or outside marriage, for health reasons? The answer, for men at least, was almost invariably no. But the problem, so conceived, was a boutique dilemma within a much more general ethics of sexuality, one that regarded all non-procreative sexuality — fornication, adultery, incest — within marriage or without, as more or less sinful. This overarching doctrine had to be weighed against the possible health benefits of discharge in circumstances where reproduction was impossible. And even in this very limited discussion, there was no mention of any of the medical dangers of masturbation that would become so prominent in the eighteenth century. Excess was always a problem — note how short the life is of the salacious sparrow — but there was no hint that masturbation was likely to be excessive, and, in any case, once one got off the moral question and returned to the medical question, excess itself depended on humoral composition. The hot, moist man could safely have intercourse or masturbate many times a day.[15]

Galen's rather limited view on masturbation in women had an even longer history and resonated even more fully through the ages. It comes in the context of clinical problems that are the result of fluid retention. Medically speaking, this sort of problem in women was more pressing than in men, for both physiological and moral reasons. On the one hand, women were cooler and hence less likely to rid themselves of excess, especially if the menstrual flow — the usual egress — was blocked. On the other, they were more restricted in their use of coition that would rid them of acrid humors; widows, wives whose husbands were away, girls after puberty and before marriage did not have the options of men and boys in similar circumstances. (In sixteenth-century England, the term "single woman" was more or less equivalent to "prostitute," and a sexually active single woman was quite simply a whore.[16])

With such limited opportunities for relief, women were thought to be liable to hysterical diseases of all sorts — that is, to diseases that originate from a sort of bottling up of what we might call sexual energies but what the ancients referred to as acrid humors or retained, irritating fluids. Galen's advice and prognosis, offered in the same text as the story of Diogenes the Cynic, is the following: first various warming treatments, then "the touch of the genitals." This will result in "twitching accompanied at the same time by pain and pleasure after which she emit[s] turbid and abundant sperm. From that time on she [will be] free of all the evil she felt." Rubbing, in short, produces orgasm, ejaculation, and relief from the symptoms of pent-up desire and pent-up "semen" gone bad.[17]

In various permutations, this prescription was the cornerstone for two millennia of medically sanctioned female masturbation, either alone or with the help of an attendant. The thirteenth-century churchman and philosopher Albert the Great went into some detail about how, around the age of fourteen, girls heat up, their thighs thicken, they are consumed with desire; the result of all of this — in the absence of emission — is engorgement and a strong urge not to be chaste. Later commentators identified a variety of consequences from this process: greensickness, a syndrome marked by the burning, irritation, and pressure from retained semen; and also as the physiological foundation of unchaste

93

behavior. By "using their fingers or other instruments until their channels are opened by the heat of the friction and coition the spermatic humor comes out, and with it the heat; and then their groins are cooled off and they are made more chaste (or continent) [...*cum quo exit calor: et tunc temparantur ipsarum inguina, et tunc efficiuntur castiores*]." In other words, in the absence of intercourse to relieve the heat of retained fluids — the genital itch — rubbing will do the trick. But coition itself is the same sort of activity: rubbing in one way is medically neither better nor worse than rubbing any other way. And afterward they become *chaster* because the pressure and irritation have been relieved. In the eighteenth century, this would be turned on its head. Real sex came to be regarded as satisfying and therefore self-limiting, whereas sex alone was seen as intrinsically unsatisfying and therefore a prelude to still more sex alone. One could not stop because desire never slackened. But in the Middle Ages, the problem was primarily interpreted not as real versus artifactual, imaginatively driven sexual desire, but as a straightforward excess of irritating material. From the doctors' vantage, once the itch was relieved it was gone. For older girls who had started menstruating, the buildup of heat was even more apparent and they had to take steps to ease the irritation; now they press their legs together, "one part of the vulva scratches the other, because delectation and pollution arise from this."[18]

There are several contexts for these views — the imagined greater salacity of women, who were by nature relatively unchecked by reason, the special problem of girls, who were cooler and less given to exercise than boys and therefore could not rid themselves of surplus as conveniently — but what we would call adolescent sexuality is not one of them. Boys are ignored — as they very decidedly were not after 1712 — because the problem is not masturbation but a distinct medical problem of pubescent heat, from which boys were generally thought not to suffer since they had other outlets.

Medieval doctors and Renaissance doctors, sometimes approvingly, sometimes not, did seem to have exercised the most salacious corners of their imaginations in elaborating the circumstances and

94

methods whereby women relieved the congestion that lack of sexual outlets might create. The laity found Galen's advice in the many self-help books that flourished with the advent of print in early modern Europe. As late as the late nineteenth and early twentieth centuries, there was a boom in devices designed to relieve medical men and their assistants from the tedium of massaging the genitals of hysterical or sexually unsatisfied women: electric vibrators, hydrotherapy machines, and hoses to direct tap water, all mass marketed in everything from needlework catalogs to Sears and Roebuck. Under the guise of a medical procedure, masturbation had a very long run indeed.[19]

The Galenic advice to women that they rub their genitals — specifically the clitoris — to relieve tension must have been commonplace even in less technological circles not interested in buying vibrators or saving themselves the trouble of using their hands. The major Catholic medical-theology guide of the nineteenth century gives as a typical case a woman who "found great relief from pains through a pressing and manipulating [of the clitoris?] accompanied by *voluptuous sensations*." This is not a *tactus impudicus* (shameless touching) that just happens to cause pollution; it is not technically pollution at all, because this isn't possible for women, the author tells us in the next section. The moral fault lies in producing venereal pleasure for its own sake; whatever reason she claims for doing it, like that it eases pressure, does not count. The old Galenic trick is totally wrong.[20]

Compared with the medical discussion of the eighteenth and nineteenth centuries, the classical tradition offers very, very little on the subject of masturbation, and then only within narrow parameters: nothing on the danger of masturbation in general; nothing on the debilitating aspects of solitary orgasm in particular; almost nothing about masturbation in women and children in any context. This is not because ancient doctors thought venery was safe, although they did not worry much about its effects on anyone but adult men. Rather, venery alone, as a category, was of no great interest to anyone and thus also not to doctors. Sidelined as an ethical question, it was also peripheral as a medical one.

95

Masturbation and the Ethics of Sexuality in
Classical Antiquity

The Greeks may not have had a technical name for what came to be called onanism in the early eighteenth century, but they knew what we are talking about. No radical conceptual chasm separates their categories from ours. On a black-figure *aryballos* by Nearkos sit three satyrs, each working his large erect penis with his hands. Two we see in profile, the other in full-frontal nudity, squatting, knees apart, holding his very large member. Terpekelos, "shaft pleasure," is the one in the middle. He is flanked on our left by Dophios, whose name comes from what he is doing, from *dephesthai*, "to knead oneself," as one might also work bread dough with one's hand; this is pretty close to a term of art for the practice it so manifestly describes. (The name Despesthai is also used in the comedies of Aristophanes to mean kneading oneself with one's hands.) On the right stands Psolas, whose name refers to the state of his penis: *psolos*, "erect," his foreskin drawn back. All three are using two hands, but other satyrs — such scenes are not unusual in vase painting — use only one hand. Word and action are unambiguous and conceptually simple. There are also later, post-Alexander figures of masturbators — grotesque, deformed, not a pretty sight. Yes, the Greeks had the concept of masturbation (figures 3.1 and 3.2).[21]

From the Romans, sometime between 84 or 85 and 103 C.E., the years during which Martial wrote his *Epigrams*, we get the words themselves — *masturbor* and *masturbator*, the direct forebearers of our terms.[22] Their referents — the actions and actors themselves — are clearly the same as their modern counterparts even if they mattered a great deal less. Their origins are shrouded in obscurity; no one knows where *masturbor* or its derivatives came from or how they evolved into the forms that were used in two, and only two sentences in the works of one man.

Man from *manus* (hand) plus *stuprare* (to defile) from *stupro* is the most common hypothesis today, one that goes back to eighteenth-century speculations, but it has not carried the day among experts, who cannot agree on how the combination was made. Alternative views are that *masturbari* and hence "masturbation"

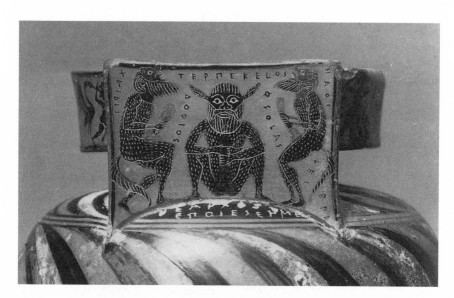

Figure 3.1. Satyrs masturbating. All three of these goat-like creatures use both hands in their manifestly crude, ungentlemanly efforts to get satisfaction. They represent the original masturbators, having been taught how to do it by the gods who took pity on their sexual frustrations. Man, it is said, learned from them. Not a very distinguished lineage! (Black-figure *aryballos* by Nearkos, New York 26.49 ABV 83 [4] from Attica. The Metropolitan Museum of Art, New York.)

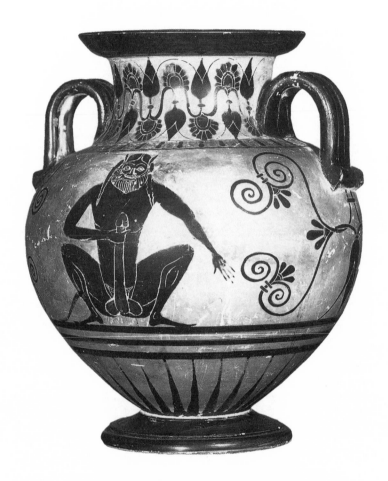

Figure 3.2. Satyr masturbating. This satyr is perhaps slightly less vulgar than those in figure 3.1, but his enormous penis is a sign, as if viewers needed it, that what he is doing is not decorous. A small penis is a sign of refinement in Greek art. (Black-figure amphora, Berlin 1671, ABV 22 [2] from Tarquinia. © bpk, Berlin, 2002. Antikennsammlung.)

come from *manstruprari*, that is, from *manu* (a form of the noun for "hand") plus *sturprum* (a noun meaning "a debauch, a defilement related to the verb *stupro*") plus *perpetrare* (the verb for "to perpetrate") or from *manus* plus *stuprare* that has somehow been reworked through *turbare* — "to disturb or disorder." No one knows and all etymologies proposed over the years are fanciful. We do know, though, that the word is extremely rare in Latin. Forms of *masturbor* are only in Martial; both times they are used in connection with the gods. The word does not seem to have been a vulgar term or it would have appeared in other contexts. Martial resurrects an obsolescent verb for mock mythologies. Latin writers, in other words, did not feel the need for a technical term to describe a morally and medically unimportant topic.[23]

Of course, the extremely limited uses of *masturbor*, *masturbari* by no means exhaust Latin allusions to the thing itself. But the absence of a technical vocabulary suggests that solitary sex was not a category that was taken terribly seriously. Writers referred to it with slang words in keeping with the generally low moral stakes in each context. Alternative terms could, depending on the context, refer both to self-stimulation and to stimulation by others — petting, oral sex, the rubbing of intercourse, one man rubbing or caressing the penis of another. *Frico*, "to rub," seems to have been the main slang term for masturbating but also had other uses; *tracto*, "to handle," and *contrecto*, "to caress," were common. There were also transparent circumlocutions: no question what the narrator did when Lydgus failed to show up for a tryst. "When I have lain for a long time tense with excitement in vain, often my left hand comes to my rescue instead of you." Likewise Priapus: "Let my hand be a girlfriend," he says dejectedly, bemoaning the fact that he has neither a naiad nor a dryad, a water and a tree nymph, respectively, at his disposal. Already in Antiquity, "hand job" has that slightly funny, slightly abject ring that it still carries today. But there is not much ethical heavy lifting here.[24]

The same moral valences seem to have dominated the "homosexual" tradition of pre-Tokugawa Japan. A servant preparing the anus of a boy destined for an old priest, for example, becomes

99

aroused as he works the clove-oiled dildo in the youth's *sun* and complains that "there's nothing to do but masturbate." In fact, since the priest is old and easily satisfied, the youth's bottom does become available, but that's another part of the story. Masturbation in Japan before the modern period, as in ancient Rome, was not much more, or less, than second-best. As an ethical problem, it was a minor kink in a much larger and more elaborate discussion of male love.[25]

The act — masturbation — existed in Antiquity; it had a name. But it had none of the resonance it came to have after *Onania*. When Greek or Roman thinkers dealt with it at all it was to make clear that it was not fit and proper for the erotic life of a gentleman; it violated some sort of sexual sumptuary law and hence it figured largely as a joke about the dismal state of one so frustrated as to be reduced to so lowly a practice. Female masturbation comes up rarely in Latin literature and only a bit more in Greek writing and art, because in the Greco-Roman world the sexual ethics and the sexual status that mattered — beyond chastity — were those of the male. Female masturbation was not morally interesting precisely because women were but imperfect men; one could not expect from them the dignity one would from a gentleman.

Solitary sex thus seems never to have mattered much in classical Antiquity because the cultural contexts that later gave it, or aspects of it, moral resonance were absent. The crux of self and sexuality lay elsewhere. Spilled semen, for example, had little of the significance it was given by the rabbis; it was not generally regarded as unclean, as it was among the Jews or at least as some Talmudic commentators were to claim. Herodotus, the Father of History and a man fascinated with the Egyptians, tells us that they, like the Greeks and unlike other, less civilized nations, are scrupulous about their sacred edifices. Priests did not have intercourse with women in their temples and did not enter a temple after having had intercourse elsewhere without first washing. But this observation is about a line between the profaneness of sex and the sacrality of the temple, between what is done in private and what is done in public. Semen in general was not polluting. When one

of the earliest known Greek poets, Hesiod, warns against exposing one's shameful parts when bespattered with seed, he refers
specifically to a place — "before the hearth." Protect the hearth;
respect decorum; keep hidden what should be hidden. Everything
in its place.[26]

Not only did seminal pollutions per se figure little in Greek
religions, but seed cast upon the ground is the start of several
origin myths. Erichthonius, the "motherless" aboriginal ancestor
of the Athenians, for example, was born in this way. Athena had
gone to Hephaistos, god of fire and of the arts, wanting him to
make her some armor. He was overcome by Aphrodite and started
to pursue his would-be client with a great passion; he finally
caught her, despite his being lame, and tried to have intercourse
with her, again under some constraint because of his handicap.

> But since she is chaste and a virgin, she would not put up with it, but
> he shot his seed onto the leg of the goddess. Then she, disgusted,
> wiped the seed off with wool and cast it into the earth, and Erichtho-
> nios was born. Athena raised him secretly from the other gods, since
> she wanted to make him immortal.

Athena was disgusted (*musakhtheisia*) at having semen spilled on
her leg — not because spilled seed was unclean but because she was
a chaste virgin (*sophron parthenos*) who had been pursued, caught,
and assaulted by a deformed stranger. The seed, cast off onto
the earth in a rag, was far from sterile. It gave birth to a king, a
parthenos, one born of only one seed, who, as a modern scholar
suggests, "lies beyond the opposition between masculine and feminine ... [and] achieves the masculine dream of the Greeks — a child
outside the limits of procreative activity."[27] Onan's sin, in other
words, founds Athens. More generally, this story of loose seed
and generation fits into a pattern of extraordinary people born in
extraordinary circumstances, of gods and heroes without mothers
in the usual sense. Aphrodite was born out of the froth from
Ouranos's genitals, cut off by Kronos and thrown into the sea.

What mattered most in the sexual ethics of Greek Antiquity
was honor and its opposite, shamefulness. A Greek gentleman

101

had to conduct a sexual life that suited his station. Masturbation would not have qualified, but no one seems to have felt compelled to point this out. Early-twentieth-century commentators in need of a classical pedigree tried to interpret Aeschines's accusation that the great orator Demosthenes used "his own body and procreative power" in some unspecified disgraceful way as a reference to masturbation, an accusation made to shame him and thus prevent him from being crowned in public for his services to the state. But, in fact, it is unlikely that Athenian citizens would have understood the charge so specifically. In a world of hierarchy and honor, any number of sexual acts inappropriate to a gentleman would have come to mind: that he had had anal rather than vaginal intercourse with his wife; that he had submitted to anal penetration, that is, that he was the passive rather than the active partner with a man; that he had made less than honorable use of his mouth — fellatio or cunnilingus. Masturbation probably never occurred to anyone.[28]

What mattered for a man of parts was *sophrosune* — temperance, control of the self. The word comes from *sōs*, "integral, safe, sound", and *phrenos*, the Homeric word for "mind" and the root of our word "phrenology"; so literally, a gentleman was "sound minded." Masturbation would certainly not have been regarded as sound minded. It was not what a temperate man did, but then neither was a host of other sexual and nonsexual activities; it was neither explicitly condemned nor even discussed in treatises on what sorts of behavior befit a temperate man. Masturbation was an easy case; it stood outside the complicated ethics of a world in which men penetrated boys of their own social class who would someday be their equals, in which whom one could love and how were matters for the most sophisticated philosophical discussion. Citizens had available attractive, dignified engagements with eros or ones that simply fell outside the moral pale, sex with common prostitutes, for example, which signified little. (The second-oldest use of "masturbation" in English captures this connection with honor. In 1623, one of the earliest dictionaries defines "mastuprate" as "dishonestly to touch one's privities.") To the Greeks, it was shameful because it was beneath one's station.[29]

Satyrs did it because that is the sort of creatures they were — beasts with big genitals, limitless sexual appetites, and little education. Of course they masturbated; what was one to expect? Not for the likes of them the subtle, modulated erotic relationships of a citizen and a boy or the matter-of-fact relief that a gentleman might find in a prostitute. They masturbated because they could not satisfy their voracious needs elsewhere or because it served as a sort of foreplay, a preparation for the raucous and unseemly coupling to which they were given. In the first case, they were less to be condemned than to be pitied. And masturbation as foreplay was a joke; satyrs, always frustrated, famously never got to the real thing. Indeed it was said that the gods first revealed masturbation to these half beasts, half men and that they were the ones who passed it on to the most humble of humans. Pan, so the story goes, was miserably frustrated because the nymph Echo — like the other nymphs he had pursued — did not reciprocate his love. His father, Hermes, took pity on his wretched state and taught him the trick through which he could relieve his frustration; Pan, in turn, taught shepherds who might well need it in their lonely lives.[30]

Slaves, too, were thought to be expert masturbators and for the same reasons as satyrs. Either they lacked the quality or quantity of sexual outlets that free men enjoyed, or, in the case of those from the East in particular, they were generally licentious. Thus in Aristophanes's *Frogs*, Dionysus imagines himself as a Persian slave left to his own devices while his master dallies on luxurious blankets with a dancing girl. Datis, a Persian slave in Aristophanes's *Peace*, is the sort of feckless layabout who enjoys masturbating in the afternoon — the ancestor of the modern wanker. In every respect, the masturbating Persian slave represents the opposite of the ideal male citizen.

Depictions on pottery of free men — as opposed to satyrs or slaves — masturbating are rare and are always of bumpkins or rustics, never of citizens. They are characters like Strepsiades in Aristophanes's *Knights*. In short, male masturbation was a joke — the butt of comedy and derision. It was certainly not a worthy thing to do; it would have been a serious lapse for a free citizen; it was treated in comedy as the easily recognizable antithesis of what was right and proper. (Aristophanes reserved his critical comedy for lapses of public ethics — excessive litigiousness, for example, or a passion for war — and put it in the mouths of the chorus and not of the most humble characters.) If art is our guide, Greek men masturbated only when they could do nothing else, and that shortage of options was itself a sign of their low status.[31] Masturbation was never the object of serious moral reflection, precisely because it fit so nicely into accepted views of how society worked.

Women masturbating — precisely because they are women — are similarly treated lightly: comic, sexually voracious creatures who cannot get satisfaction elsewhere. Lots of images on vases show one or several women, each to herself or one with another, working an *olisbos* in her vagina and a second one in her mouth or anus. The women without men in *Lysistrata* use a "leather assistance" eight fingers long; to "skin the skinned dog" seems likewise to refer to masturbating in lieu of the real thing. Invariably phallic, this is a male erotic fantasy that confirms the centrality of heterosexual intercourse through its temporary displacement. (Of course, the women in *Lysistrata* were withholding themselves to put pressure on their men; there was power in the dildo.) Solitary pleasures for their own sake were not an option (figures 3.3a and 3.3b).

Latin literature has references to masturbation in more genres than Greek, but most contexts are still either comic or pathetic. Of course, Roman philosophers and doctors in more sober moments condemned excessive sexual pleasure, however derived. Control and moderation were the ideals a gentleman should strive for, and any deviations were unworthy of his status. Thus Cicero says, "Just as those who are carried away with delight when they enjoy sexual pleasures are base, in the same way, those who lust after them with a feverish soul are disgraceful." The first-century Stoic philosopher Musonius Rufus explicitly condemned all sexual practices outside marriage and countenanced sex within marriage only when pleasure was not its main purpose. We are here well within the world out of which the Christian ethic of marital sexuality will emerge. Reading backward from a modern

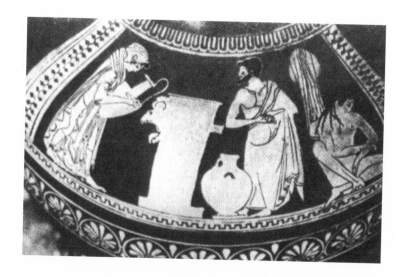

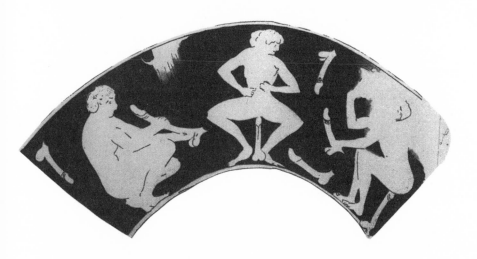

Figures 3.3a and 3.3b. Women masturbating. Pictures of women masturbating in Greek Antiquity are extremely rare. Perhaps the woman's left hand in the scene at a fountain is playing with her genitals as the man and the woman carrying a jug enter the scene. Depictions of women with dildos are less about masturbation than about what women are thought to do in the absence of the real thing. (Top: hydria, Leningrad, Stephani 623, ABV 34, 26; bottom: cup [after Gaston Vorberg, Glossarium eroticum 409], Once Castellani Collection.)

perspective, we might interpret these comments to cover masturbation, but it was, in fact, not mentioned. Solitary self-indulgence
was so far beneath contempt that it would not bear mentioning in
a serious moral treatise.[32]

It does figure as a breach of decorum, a more or less comic fall
from status, in other literary forms. Martial's masturbator speaks
in a voice of mock self-pity. "Friends have all in common," the
poet says ironically at the beginning of a list proving just the opposite. "*You* wear an exquisite toga made of the finest wool," he
says addressing Candidus, "*I* wear one which the straw dummy
thrown into the ring to enrage a bull would not wear; *you* have a
fine mantle, *I* have one that is worthless; *your* Libyan tabletop is
supported by ivory legs, *my* beech tabletop is supported by tiles.
You have at your disposal a train of slaves that might vie with Illian
cinaedus; *I* have to masturbate." (Literally, "My hand comes to my
assistance in lieu of Ganymede."[33]) This is basically the same joke
as in Aristophanes; only those too poor and pathetic to afford a
prostitute or slave boy are reduced to masturbating. They are, at
least for the moment, ridiculous. (On plenty of occasions, Martial
— or in any case the poet — does get the boy.)

Almost invariably in elite Latin literature, as in Greek, masturbation is the stuff of jokes, exaggerated claims, and cruel teases,
nothing more or less: "She is so sexy she'd make a saint masturbate"; "the girl from Gades," a famous Phoenician colony beyond
the pillar of Hercules, has "so tremulous a wiggle, so seductive an
itch that she would make a masturbator of Hippolytus," the bastard
son of Theseus and the Amazon queen Hippolyta who in Greek
mythology is the man of perfect purity who dies because a willful
woman, frustrated by his chastity, arranges, through a series of
events, to have sea monsters sent by Poseidon to scare his horses
until they are out of control and kill him. And, too, there is the
"too old for anything better" bit of pathos: with dribbling nose,
toothless gums, and shaky limbs, offensive to his wife, children, and
himself, and having long forgotten the real pleasures of the flesh,
the old man is reduced to caressing himself.[34] There is a point to this
kind of humor; there is even a sting; but there is little moral gravity.
We are at the beginning of a very long tradition of locker-room rap.

One makes fun of the frustrated masturbator. Ovid, for example, tells of Priapus, who sneaks up on the nymph Lotis with the intention of raping her; he is foiled when the braying of an ass awakens her, and he is left with "his obscene, excessively large — theatrically large — member at the ready [*obscena nimium quoque parte paratus*]." Meanwhile, by the light of the moon, everyone laughs at him. Chaucer celebrated this frustration — the very old, bitter object of masturbation jokes — by leaving him permanently with "sceptre in honde." So the Greek comedic tradition of randy satyrs and large-membered gods who penetrate donkeys and masturbate lives on, not as the subject of serious reflection but as a reminder that being caught with erect penis in hand is, at the very least, a bit embarrassing. It is decidedly not dignified.[35]

The ribald comedy of masturbation finds new voice in late-medieval secular epics, as grotesque parodies of role reversal and bodily excess. In one such German poem, a girl named Matzli waits in a stable. She is horny; there is a suggestion that she is a parodic Virgin Mary; she is the perfect antithesis of the beloved in courtly romances — dark, ugly, hunched, and eager for sex instead of fair, beautiful, shapely, and chaste. Her lover, an equally parodic inversion of the chivalric hero, is about to fall through the roof. But meanwhile the "lady" in the stable sits, regards her white legs, and as "she looks down at her deep brown twat [*Mutze*] there began a pulling and rubbing and hitting and teasing and probing ...in the hairy tuft so that you never heard such moaning." After this masturbatory orgy, she starts talking to her cunt (*Futzen*), piling obscenity on obscenity: "God give you the misery, suffering, and trouble that I have had to endure in my heart because of you." This has no classical roots; we have no such scenes with women in Antiquity and very few afterward. But it is in keeping with the tradition that masturbation is something uproariously grotesque that peasants or those sexually less fortunate than oneself do, something from which the reader can derive a knowing, salacious chuckle.[36]

Martial's joke about masturbation as second-best and the masturbator as a lesser man for resorting to it also echoes through the ages: especially among the classically educated. (It finds resonance too in other traditions. A major eleventh century Arabic philological work, for example, offers extremely precise terms for sexual acts that really mattered — fornication — and treat male masturbation as a joke — "marrying Hand, daughter of Arm.") Alexander Pope is mocked because he is afraid he will be raped by Lady Mary Montagu, and it is said that he much prefers self-abuse to women; maybe, writes another enemy in the most scurrilous of the many attacks on Pope, his retirement to his grotto has given him a "Dis-relish for the Sex [women]," but "no doubt he has found some other amusement, equally entertaining to him in his solitude," that makes him less worried about "losing the favour of the ladies." John Dryden's satire has much the same message and tone as the Latin ones we have quoted. Sex with oneself is a poor and eminently mockable substitute for the real thing. The young squire in one poem is abject and pitiable because, for whatever reason, he can't get with the program of appropriate male heterosexual behavior. But he — and it is almost always a he in this tradition — is not doing anything that is morally suspect:

> (Pleased with some sport which he alone does find,
> And Thinks a secret to all humane kind;)
> Till mightily in love, yet half afraid
> He first attempts the gentle dairymaid
> Succeeding there and led by the renown
> Of *Whetstones Park* he comes at length to Town.

Whetstone's Park was a notorious haunt of prostitutes; our "wild gallant," in short, graduates from his solitary sport, to dairymaids, to prostitutes, and then to wives of citizens.[37] Or, he never quite makes it. The abject protagonist in Rochester's "A Ramble in St. James Park," "Deluded of his assignation / (Jilting, it seems was then in fashion)," "would frig upon his mother's face / Whence rows of mandrakes tall did rise / Whose lewd tops fucked the very skies." (Women fare better in Rochester's poems; in any case their masturbating does not make them into losers or clowns. Cloris in her pigsty might dream of being raped but her reveries have a happy ending: "frightened she wakes, and waking frigs /

Nature thus kindly eased / . . ., her own thumb between her legs / She's innocent and pleased." The dedicatee of "On Cary Frazier" was given twelve dildoes by her parents but decides, "she loves nought but living pricks / And swears by God she'll frig no more." The whole joke in "Signor Dildo," is that women, unlike men, have serious substitutes at hand — "As ever was candle, carrot, or thumb." Rochester remains reliably phallic; no hint of the clitoris in all his female frigging.)[38]

The classical tradition of more or less tongue-in-cheek self-mockery combined with self-importance also had a very long run. One wonders how many poems there are to be discovered like the sonnet of a seventeenth-century Danish military man praising masturbation, not all too seriously. In gratuitously repeated rhymes that give the poem a circularity which mirrors the activity it describes, a soldier announces that "to while away time and trouble / I go to my treasure, which stands ready to use / down in place between my legs." His hand knows "how to stiffen the tool," which he then works "with a rhythm up and down as long as I am able." He enjoys his pleasure and in the end he "becomes, as before, the conqueror of my passion / See here my heart's desire, see here my whiling of time." This is the jest of a man who does not take solitary sex terribly seriously: an easy, amusing way to get off without much trouble. Little more. (It is also one of the first allusions to masturbation as a waste of time, which by the nineteenth century would be no joking matter.)[39]

There is one *locus classicus* in the literature of Antiquity that does seem to make more of masturbation, but again the issue is status and honor, not solitary sex as an ethically specific way of satisfying desire. In the second mythological occasion in which Martial uses the word *masturbor*, he backs off from a real attack just when modern readers might expect him to nail home his point. The poet's tone does not promise anything too serious: "Ponticus, do you think it's nothing that you only fuck with your left hand as a handmaiden and make it the girlfriend of your lusts?" This is a great crime, the poet continues, because a man as great as you should beget heroes. Martial is trying to flatter his friend into procreation: "Horatio fucked just once and bore three

children; Mars once and the chaste Illia bore him twins." If either
had masturbated, all would have been lost. Modern readers might
expect a general condemnation of what Ponticus has been doing,
if only because it is shameful. But the verse ends with the poet
asking his friend to imagine the brilliant offspring he — a man
capable, like Horatio and the god Mars, of begetting heroes —
might lose.[40]

In the end, it comes back to a question of rank and decorum.
Masturbation in classical Antiquity and in the long tradition to
which it gave birth was basically a violation of a libidinal sumptuary law. A gentleman ought not to, indeed ought not need to,
masturbate, given the options he had available: slaves, boy or girl,
prostitutes, women of the lower orders. Arguably — the much-
cited case of Diogenes comes to mind — it was better to masturbate than to evacuate semen in a more arousing and engaging way.
That is, from a purely medical perspective of elimination, solitary
sex might be healthier than sex with someone because a man was
less likely to be aroused if he got rid of the excess alone. But generally, any number of ways was thought more appropriate to a
man of substance and education.

Antiquity did have its physiognomic equivalent of one variety
of the eighteenth- and nineteenth-century masturbatory wreck.
He was the *cinaedus*, the unmasculine man who did not walk, talk,
or look as he should; he was a bit epicene, mincing, shifty-eyed.
But however he came by his effeminacy — through birth or improper education — no one claimed that self-abuse had made him
that way.[41]

Wherever one looks in Greek or Roman discussions of what is
right and proper sexually, masturbation figures only dimly. What
mattered were the regulation of eros within marriage and with
others outside it, the moderation of venereal and other pleasures
more generally, the choice of partner appropriate to one's status.
Women, boys, and girls were largely irrelevant in all this. And sex
with one's own hand was a lapse of propriety, not, as it would
become, a matter of life and death.

Onan and Masturbation in the Jewish Tradition

The situation here is different from how it was in the last section. There, it was clear that the Greeks and the Romans had a concept of masturbation similar to ours but that they regarded the act itself as not especially problematic or interesting, morally or medically. Hebrew, however, has neither words for masturbation nor euphemisms and circumlocutions that are anywhere near as specific as they are, for example, in Latin. That, in itself, might not be telling. One might claim, as many do, that homosexuality existed before the word "homosexuality" was coined in the late nineteenth century. We never really know what the absence of a word in a culture means. Perhaps the culture lacked the concept; or perhaps the practice was so commonplace that no special word was needed. But the problem here goes beyond the lexical.

Even if masturbation did exist in Jewish thought about sexuality, all the conceivably relevant original texts are, from a modern perspective, remarkably limited in their range and extent. The modern scholarship on the subject is tiny, and even the most careful, brilliant, and well-informed scholars who set out to understand sex in Talmudic culture have nothing to say on the subject. If, as Augustine charged, the Jews are indisputably carnal, masturbation seems not to have figured among them as a problem of carnality.[42] What references we have all address exclusively adult males of procreative age, that is, married men of the covenant, an odd population to target on a form of sexuality we associated with children and adolescents. There is nothing pertaining to women, and when we think there just might be, we are quickly disabused. Tamar, Onan's wife, is said by the rabbis to have "exercised friction with her finger," which explains, they say, how she conceived the first time, the time with Judah, the father of Onan. But they were not thinking of masturbation; they wanted to account for the fact that she was not a virgin, because a virgin was thought unable to conceive. But, another rabbi points out, "were there not Onan and Er," that is, had she not, in fact, already had intercourse at least twice? No, not really, is an alternative interpretation, because "they indulged in unnatural intercourse," that is, anal intercourse.[43] We are well off the masturbation track with

111

respect to women. There are no comments on boys and girls that could be read as pertaining to warnings about self-abuse.

But the main reason it is so hard to find masturbation, as we understand it, in the long Jewish tradition of biblical and legal interpretation is neither lexical nor sociological. Rather, it derives from a conceptual chasm that separates our world from the worlds of the Old Testament, of the second- through sixth-century rabbis who produced the Talmuds and midrashim, and of the writers in the Kabbalistic tradition of the eleventh and twelfth centuries. Masturbation fell entirely outside the interests of the redactors of Genesis. It fell between two questions of enormous interest to the rabbis: on the one hand, a great complex of issues about semen and its proper uses; on the other, a narrower set of questions about arousal itself, as manifested in the penis and as something that might lead to abuse of semen. Willful self-arousal by men or women, boys or girls to attain orgasm — that is, masturbation, sexual pleasure for its own sake, "yielding to filthy imagination...endeavor[ing] to imitate and procure...that Sensation, which God has ordered to attend...for the Continuance of our Species" — as *Onania* defined it — had no place in this scheme; it shared something of each category but in itself fit into neither of them. The Kabbala would put semen in such a different universe from ours — one in which, out of place, it could set loose demons and cause souls to wander — that it simply will not translate into the modern concern about masturbation.

I will begin with Genesis 38.8–10, where it is said that Onan "spilled his seed upon the ground" and that this so displeased the Lord that He struck him dead. I do this not because we know that Onan masturbated, which would make his act the true ground zero of solitary sex, but, quite to the contrary, because we do not know what he did. Or, rather, because there is no hint that he masturbated in the Old Testament and because later generations of rabbis have offered varied accounts of just how he managed so to offend God that it cost him his life. These verses not only were open to several interpretations but also were adduced in commentary on a complex of related questions having to do with semen and arousal. Tracking Onan will show

how nearly impossible it was for Jewish tradition to think the idea "masturbation."

But first, a fuller context for the poor lad's fate. In the previous chapter, Genesis 37, Jacob's youngest son, Joseph, is herding sheep with his brothers. They are jealous of the favor he holds in his father's eye; they conspire to kill him; two of them, Reuben and Judah, have second thoughts and convince the others of a compromise: cast Joseph alive into a pit. They go for it. Joseph is soon rescued and sold into slavery in Egypt, where great things await him; his story is taken up again in Genesis 39. But meanwhile the brothers soak his coat in goat's blood and bring it to their father as evidence that a wild beast has killed his beloved youngest son. Jacob is in mourning and Joseph is in Egypt as the next chapter, Genesis 38, begins.

It is an interlude that tells a strange story of failed, and then successful, procreation, of a near disaster in the royal lineage of David and ultimately of the Messiah. The central figures are not Onan or his brother but their father, Judah, and their would-be wife, Tamar. Judah has by now married a Canaanite woman, a foreigner, the daughter of Shua. She has borne him three sons — Er, Onan, and Shelah. When the eldest, Er, is old enough to marry, Judah finds for him a wife: Tamar. (In other versions of the story, she is also a stranger.) This takes us up to 38.6. The next thing we learn, in 38.7, is that God has slain Er, Judah's firstborn, for some unspecified failing: that "he was wicked in the sight of the Lord" is as much as we get. Judah then orders his second son, Onan, to "go in unto thy brother's wife [Tamar], and marry her, and raise up seed to thy brother." Under the ancient kinship rules, the so-called obligations of levirate marriage, Onan has not only to marry his dead brother's wife but also to sire children on her body in his brother's name. In other words, Onan's father asks him selflessly to help continue someone else's, Er's, and, of course, also Judah's, lineage.

This is critical. The proper succession of generations and of paternity will loom large both in Jewish and in Christian exegesis of Genesis 38.8–10 because from the child of Tamar would eventually grow the "root of Jesse," that is, King David's father and later a powerful element in messianic prophecy. "The generations of Jesus Christ, the son of David, the son of Abraham," so begins the first of the synoptic Gospels (Matthew 1.1–17); "Abraham begat Isaac and Isaac begat Jacob and Jacob begat *Judah* who begat Phares and Zara of Tamar," it continues. Then, the ninth generation after Judah, Jesse begat David, and three times fourteen generations from Abraham we arrive at the birth of Jesus Christ. Er and Onan are conspicuously absent from the genealogy.

Onan, in short, refused to play his part in this succession. Verse 38.9 tells us that he "knew that the seed should not be his; and it came to pass, when he went in unto his brother's wife, that he spilled it on the ground lest that he should give the seed to his brother." In verse 38.10, we learn what happened because of his action, or inaction: "And the thing which he did displeased God and he slew him." The Vulgate translation of the fourth-century scholar and Father of the Church Saint Jerome follows the Hebrew fastidiously and makes very clear why Onan refused his father's request: "Lest a child should be born in the *name* of his brother [*ne liberi fratis nomine nascerentur*]." This was the standard text for Christian interpretation for more than a millennium and leaves no ambiguity about Onan's motives. It does not specify, however, what exactly he did.

This is all we know of the two brothers and their sin or sins; there was much debate whether they were struck down for the same or different reasons. In the story, Judah himself is not sure why they died. Shelah, the third son, is too young to marry, and so Judah asks his daughter-in-law to go back to her father's house and live there as a widow. Perhaps he thinks that having her out of the way will prevent this strangely dangerous woman from ever marrying his last son; perhaps he hopes that by the time Shelah comes of age, sleeping with Tamar will be less fraught. Verse 11 says only that he asks her to leave until his third son has grown up and that he fears this son, too, will die. In any case, events intervene, and the real story of the chapter commences.

Judah's wife dies, and when he is comforted, he goes with some companions and their sheep to the lands where Tamar dwells. She hears that the widower is coming into her neighborhood, disguises herself as a harlot (sacred prostitute is the usual gloss), and easily seduces him. He promises her a kid goat for her services, and she, clever as she is, asks for, and receives, a security deposit: to wit, his cord, signet, and staff. He leaves these with her; she takes off her harlot's veil and goes back to her widow's weeds.

True to his word, Judah sends the kid goat to redeem his collateral. But his servant cannot find the woman to whom it is owed; everyone denies that any harlots have been in the neighborhood, and, lest he be made the butt of jokes, the servant gives up and decides to keep Judah's goat. Whoever has Judah's ring, staff, and cord can keep them. Three months later, Judah's daughter-in-law appears, pregnant. Judah demands that she be brought to him, as an errant member of his family, so that she can be burned for harlotry, even though he has sent her back to her own father and presumably relinquished authority and the right to punish. When Tamar appears, she reveals that she is pregnant by the man who owns the staff, cord, and signet she carries with her. Judah acknowledges that she has been the more righteous of the two; he, after all, has failed to give her to Shelah, his youngest son. And he resolves never to lie with her again. She bears twins — Perez, through whom the sacred line will be continued, and Zerah, who comes out with a scarlet thread on his hand — and that is the last we hear of Tamar. We do not know whether she eventually marries Shelah or not. Readers learn more about the royal lineage of Perez much later — in Ruth 4.18–22 and in 1 Chronicles 2.3–15 — but Genesis 38 ends with the twins' birth; the Joseph story resumes in the next chapter.[44]

This is a manifestly strange tale and cries out for interpretation; much of it is outside our brief. But even with a more limited agenda, we will have difficulty translating the language of alternative versions of the Onan story, of Talmudic commentary on it and related topics, and of later commentary into words that reflect what we mean by "masturbation."

The world in which Onan failed to sire a son in the body of his dead brother's wife lacked a vision of an afterlife. It was an agrarian society in which planting seed can be taken almost literally, as assuring the continuity of not only a living thing but a community and in this case a lineage. Onan was denying his brother the only immortality he would ever have. This near-murderous act is immensely concrete and reprehensible quite apart from the later messianic interpretation of his failure to plant his seed in the family garden of the Messiah. How he failed to do his duty is irrelevant and unspoken.

A bit more abstract than the absolutely specific account we get in Genesis is that Onan, by failing to sire a son that would count as his brother's, violated the so-called levirate law. If not a masturbator, he was at the very least an irresponsible adolescent who refused to play his part in maintaining the continuity of generations. But the wickedness of this kind of lapse was, in later biblical contexts, not so great and the specific means by which Onan shirked his duty are never mentioned. In Deuteronomy 25.5–12, the obligation to marry a dead brother's widow is the subject of a ritual in which she, in front of the elders, spits in the face of the surviving brother who refuses to marry her, pulls off his sandal, and says, "So shall it be done to the man who does not build on his brother's house." Nothing more seems to happen to the selfish sib; nothing about spilled seed. In the Book of Ruth, this exchange is already regarded as a quaint custom of former times. The "next of kin" who refuses to marry the widow Ruth escapes with his body, honor, and excuses all intact. Having been rejected once, Ruth seduces Boaz, a more distant kinsman, and the messianic line is back on track. (Boaz is the sixth generation after Perez, Judah's son by Tamar and the great-grandfather of David.) Again, the succession of generations and the proper transmission of semen matter a great deal; how specifically that transmission was occasionally averted is not part of the story.[45]

Levirate marriage, the specific context of Onan's failure, is, however, but a special case of the more general prescription in Genesis 1.28: "And God said to them, be fruitful and multiply." Minimally, this enjoins marriage and the bearing of children. At the cosmic level, it marks out a sphere in which God's plan for His creation meets human flesh. This will be an immensely rich area for interpretation, but masturbation has no place in it except by inference.[46] The Talmudic masters draw no explicit connection between the prescription to be fruitful and multiply and the proscription against needlessly spilling seed. The sticking point seems to have been in the purchase of "needlessly," and in that discussion our vice again falls into an empty space between two exigent issues.

In somewhat later but still pre-rabbinic texts, Onan's failure is mirrored in God's relation to His creation and to His chosen people, on whose bodies the covenant is inscribed through circumcision. This is related, of course, to the levirate-marriage question and the prescription of Genesis 1.28 but bypasses onanism entirely. Continuing a lineage matters deeply, and the re-telling in other sources of the Genesis 38 story sometimes reflects on Judah and his family's difficulties in this regard. Masturbation is irrelevant in this interpretive strand as well. In one version, Judah's sons and his wife died as punishment for his responsibility in selling Joseph into slavery.[47] The Testament of Judah lays all the blame on patriarchal failure and the domination of women. Er was a mama's boy who disdained Tamar because she was not a Canaanite like his mother. Onan likewise refused her at his mother's urging. This account of the brothers' motives from the Testament of Judah is slightly implausible, because the same text says that Er, if not Onan, picked his wife himself. Er, at least, died because he refused intercourse entirely; Onan then is struck down because, as in the Bible, he spilled his seed on the ground. Alternatively — so goes the story in Jubilees — Er wanted to marry a Canaanite like his mother, but his father picked a bride for him from another nation. Here the story is consistent; Er rebels against his ineffectual father's choice of a bride. And Onan did what he did to avoid having a son who would take his brother's name. Vicissitudes of "the dysfunctional family of Judah" and interpretations of the kinship rules they did or did not follow are critical in understanding the meaning of semen but have nothing to do with masturbation.[48]

Biblical accounts of pollution in which we might hope to find some earlier, recognizable ancestor of our modern "self-pollution" yield little by way of a genealogy. In general, semen was a serious source of pollution, a "Father of Uncleanness," but the degree of uncleanness it conveyed differed according to circumstances. On the one hand, abnormal discharges of semen — from a urethral infection, for example — were as polluting as menstrual blood: hence the Talmudic questions about examining one's penis for their telltale signs, which we will talk about in a moment. Like a menstruating woman, a *zab*, a man who has a genital discharge is unclean for seven days, and anything he touches, as well as anything that any of his bodily fluids touch, is unclean and can in turn convey uncleanness. Leviticus 15.1–15 gives the sordid details. On the other hand, nocturnal discharges of the ordinary sort also rendered a man unclean, but only for one day and not as powerfully. As Deuteronomy 23.10 prescribes, any man "that is not clean by reason of what chances to him by the night" must leave the camp for the night and ritually bathe before he returns after the next nightfall. (This was later interpreted to refer not to the war camp but to the temple.) Finally, semen spilled in ordinary intercourse polluted: the semen emitter was unclean for a day and conveyed his uncleanness to foodstuffs but not to their containers or to persons. And the woman who was his partner was also polluted: semen itself and not the act mattered; vaginal intercourse without emission did not pollute. Why women were rendered unclean when, in principle, only external contact disturbed purity was a great mystery, thought the rabbis, put there by God to keep them from thinking that they had figured it all out. In all this, masturbation played no part, nor did morality map nicely onto the clean and the unclean. Certainly, this system conveyed a sense of what was decent and what was not. But semen spilled in perfectly innocent and indeed commendable acts — reproductive intercourse — polluted.[49]

Moreover, spilling seed is not wrong under all circumstances; that would be too simple. In general, the rabbis did not regard sexual pleasure within marriage as problematic and debated the point largely as a question of decency and decorum. Rabbi Eliezer, the same one who elsewhere worried about the danger of a man holding his penis while urinating, explains that men are permitted, under some circumstances, to "thresh within and winnow without," that is, practice coitus interruptus. But what about

Onan and Er, who died for precisely this? other rabbis respond. His answer: it is allowable, for example, when a woman is nursing and a new child might deprive another who still needs it of the breast. Er and Onan did more than simply threshing without. Specifically, they spilled their seed in an "unnatural" (she-lo keᵉ-darkah) way as opposed to the "natural" (kᵉ-darkah) one of withdrawing during vaginal intercourse. Some rabbis whose views are collected in this Talmudic tractate interpreted Er's deadly offense — and perhaps also Onan's if one believes they did the same thing — as "corrupt[ing] her ground," meaning that he had anal intercourse with her. Still others were shocked by this suggestion, although it is found in the oldest of the midrashic commentaries, the Genesis Rabbah, which says Er "ploughed on roofs" a circumlocution that the editors glossed as "unnatural intercourse." Still others — for example, Rabbi Yohanan — thought that anything sexual within marriage was fine, including, presumably, anal intercourse, but that "whoever emits semen purposelessly is liable to the death penalty." It would seem that the rabbis generally regarded the Onan story as a cautionary tale enjoining procreation, with some exceptions, as long as intercourse was "natural," although some allowed even unnatural acts as long as the intention was to fulfill legitimate sexual desire.[50] Masturbation does not fit in here. But Onan appears in another context that suggests that maybe the rabbis did after all have our vice in mind.

In the tractate Niddah 13a–b of the Babylonian Talmud, the rabbis comment on the view that "every hand that 'checks' [the genitals] frequently — if by a woman, it is praiseworthy, but if by a man it should be cut off." The context is the previous folio's clear prescription that a woman who does not have regular periods must examine herself often lest she not notice that she has begun menstruating and hence become unclean. It is a difficult passage to fit into our history of male masturbation because it links two quite separate themes. Much of it is about spilled seed, which is, as we have already discussed, both polluting and non-procreative. Specifically, it is about spilling seed by checking the genitals, touching the penis, which is reprehensible for all the reasons we have already noted. But seemingly linked to these concerns are the questions of arousal per se and of purposeless emission of semen through self-arousal as especially horrible. One reason for the muddle is historical: the juxtaposition of these two themes is the result of joining different traditions in the Babylonian Talmud through a bit of editorial carpentry. Earlier rabbis operated within a Greco-Roman world that regarded self-arousal as a violation of sexual self-control and of self-possession, although not an especially interesting one. It was not a good thing but fit, as a relatively minor issue, into a larger whole. Later sources, drawing on different traditions, worry more about spilled seed. It is the editor(s) who, by combining the two, made this section of the Talmud read as if it were a powerful condemnation of non-procreative emission and, arguably, of masturbation, specifically and exclusively male masturbation, that is, touching the penis until it becomes aroused and ejaculates.[51] But the difficulty may also be the result of our trying to read what we regard as autoeroticism into a complex text that is born of concerns very different from ours.

The rabbis' discussion begins by arguing about whether a man who has a genital flux, and is thus as unclean as a menstruating woman, is allowed to examine his penis and, if so, how: with a splinter, a potsherd, a rag, a thick rag. There is much to be puzzled over here, but for our purposes the critical pronouncement is Rabbi Eliezer's: "Anyone who holds his penis when he urinates is as though he brought the flood into the world." The reference to the flood is portentous for our purposes. The verb used for "Onan *spilled*," *shaḥat*, is a strong one. It is the same verb used in Genesis 6, at the beginning of the flood story — "all flesh had corrupted their way upon the world." It appears again in Exodus 32.7, where God says to Moses that his people had "corrupted themselves" or "acted perversely" by making the golden calf. This puts what Onan did, linguistically at least, in the big leagues of evil and offers a rationale for why Rabbi Yohanan might hold that wastefully emitting semen, as Onan had done, is worthy of the death penalty.[52]

Most of the *sugya* — a chapter of the Talmud, discussing a particular topic — is devoted to discussions of Rabbi Eliezer's claim. Several questions are raised: whether, for example, examining the penis with a soft rag after ejaculation is likely to produce further ejaculations; if one does not hold one's penis while urinating and spills urine on one's cloak, might not people think that one is unclean or that one has a hole in one's scrotum that would make it impossible to father children? The rabbis also comment on the importance of specific circumstances of urination: arousal, and hence wasteful emission, are less likely if one urinates from the parapet of a synagogue, because both the danger of heights and the awesomeness of the place mitigate it; arousal is less likely in the presence of one's teacher; a married man is in less danger of arousal because, presumably, his desire could be lawfully satisfied. The last is Rabbi Nahman's view.

But among those offering views on needless emission, some suggest that arousal, self-arousal through holding the penis, is itself the problem, quite independently of whether semen is lost or not. In the midst of the urination debate, Rabbi Ammi likens the spiller of seed to one who worships idols, referring to Deuteronomy 12.2, where the Israelites are commanded to destroy all places where the people they had supplanted once had worshiped their gods. This might not be promising for our history except that very soon the question is posed: Why is it written that "he who deliberately makes himself hard should be banished" rather than that "it is forbidden [to make oneself hard]"? This is the nearest we come, I think, to masturbation as we understand it. The phrase reads literally, "Anyone [clearly 'he'] who brings his bone [penis] to the hands of impure fantasy [or heated imagination] is to be excommunicated." The prohibition is in the stronger form because he "incites his evil inclination himself." Such a person has no inner moral beacon; he responds to dictates of the moment. As Rabbi Ammi said, tell him today to do one thing, he goes off and does it, and tell him tomorrow to do another, and he likewise complies, and the day after tell him to worship an idol, he will do that too. In fact, self-arousal is a form of idolatry. In other words, "he who offers his penis into the hands of thought," who "incites his evil inclinations himself," is given to the craft of doing evil and specifically to an evil very akin to idolatry, of taking a graven image to be a god and that god as a substitute for the true God. This brings us very close to identifying Onan as an onanist. "Some say," in the words of Rabbi Yosi, "anyone who incites himself lustfully is not to be brought into the precinct of the holy one," the case in point being Genesis 38.10: "What he did was displeasing to the Lord." If we combine these comments with views expressed elsewhere on the imagination, it begins to seem plausible that the rabbis really were worried about masturbation as we know it. In general, and not just when it embraced sex, the imagination was deeply problematic: "Imaginations are more injurious to health than the sin itself." Idolatry is by its nature phantasmic; it regards other, false, gods as if they were real, as if idols were the true God. Thus self-arousal — from touching the penis while urinating to deliberately making oneself hard — is an instance of the misuse of the imagination that in almost every other context is also deeply suspect.[53]

But just when we think we recognize the vice whose history we are tracing, we are brought up short. Immediately after Rabbi Yosi's citation of Genesis 38.10, Rabbi Eliezer is reported to have asked, "Why is it written, 'Your hands are full of blood'? (Isaiah 1.15) These are those who commit adultery with their hand." Aha! But this is followed by a Tannaitic authority, who specifies that "you will not be subject to adultery, whether committed by hand or *by foot*." Next is the observation that "converts and those that play with children delay the Messiah." Spilling semen, and not specifically masturbation or self-arousal, seems to be the issue again. To be sure, "masturbation" is given in the translation as one way to "play with children," but the Hebrew refers only to those who do it "between the legs," meaning, perhaps, those who engage in intercrural sex? The two other instances of those who "play with children" are sodomites, who are liable to stoning, and those who marry girls below childbearing age. Non-procreative sex is the issue once again. Back to semen and how it is spent. We are again very far from our subject.

In the later medieval mystical tradition, all of this took on different meanings again, in many ways stranger and even less akin to the vice we know than the commentaries of the rabbis. In the Kabbala and the mystical tradition more generally, for example,

violations of levirate-marriage rule came to be regarded as especially horrendous, because marrying a deceased brother's widow
helped his soul to come to rest. In other words, a brother's failure
to sire children in his dead sibling's name was tantamount to condemning his spirit to a horrible limbo. But this is another world
entirely from that in which masturbation came to play an important part, one in which Adam's loose semen was regarded as the
source of "spirits, demons, and Liliths" and any man's seed could
give rise to demons. We enter now the realm of metempsycho-
sis, the transmigration of souls. Ramban, the medieval rabbi, biblical exegete, and mystic Nachmanides, glosses "Onan *knew* — as
opposed to *said* — that the seed would not be his" to mean that
he knew his brother's soul would become incarnate in the seed
and willfully kept this from happening. How this worked, Nachmanides thought, was unknowable; generation is one of the great
secrets of the Torah. So, spilling seed to deny Er progeny was not
half the problem; by needlessly emitting his seed, Onan not only
kept the transmigrating soul of his brother from being embodied
but aborted the whole procreative process, which is itself a small-
scale version of the divine plan. Nothing is worse than spilling
seed. "The murderer," says the Zohar, based on a reading of Genesis 38.10, "kills another man's children but he [he who does like
Onan] kills his own, and spills very much blood." Here spilling of
seed to prevent conception or for pure pleasure is almost irrelevant in light of the cosmic harm such an act perpetrates. Masturbation would, of course, be unthinkable in this minority view, but
perhaps because it is so far beyond any conceivable evil, it need
not be spoken of. If a wet dream is tantamount to murder, willful
ejaculation outside a procreative context is outside language. With
Jewish mysticism of this sort, Onan's deed and his fate take on
meaning well beyond any we would recognize as the solitary vice
of boys and girls, men and women.[54]

If generation represents one of the deepest mysteries of the
universe, then "destruction of seed" or "purposeless emission"
has a range of reference outside anything that the modern Onan
dreamed of. In some writings, "destruction of seed" refers to
ordinary heterosexual intercourse in which mundane, all-too-

corporeal pleasure takes over. The act is procreative but idolatrous; the children so conceived have the souls of non-Jews. An
elaborate ethics of marital sexuality is at work here, just as it is in
much Christian moral theology, and it overwhelms the merely
masturbatory insofar as self-arousal is relevant to these texts
at all.[55]

This brings us back to where we began this section: Did the
rabbis think about masturbation, and what did they think of it?
Plainly, they would not have regarded it favorably. Perhaps they
remained silent because it was so horrible, a secret whose name
could not be spoken. More plausibly, I have suggested, what we
think of as masturbation did not fit their conceptual categories:
idolatry, pollution, and procreation. Gratuitous, self-generated
pleasure would certainly have come under the rabbis' proscriptions of idolatry in all its forms. But discussions of this topic
turned so quickly to the ejaculating penis — or the penis in danger
of ejaculations — in a variety of circumstances that much of what
we mean by "masturbation" is left to be imagined: it never comes
into clear focus. Similarly, discussions of pollution and generation
have other purposes. Only when what was sinned against was no
longer the divine order but what Emile Durkheim would see as
its replacement — Society — did sex alone come into its own.

Christianity and Solitary Pleasures
The status of masturbation in the writings of Christian commentators and preachers is not as iffy as it is among the rabbis. There
are words for it, although for centuries there was a lexical slipper-
iness, which suggests not so much modesty as disinterest. By the
twelfth century the vocabulary of sexual sin had become more
precise, and masturbation by and large was settled into the second-order position among vices that it would hold until the eighteenth century: a harbinger of something worse, a practice that
kept very bad company, but not something anyone worried about
very much. Concupiscence and the soul's estrangement from
God, nowhere more evident than in the body's unruly, demanding genitals and its more diffuse sexual desires, defined the parameters of Christian anxiety. Celibacy in orders and modesty

124

within marriage were its great practical concerns. At the practical level what mattered were those aspects of sexuality that most threatened a godly order: incest or concubinage or bestiality or sodomy or fornication or adultery. The silent and inward vices mattered only in very specific contexts until the problem of the individual's relation to the social order came to loom large in our era. Before, the ethics of social sexuality were of almost exclusive concern, while the ethics of solitary sex went largely unnoticed. What one did alone might have been wrong and blameworthy, but it did not threaten anything fundamental.

Onan, that is to say Genesis 38.8–10, had relatively little purchase in Christian exegesis for centuries. These verses were not generally adduced as authorities in arguments against birth control, for example, until the twelfth century. There is no mention of "spilling seed upon the ground" — coitus interruptus — in any penitential (reference guides for priests, that helped them evaluate the sinfulness of a wide range of behaviors and to assign to each offense the appropriate level of penance) until the early ninth century, and then it was not associated with Onan. Saint Jerome inveighs against contraceptive potions but not against the sin of Onan.[56] Even in later medieval secular sources where the reader might expect to find some account of what exactly Onan did, and why it was wrong, there is nothing very helpful. A fourteenth-century book on the subject of marriage, written by a French knight for his daughters, is explicit on fornication, adultery, and much else but says no more about Onan's sin than that it was "pervers."[57] To a great extent, the history of Onan before onanism, from the tenth century forward, is the story of Christian — Catholic as well as Protestant — attacks on birth control and abortion. "Onanism" as a term of art in Catholic moral theology *means* coitus interruptus. This is an important issue but one that engages a social question — the purpose of marriage, the obligation to procreate — not a matter of individual desire, much less masturbation as a private vice.

By and large, when Genesis 38.8–10 was noticed, it was in an allegorical context. Saint Augustine, for example, in *On the Pentateuch*, interprets Onan as a type — as the sort of person who fails to do what he can to help those in need. He uses exactly the same words in *Against Faustus*, where we might have expected something else. (In this polemical text, he condemns the Manichaean use of coitus interruptus as a way of preventing God in the seed from being bound in the flesh — the first such condemnation of the practice by a theologian in the West — but says no more about Onan than he had in a different exegetical context.) Onan's offense is thus less spilling his seed, which Augustine had all manner of other arguments against, than failing to come to the aid of his dead brother. This was the Venerable Bede's view as well in the late seventh century, who regarded the boy's refusal to sire a son for his dead brother as Judah had asked him to do as exemplary of his uselessness, of his being — to use modern terms — a feckless, irresponsible adolescent. Or worse, Onan spilled his seed not simply because of a lack of public-spiritedness but because he actively hated his brother. So Saint Ephraem the Syrian had argued in the fourth century. Before him, the first-century Jewish legal scholar Philo of Alexandria had likewise thought that Onan sinned primarily against philanthropy; unlike Abraham and Hannah, the mother of Samuel, he was a narcissist when it came to procreation. He basked in self-love and the narrow perspective of the self; they lived for the ages and God's plan.[58] All of this may seem to prefigure how masturbation came to be understood much later as the vice of irresponsible teenagers, unknowing children, or anomic adults, but in context it has little if anything to do with our subject. Nor would it later when this exegetical tradition was carried over into Protestant commentary.

Martin Luther regarded Onan as a "malicious and incorrigible scoundrel" and his sin as "more atrocious than incest and adultery," because, he said, "it was a most disgraceful crime to produce semen and excite the woman and to frustrate her at that very moment." This gloss, as well as other letters Luther wrote on Genesis 38.8–10, is unconcerned with masturbation and very much focused on misguided Roman Catholic views on celibacy and on chastity within marriage and, conversely, on the importance of sexual love between man and wife in Protestant teaching. But more is at stake. First of all, Onan frustrates the coming of the

Messiah; the whole chapter, Luther tells us, as does modern scholarship, is really about Tamar, "for she is the Mother of the Savior." More immediately, Luther, like Augustine, interprets Onan allegorically as the type of someone who refuses to provide the help that law, custom, and love demand of him. The levirate obligation that Onan shirked was admittedly burdensome: "It seems impossible to love with chaste and conjugal love a woman one does not choose or desire." ("Unless," Luther adds, "this is done in mad lust.") It is perhaps an even greater burden to "serve another by raising up and preserving descendants and heirs, to beget children for others." But such is the test of love that God sets; the law to marry one's brother's wife so that *he* may have children "includes the most ardent love." Onan, "that worthless fellow, refused to exercise it." Unclean as spilling seed upon the ground might have been, the great moral disruption was the failure to do what love and duty dictated.[59]

John Calvin is one of the rare major figures in the Christian tradition to associate masturbation with what Onan did or did not do. But as with the rabbis, there is a grinding of categories, a Borgesian collection of seemingly disparate things. Masturbation is but one example of another, more general evil: "extirpating the hope of posterity" through a willful act of contraception. This is very much in the Roman tradition of defining the sin of Onan as coitus interruptus. But there are other moral failings in what Onan did not do. In the first place, he violated what Calvin thought of as a precept of "civil government" that God had given to the Jews. It was a "dutie of humanity" to do what one's father ordered and, more important, to do one's bit in overcoming the horrible curse of barrenness that threatened to erase the memory of those upon whom it fell. The Jews, Calvin says, did "account it a great courtessie to get some name unto those that were dead whereby it might appear that they had lived." To refuse to continue his brother Er's line is essentially to obliterate his name and, with it, any trace of his existence. Only when he is done with this argument does Calvin turn to what became "the sin of Onan" after 1712 — "the voluntary effusion of seed, without company of man and a woman." This, he said, was a monstrous thing but he

127

scarcely pauses. Coitus interruptus is "doubly monstrous" in that it is "to kill a child before he is born"; in withdrawing before emission, Onan did what he could to "destroy part of mankind." How he ejaculated is immaterial. And finally — Calvin shifts to address women for the first time in this exegesis — he declares that abortion is worst of all. Using medicines to kill a child in the womb "is justly accounted a fault not to be pardoned; with the same kinde of sinne did Onan defile himself." In other words, God punished Onan with death because he practiced a sort of abortion before the fact; he prevented a birth. Onan, in Calvin's view, is thus culpable both for what he did not do — follow the commands of his father, through whom civil society spoke — and for what he did do — take the first step in a cascade of sins that ends with abortion and murder. The bottom of the slippery slope points to its beginning.[60]

Iterations and variations on these Roman, as well as Luther-an and Calvinist, views made their way into Protestant exegesis in the century before *Onania*. Of course, they were part of the cultural lens through which the new onanism was greeted but they contributed little to making it the "trouble and agony of a wounded conscience" that it became. One bishop of Llandaff in the late sixteenth century, for example, thought that Onan was one of those spiteful and envious sorts who would rather "hurt themselves than pleasure another." Another Anglican prelate in the seventeenth century, Symon, lord bishop of Ely, thought, like Luther, that Onan's selfish disregard for his brother's interest was compounded by the fact that he acted against the divine promise, made to Abraham, that the multiplication of his seed would lead to a great nation; more specifically, he delayed the coming of the much-longed-for Messiah. We find the same views in the seventeenth-century Puritan tradition: "an unkinde, and most un-natural fact, to spill the seed which by God's blessing should serve for the propagation of mankinde"; and it is all the worse in Onan's case, where the seed was destined "for the propagation of the sonne of God according to the flesh," wrote Henry Ains-worth. At a time when so much divided religious communities in seventeenth-century England, there was little division over why

Onan was bad. The learned and prolific Puritan divine George Hughes glossed "that he spilled his seed on the ground" as (1) "uncleanness," (2) "selfe-pollution," (3) "destruction of future seed, which God ordered produced." Hughes is very precise in numbering his lists. Self-pollution and uncleanness seem to refer generically to the act of emitting semen somewhere other than in a woman's vagina. But this is largely beside the point. It is the second part of the verse that really interests Hughes: "that he might not give his seed unto his brother." "Herein," he warns, "is the greater sin," because "it was aimed in envy to his brother." First in the list of what readers were to learn from the whole episode is that wicked creatures are selfish and "unwilling to seek any good but their owne."[61]

More generally, in various allegorical interpretations it is a cautionary tale about human resistance to God's plan for the world. The Onan that emerges from these exegeses is a disobedient, irresponsible adolescent who did not do what he was told, who managed still to have an orgasm while frustrating the pleasure of his partner, and who, unbeknownst to him, threw a spanner into messianic genealogy. Here was a twelve-year-old boy — this is Luther's and Nachmanides's estimate of his and Er's age — who refused to take his place in the procreative, patriarchal order of the world. [62]

Much in his story would fit well into the modern account of masturbation as a rejection of civilization and the reality principle, but to read it back before the eighteenth century would be anachronistic. In the first place, it is difficult to translate much of anything that Onan did into the lives of girls and women, not to speak of very young children, who constituted a large part of the eighteenth-century world of solitary sinners. Moreover, none of these discussions describes *how* Onan spilled his seed upon the ground, and no one seems to care very much. Masturbation is at best implied, and only in some texts; interfemoral ejaculation, for example, would have been just as bad and indeed is conflated with what we take to be masturbation in various medieval penitentials and Jewish commentaries. Finally, Onan was decidedly not guilty of taking pleasure in his sin and certainly not a secret or a solitary pleasure. He has no interior life in any of the interpretations we have surveyed beyond being selfish, recalcitrant, and perhaps idolatrous if we credit rabbinic accounts of sexual arousal as pertaining specifically to him. Missing in discussions of his crime is the hugely complex, subtle analysis of the flesh — of desire, passion, and concupiscence — that characterizes much Christian teaching on sexuality. Missing is any sense that what Onan did is both a sign and a cause of a deep-seated malaise, one that, in its secular form, seemed to wreak such havoc in modern times.

There is one great exception that does link Onan's sin to the psychology of desire: the *Conferences* of the fifth-century abbot John Cassian. They constitute one of the most penetrating and moving meditations we have from the early Church on the cavernous spaces of the human soul. But they also very quickly move beyond the problem of Onan and what would come to be called onanism into quite another register. Cassian writes for monks who had isolated themselves in the backwaters of Gaul to escape the weight of the desire that would be the glory of the eighteenth-century secular society that gave birth to *Onania*. Onan's sin for Cassian is but a small example in a wide-ranging discussion of sins. Sexual failings are just one of eight principal vices against which his auditors must be wary. Fornication is linked explicitly to gluttony, which seems to shelter more of the failings and more of the social consequences that came to be associated with masturbation than does the more explicitly sexual vice of fornication. For the gluttonous monk, "burning pricks of lascivious and wanton desire are aroused." He wants to eat early and as much as possible; he will eat anything; he desires ever more refined and delicate foods, which "fastens the inextricable bonds of avarice on the necks of its captives"; these profoundly antisocial wants produce and are symptoms of an illness of the soul; the monk wants to flee the monastery, to return to the world where the inner reaches of the soul are not under such intense scrutiny. Gluttony enslaves through a corporeal avarice, and avarice, in turn, is a form of slavery to idols, a form of idolatry that, as we saw, the rabbis occasionally associated with Onan.[63]

For centuries, this would hold true. Not lechery but gluttony, not emblematically a lady riding a goat but a youth riding a wolf, bears the psychological weight of that never-ending, always un-satisfied addictive desire that the eighteenth century associated with the secret vice. Brueghel's visual epitome of gluttony is a woman drinking voraciously. The *Ancrene Riwle* (Ancient rule) speaks of it in a way that is almost interchangeable with Enlight-enment attacks on masturbation. The "sow of Gluttony," it says, "has young with these names": "too early...too voraciously, too much, too often." Only the fifth, — "too delicately," would not apply to the vice we are tracking.[64] Gluttony is the sin of excess, of an overpowering appetite, of taking more than one needs. It was perhaps not as serious as the mortal sin of unnatural sex, but it was much closer to what onanism came to mean in modernity.

That said, Cassian's exposition of fornication under the head-ing "lechery" is one of the rare instances before the eighteenth century of an unambiguous connection between Onan and mas-turbation. It is worth a closer look, if only a fleeting one, pre-cisely because Onan has only a cameo appearance before the main actors come onstage.

There are, Cassian says, three kinds of fornication, just as there are three kinds of gluttony: "The first takes place in the union of the sexes [*per conmixtionem sexus*]." His monastic hearers would recognize this immediately; it means any form of sexual inter-course. For the lay readers who came upon Cassian outside the cloister, this definition would need to be filled in. Some sorts of sexual relations between a man and a wife escaped the Church's condemnation of fornication; others were thought so lascivious as to constitute fornication within marriage. Where and how to draw this line became, over the next millennium, a hugely con-troverted question. But Cassian does not take it on.

"The second [kind of fornication]," he continues, "occurs without touching a woman [*absque femineo tactu*] and for it we read that Onan, the son of the Patriarch of Judah, was struck down by the Lord." Cassian clearly does not mean coitus inter-ruptus: he cites 1 Corinthians 7.8–9, which addresses widows and the unmarried, for whom warnings about contraception would presumably not be relevant but who might be tempted by contemporary medical advice regarding the therapeutic benefits of masturbation. We are talking here about fornication *alone*. Finally, Cassian addresses the fornication that "is conceived in the soul and in the mind, and about which the Lord says in the Gospel: 'Whosoever looks at a woman with lust has already committed adultery with her in his heart.'" All three must be extinguished, he says, and moves on, after one more paragraph on this subject, to outline three kinds of avarice, a sin he links with the gluttony-fornication duo. And this is all that Cassian has to say on the subject of Onan and solitary sex at this point.

When he returns to this same taxonomy of fornication in a more extended, more psychologically probing analysis in his twelfth conference, "On Chastity," neither masturbation nor its first famous would-be practitioner is so much as mentioned. At stake is not purity of action, which in the context of a group of monks secluded in a monastery is, in principle at least, relatively unproblematic, but purity of the soul. This is an altogether different story. "I have not known woman," Cassian elsewhere quotes Basil of Caesarea as saying, "and nevertheless I am not a virgin."[65] Fornication, in the sense that interests Cassian in the twelfth conference, is not so much an action — something sinful that one does or does not do — as a state. It is the condition of unchastity, of uncleanness of the soul, from which only a divine gift can deliver the monk who has done everything within human power to attain purity.

As in the fifth conference, Cassian begins with the mundane, with fornication "that occurs in carnal union." Second is, again, fornication of the sort that occurs "without even touching a woman," but this time he clearly does not mean the sin of Onan. He means "member impurity," not a willful act but something that "creeps up on those who are sleeping or awake, without even touching a woman, due to the negligence of a heedless mind." It is the sort of impurity, he goes on to specify, that is spoken of in Deuteronomy 23.10, where it is written that "if there is among you a man who has been polluted in a dream [*homo qui nocturno pollutus sit somnio*] he shall leave the camp and shall not return until he has washed himself." (See above, p. 118.) Masturbation, if it is anything, is the act not of a "heedless mind" but of one that wills arousal and what follows afterward. Finally, there is again Cassian's third sense of fornication. It is a secret sin but not *the* secret vice of another time and place. It is, instead, a sin that "grows in the recesses of the soul," not a sin of passion, much less solitary sex, but a kind of fornication that is a state of the soul: the state of wantonness.

There follows a brief discussion of avarice — a vice of idolatry — in which one is enslaved to idols, preferring "the love of worldly goods to divine love." Some of this will, in transmuted form, appear in eighteenth-century attacks on masturbation; some of it might remind us of what the rabbis said about the imagination and false gods. Cassian is not interested in what one does or does not do or what one does or does not allow oneself to fantasize. This would be too easy. In fact, one can no more give up fornication by giving up carnal knowledge than one can cease being avaricious by giving away one's money. To forswear avarice is to be rid of the *desire* for money. The "fire of fornication" can only "be extinguished in the same way."

The problem of fornication is, in this sense, tied to seminal pollution, but only because unconscious, unwilled ejaculations are manifest signs in the body of what might otherwise be hidden in the soul. Wet dreams were evidence that all was not right in the deepest recesses of a monk's being. There was in Antiquity a complicated and much-debated physiology and psychology of nocturnal emissions that could be brought to bear on such events, but basically they were thought to be a response to remembered images, the real version of which would stimulate sexual feelings in the dreamer were he awake. There were, it was thought both in Antiquity and in the medieval medical traditions, material ways to prevent these lapses. One did things to reduce the surfeit of fluids in the body; one slept in postures less likely to heat the blood. But this, Cassian makes clear, ignores the fundamental issue. Just as giving away one's money would not wipe out avarice, neither the "rigors of abstinence — namely hunger and thirst, along with vigils and constant work and an unceasing pursuit of reading" — nor castration would ensure the "perpetual purity of chastity." God does not ask anything so rigorous of those who would avoid fornication;

indeed castration is forbidden. What matters is that all and any disciplines will not avail the monk without "the bounty of divine grace." A monk can only admire a God who "cools the fire of his lust . . . so that he is no longer subject to the least erotic excitement of the flesh." The benign neglect of demons helps; a monk who was clearly neither prideful nor gluttonous was advised that he could take Communion — indeed was obliged to do so — despite having had a nocturnal emission just before Sunday Eucharist, because it was the work of demons seeking to confuse him.[66]

This is a far cry from simply not doing something: not committing impurity, not masturbating. Only those who renounce any faith in their own virtue or outward capacities *and* who open themselves to the mercy of the Lord will proceed successfully through the stages of chastity. Without prayer, "the hard ways of the Lord" will yield little. Cassian proceeds to lay out steps in this difficult journey: first, safety from carnal attacks while awake — easy, one presumes; second, a mind that does not "dwell upon pleasurable thoughts"; third, "not to be moved by desire, even ever so slightly, by looking upon a woman"; fourth, to prevent "any movement of the flesh, however simple, while awake"; fifth, to take no pleasure in, or give even the subtlest assent to, the stirrings one might feel when one reads about human generation. One must calmly think of such things as an unavoidable part of human nature, and they should evoke no more powerful a recollection than talk about "bricklaying or some other task." (This is like Augustine's speculation in Book 14 of *City of God* that sex in paradise was no more overwhelming than raising one's arm.) Sixth, and last, the monk is "not [to] be deluded by the alluring images of women even when asleep"; the unconscious mind learns to hate what it once found pleasurable.

We are here, as Cassian says, "placed at the boundaries of flesh and spirit [*ad confinia carnis ac spiritus*]." In this liminal zone, nocturnal emissions are, in a curious way, what masturbation became — a secret vice — but for very different reasons. The monk who suffers them — or in any case who suffers them with any titillation, for whom they are anything more than "nature at work," the release of "excess moisture during sleep" — has a dark place, a

134

hiding place, a place unobserved, which is revealed when his guard is down. Ejaculation other than of the most purely physiological sort, other than as a form of elimination like micturition or sweating, is a sign "of some sickness hidden inside, something in the innermost fibers of the soul." Conversely, through God's grace and through constant humility and submission, the monk might come finally to a state where "he never sees himself in secret as he would blush to be seen by men." He bathes in "the sweet light of chastity."[67] The secret vice is thus infinitely less mechanical than it became in 1712 and reveals dangers to the soul that are quite different from those onanism posed to the Enlightenment psyche.

At this exquisitely fine level of attention to the unruliness of the flesh, and in other monastic writings as well, talking about masturbation would be like worrying about open-string bowing in a master class with Pablo Casals. One can assume that so basic a technique has been mastered; the discipline required to prevent spilling seed in one's sleep without a hint of pleasure is of a different order from what was being asked of men and women, boys and girls by those who first brought a new "trouble and agony of a wounded conscience" to their attention in early-eighteenth-century London.[68] Cassian's brilliant Conference 22, "The Illusion of the Night," is from another world than the illusions of the day upon which *Onania* and its successors dwelled.[69]

So much for the limited purchase of Onan and his sin. More generally, the history of masturbation in the Christian era before modernity falls into three stages. First, there is what Christianity inherited from classical Antiquity, a continuation of the sexual ethics we have already discussed. Alternatively, in the first centuries of the new Christian era, the heroic age in which a new regime of sexuality and the body was being created, there is almost complete silence on our topic. It simply did not register. Then, between roughly the seventh and the twelfth century, we catch glimpses of what may be a prohibition on masturbation: cautious, linguistically ambiguous, mixed up with other minor infractions, seldom if ever severely punished. Finally, around 1100, our vice became linked with some very serious sins: the company of sexual acts contrary to nature like bestiality and sodomy. But it was decidedly the most innocent of the bunch and in fact received far less attention in the succeeding ages than its essential wickedness would lead us to expect. As before, however, masturbation remained peripheral, scarcely noticed in a crowd of other sins, many of which were, in their essential qualities, less serious. Sex with oneself never attained the notice that its status as a sin *contra naturam* would suggest.

The gentlemen of late Antiquity who formulated the new religion took much from the pagan medico-ethical world around them. Stoic and Cynic doctrines that regarded sexual pleasure as an unfortunate accompaniment to reproduction, an unpleasantness necessary for the process to work but nothing more, something that *askesis* could keep in place, were translated into Christian terms. Classical regimes for managing the intimate connection of the body and the soul found new voices in Christian late Antiquity and persisted in secular manifestations well into the Renaissance. Montaigne, for example, says that the counsel to have sex "that simply satisfies the body's need, that does not stir the soul," is a bit too rigorous. But he thinks there is something unseemly, something deeply inappropriate, about sexual passion in marriage: "Few men have married their mistresses and have not repented of it"; "I see no marriages that sooner are troubled and fail than those that progress by means of beauty and amorous desire."[70] He quotes Aristotle approvingly to the effect that a man should touch his wife "prudently and soberly." In this long *durée*, both in its rigorous Christian inflections and in the softer tones of neoclassicism, sexual ethics concerned itself with the relationships of men and women or, in Antiquity, of men and boys. Masturbation was scarcely visible on the moral horizon.

In the great shift from the second century of Marcus Aurelius to the sixth century — when the political and economic structures of urban life changed so deeply, when the place of the person and the body in relation to the community was transformed — solitary sex was an irrelevant issue. This was the age of heroic virginity and sexual renunciation, the age when marriage — and procreation itself — could be regarded as, at best, a shield against concupiscence or an admission that this world would not end quite as soon as had once been hoped. *Voluptas*, the capacity for sexual pleasure, and, more generally, the impossibility of singleness of heart, of the capacity to master a will that was concupiscent to its sinful core, bore down heavily on those creating new, Christian communities — monastic or secular.

In this world, moderating sensuality and maintaining chastity within marriage and refining celibacy among those who vowed renunciation mattered deeply. Amid these mighty engagements with desire, masturbation was almost unnoticed. We have already encountered John Cassian's writing on the struggles of celibate monks with the seemingly unyielding impurity of fallen man. Saint Jerome's poignant struggles are another famous example. His mind "burnt with desire in his frigid body"; he saw "maidens in the dances." His body was "haggard from fasting," "companion to scorpions and wild beasts," dirty, dressed in sackcloth. This athletic asceticism, this struggle with the flesh, overwhelmed the particularity of masturbation. More important, the solitariness of the solitary vice had little resonance. Sensuality alone was but a species of sensuality generally; the dangers of a collapse into solipsism were unimaginably distant in a world in which *Gemeinschaft* bore heavily upon each and every individual.[71]

If we put aside for a moment the problem of ascetics and those committed, more or less strongly, to celibacy — that is, of single adults — the great arena of struggle against sensuality was marriage. This struggle provides the context for the more or less benign neglect of masturbation, however it was classified, in Catholic moral theology and pastoral care until the modern period. The unmarried young, those we think of as adolescents, figured little in thinking about sexuality before the eighteenth century.

The medieval Church inherited a powerful tradition from the Fathers that holds that the union of man and wife is little more than an excuse for sin. Marriage had, as Augustine put it with ruthless simplicity, only three goods: *proles, fides, sacramentum* — procreation and the education of children; faithfulness, both sexual and in all one's duties; and sacrality, referring to the indissolubility and sacramental nature of its bond. Within so rigorous a model, only procreation justified the sexual pleasure that inevitably occurred during coition and that was regarded as a necessary part of generation. To pay the marital debt — or to ask for payment of the marital debt — for any reason other than having children was sinful. If demanded and paid as a remedy against incontinence and fornication, the sin was only venial. If for pleasure alone, it was mortal. A complicated calculus thus governed the marriage bed. It was better, for example, to commit a minor sin to be saved from a major one: a man might lawfully demand access to his wife when he knew she was not fertile or when she was menstruating if he did it so as to help himself resist sex with a prostitute.[72]

Some important theologians and bishops were even more deeply pessimistic about the possibility of innocent marital pleasure. The most famous of the decretalists (experts on that part of law that expounded on papal decrees or other authoritative statements of doctrine), Huggucio (Hugh of Pisa) in the twelfth century and his pupil the future Innocent III, reached the outer boundaries of orthodoxy by arguing that *every* act of sexual intercourse was sinful and guilty: *culpa et peccatum.* "It always occurs with excitement and pleasure which cannot be without sin." Under the tightly controlled circumstances of the most instrumental marital intercourse imaginable, expressly undertaken for procreation, it might be only a venial sin, but a sin nevertheless. To take this line of reasoning any further would have been to risk Manichaeanism — the heretical view positing a radical duality of flesh and spirit — and most churchmen did not go so near the brink.

But in general, the more pleasurable the sexual act — less because of the pleasure itself than because of attendant excitement and loss of reason — the more sinful it was. The faithful heard echoes of the rigorist position for at least the next five centuries as it filtered its way down to sermons. Indeed, unnatural sex with one's wife — for purposes of either pleasure or non-procreation — was as bad as sex could get. Bernardino of Siena, the Franciscan preacher and reformer of the early fifteenth century, may have been over-reading his legal authorities, but he did say that in a hierarchy of transgression, sex with a prostitute was a

mortal sin; and sex with a nun, with one's mother, or with someone else's wife was an even worse mortal sin; but sex with one's
wife in an unnatural position was the worst of all. A husband who
insisted on taking his pleasure within marriage, thought Burchard
of Worms, was four times worse than the bachelor who sought it
from prostitutes. And a woman's committing adultery was the
most heinous and punishable offense of all.[73]

Radical as these views might seem, they were building on a
long history of suspicion: the idea that marital sex could not be
enjoyed without sin, was already clearly articulated by Gregory
the Great in the seventh century. Masturbation does make a cameo
appearance in this discussion, but only because it might lead to
something worse — to a passionate desire for one's spouse and
the strength to fulfill it! The gloss to Raymond of Peñafort, for
example, cites Huggucio as the authority to condemn as a mortal
sin the actions of a man who provokes himself with his hands or
through warming drinks so "as to more often copulate with one's
wife."[74] Autoeroticism, in short, is bad because it might lead to
what we take to be normal sex.

A man might, for example, make an adulterer of himself by
being "too ardent a lover" with his wife. "Nothing is more vile,"
says Raymond, "than to love your wife in an adulterous fashion."
By the thirteenth century, the high tide of rigor had passed, but
questions about marital sexuality remained at the core of confessional practice. For the next six centuries, the intimacies of the
marriage bed were under intense scrutiny and became the arena
for generating pervasive guilt: "If one is too immodest in touches,
embraces, kisses, and other dishonorable things it might be
mortally sinful," says one confessional. Had the couple "intended
minimally the good of offspring"? asks another. Could one cease
intercourse without ejaculation — *amplexus reservatus*? Could one
have it during pregnancy or menstruation, or without going all
the way, *a tergo* — rubbing without penetration? There were questions about positions and times of the year and times of the week.
And there were questions about putting off intercourse: Would
denying payment of the marital debt increase the desire of one's
partner and put him or her in greater danger? "These were," as

the leading authority on the history of sin and guilt puts it, "so many questions that married people had to ask themselves."[75]

Less rigorous theologians right through the Counter-Reformation had to deal with these views; in a fundamental way, sex within marriage had to be excused. Positions did soften, perhaps as a response to the depopulation that followed the Black Death; from the late thirteenth century on, the pleasures of marital intercourse, at least as an intermediate good, did find some defenders. Under certain circumstances, intercourse per se was perhaps not sinful. But it was always under a cloud, always at the brink of perdition.[76]

Sex with a prostitute, though less fraught, was nevertheless very much in casuistic play: Ought it to be condoned because it prevented worse sins? Would payment be morally neutral even if the underlying act, fornication, was not? Is payment morally mandated after fornication with a whore even if soliciting fornication for money is a mortal sin? Ought money gained for bad purposes be accepted for alms or at the altar? (Yes, it was generally felt.) By the sixteenth century, in a general climate of reform, prostitution itself, or rather the sexual activity of young unmarried men with prostitutes, had come to be much less tolerated. As simple fornication came under increasing attack, as both the Protestant Church and the Church of Rome struggled to put their imprint on marriage, prostitution and concubinage lost the de facto acceptance they had enjoyed before. Sodomy, as a sin among the supposedly celibate clergy and in monastic communities but also in some secular contexts, came under increased vigilance. In short, all manner of sex for two was much discussed, reformed, and, on occasion, repressed. But there was largely silence regarding sex alone, and when that silence was broken, it was usually as a prelude to discussion of some more serious sin.[77]

This means not, of course, that masturbation was ever morally neutral in Christian Europe but that it was, considered as a freestanding act, not regarded as an especially problematic form of *luxuria* or in any other way especially threatening to the individual or society. (With respect to girls, the silence is almost total.) Other concerns about sexual matters seemed always to deflect discussions of masturbation in more exigent directions.

This deflection is especially evident before the twelfth century, when it was, in fact, scarcely noticed at all. What evidence
we have for it comes largely from penitentials — books that offer
modern readers a view into the difficulties the Church faced in
building a Christian culture, and a Christian sexual morality in
particular, in the West. They also allow us — by the admittedly
treacherous process of working backward from the severity of the
penance to the severity of the sin — to gauge the seriousness with
which various offenses were regarded.[78]

One thing is clear. Between the late sixth and the twelfth century, there was no word, no class noun, for masturbation. Again,
as in our discussion of the Jewish tradition, it is difficult to say
what this lexical silence signifies. I think that the creators of
a Christian sexual ethics thought in more general categories of
action than we do, and for these they used general-purpose verbs
— "to fornicate" (*fornicare*) or "to violate" (*violo*), for example —
which covered a whole category of sins that they then specified
contextually.[79] In any case, they had both technical Latin words at
their disposal and generally accepted circumlocutions, like *amica
manus* and did not use them. And if our sources seem to speak to
our sense of the solitary vice on some occasions, they are mad-
deningly obscure on others. Masturbation was not, it seems, a
category of sexual sin worth sustained precision of language.

The degree of clarity in penitential references varies. Sometimes there is no mistaking what the priest was being asked to
consider: "to fornicate by himself [*se impsum fornicaverit*]" or he
"has violated himself with his own members [*propriis membris se
ipsum violaverit*]" seems to refers unambiguously to masturbation.
The *Canons of Theodore* specifies a penance for a woman who has
"had coition alone with herself [*sola cum se ipsa coitum habet*],"
which may refer to masturbating using an object or to the act as
practiced with the hand or in some other way. In this case, the
transgression is a species of fornication and follows the penance
for a woman fornicating with another woman. The severity of the
penance — three years — suggests that the penitential is interested
in homosexual fornication and not in the normally far more lightly punished masturbation. In this text, as later in works directed

at monks, nuns, or priests, the author raises the subject of masturbation as a prelude to an extensive attack on what we would call
pedophilia or homosexuality.[80]

In other instances, we cannot be sure what a penitential really
means when it might be referring to masturbation. For example,
"whoever pollutes himself [*qui se ipsum quoinquinaverit*]" may well
refer to a masturbator, but there are other ways someone, clearly
a male in this case, might pollute himself.[81] Penitentials discuss
the nuances of moral culpability for wet dreams and nocturnal
emissions without dreams more extensively than they address
anything that might be construed as onanism. Maybe an emission
"if in one's thighs [*si in femoribus*]" was the result of masturbation,
but the phrase could, and often did, refer to intercrural sex, that
is, a "homosexual," not a solitary, act.

Finally, there are cases where the offense is designated so
generally that we modern readers are at more of a loss. "*Mollicies*"
(softness, effeminacy), for example, is often, perhaps rightly,
translated as "masturbation." But whatever the referent, it is clear
that the sin in question was part of an intricate taxonomy of permitted and forbidden acts in which solitary pleasure was, at best,
an insignificant species.

A case in point: a passage from Theodulf's *Second Diocesan
Statutes*, the work of a learned eighth-century Spanish Visigoth
who figured prominently in the court of Charlemagne and became bishop of Orléans in 798, seems to be a discussion of the
vice we are tracking. The work is not a penitential but was intended as a way to instruct priests in their dealings with wrong-
doers; it was meant as much as a list of admonishments as a
catalog of punishments. It says:

> Likewise, "masturbation" is called uncleanness either on account
> of the touch or sight or memory of a woman, or because of some
> pleasure occurring to him when awake, or if he exercises impurity
> between his own thighs, alone or with another.

The Latin text will make clear just how difficult it is to map
our modern classification of sexual acts onto that of another age:

142

Simul etiam vocatur immunditia mollicies vel propter tactum vel visum vel recordationem mulieris, vel aliqua delectatione accidens vigilanti, vel qui inter femora sua impuritatem solus cum ipso vel cum alio exercet.[82]

None of our words for sexual acts covers what Theodulf called "immunditia mollicies," literally "unclean softness or effeminacy." "Masturbation," the translation used by the leading modern authority, does not begin to serve the purpose. "Simul," "likewise," in this passage (meaning, explicitly in this text, having relations with a woman in an unnatural way) refers back to the sin of Onan in the strict sense, that is, to Onan's entering his wife, and then spilling his seed on the ground: coitus interruptus. So "immunditia mollicies" is definitely not the sin of Onan as it was understood after the eighteenth century. Nor does "mollicies" seem to mean a species of unnatural sex, as it did for Saint Thomas Aquinas when he classified the vices of *luxuria* that are against nature. The statute had already dealt with "irrational fornication" (*De irrationali fornicatione*), which referred to incest, bestiality, and "homosexual" acts: sexual relations with a blood relative, with a mule, with a male.[83]

What, then, is a *mollitia*? What are "mollities"? In classical Latin, the adjective *mollis-e* referred to the condition of softness — the opposite of the hard real man — and also to the moral condition such softness suggested: wantonness, voluptuousness, effeminacy, unchasteness. The body of the soft, yielding weak man was the sign of a personality to match. Saint Jerome used a noun version of this adjective to translate the much-discussed and completely obscure *malakoi arsenikoi* in the Greek version of 1 Corinthians 6.9. In this verse, Saint Paul specifies precisely which kinds of sinners, against sexual norms in this instance, would not inherit the kingdom of God: "neither fornicators, nor idolaters, nor adulterers, nor effeminates [*molles*], nor abusers of themselves with mankind," in the words of the King James Version. No one knows what the original Greek words meant. *Molles* for Saint Jerome probably referred to the painted young man of ambiguous sexuality who was also known as *cinaedus* in late Antiquity.

143

Thomas Aquinas, who did so much to make *mollities* the term for masturbation in his passages on unnatural sex (see below, p. 152), has a separate section of the *Summa theologica* (2.2.138.1) on "softnesses" in which he discusses effeminacy — in the old sense of the word as well as excessive fondness for pleasure, playing here on the connection between softness and moral laxity. Masturbation is not mentioned.

Later Protestant translators would follow in the footsteps of Jerome and Aquinas in their more general views. The English translation of John Calvin's commentaries on this verse uses "weakling," which it derives from Tyndale's 1534 and Cranmer's 1539 translations for the *molles* of the Vulgate. Calvin glosses the word to mean "those who, though they do not commonly give themselves to lust, yet not withstanding they do betray their impudence by their unchaste talk, effeminate texture, by their apparel, and by other debaucheries." The Geneva Bible uses "wantons" for Jerome's *molles*; the King James Version, as we saw already, and the Rheims translations use "effeminates."[84]

So, could *mollicies* have meant "masturbation" for Theodulf back in the eighth century? We do not know. Whatever it is, it "is called uncleanness either on account of the touch or sight or memory of a woman, or because of some pleasure occurring to him when awake, or if he exercises impurity between his own thighs, alone or with another." The sin in question seems to involve an emission occasioned by one of several circumstances. The first phrase could refer to a nocturnal emission induced by the thought or memory of a woman; whatever this form of uncleanness might be, the text contrasts it with what seems to be an inadvertent ejaculation — a *delectatione accidens vigilanti* — that happens while awake but not on account of thinking about or touching a woman; then there is impurity between his own thighs, alone or with another, which might refer to masturbation when alone and intercrural "homosexual" sex if with another man. The generic "unchastity" as a translation for *mollicies* would fit this list better; certainly "masturbation" is much too narrow. But the rhetorical force of this list is clearly to emphasize that uncleanness, however it occurs, is reprehensible. The question that remains is whether masturbation is a particularly sinful or revelatory kind of uncleanness.

And the answer seems to be that it is not. Even if it were possible in all of these instances to specify "masturbation" as the sin in question, we would still be in a moral backwater. In the great campaign to ensure clerical celibacy, monastic chastity, and the moderation of the sexual pleasures of the marriage bed, the penitential's interest in masturbation was minimal and the penances exacted small. Burchard of Worms, a major late-tenth-, early-eleventh-century figure, was far clearer than most in specifying what we understand as masturbation, but he thought little of it: ten days of mild penance if a boy did it alone; three times that if in company. *The Penitential of Cummean* is only slightly more severe but considerably more obscure: older boys — twenty is the upper age limit — who practice manual pollutions shall do twenty to forty days of penance. ("Pueri ante xx annos se invicem manibus coinquinantes.") Children imitating coition get about the same: twenty days. A monk who pollutes himself through his violent imagination does only seven days of penance; a man who pollutes himself with semen ("Vir semetipsum coinquinans") gets a bit more — one hundred days for the first time with added penance for repetition, although it is not specified how the pollution came about; a boy of fifteen or younger gets forty days. If masturbation was a sin, it seems to have affected men and older boys only; among the many horrible lapses to which concupiscence leads fallen man, it meant little.[85]

The sins that mattered were the ones that threatened the institutions God had ordained to contain lust: marriage for the majority, celibacy for a few. The layman who violates his neighbor's wife is to do a year's penance; he is enjoined from having sex with his wife if she is barren and also should abstain from intercourse during at least three forty-day periods around holy days. Violations of celibacy for priests or those in orders are clearly regarded as terribly serious: a monk who befouls the lips — oral sex — gets four years of penance, incest merits three, and sodomy seven. A bishop who fornicates merits twelve years' penance and is degraded. The higher the standing of the monk or priest, the more

145

likely his offense is to lead to scandal, the more socially disruptive the action, the tougher the penalty. Masturbation was a side issue in this context. Likewise, it mattered little in the struggle to confirm marriage as a defense against concupiscence or in efforts to make monks and priests stick to their vows of chastity. If defilement or pollution (*coinquination*) were the generic category, masturbation would be one, relatively minor subspecies.[86] It is one of a hodgepodge of pollutions, all subject to relatively short penances, all of which are much less severe than sexual offenses that threaten the collapse of institutions dedicated to chastity and community good order.

The important penitential of Theodore of Canterbury (archbishop 668–690) gives a good sense of these two constellations of sin, both relevant almost exclusively to the male clergy. With respect to pollutions he offers this list:

> "If the presbyter by the imagination sheds semen he shall fast for a week."
>
> "If [the presbyter] by the hand touching" — this presumably *is* masturbation — "he shall fast three weeks."
>
> "The priest who pollutes [*coinquinabitur*] himself by touching or kissing a woman is to do penance for forty days."

A presbyter who kisses a woman through desire — and presumably does *not* pollute himself — does the same penance as for masturbating, for touching himself and ejaculating: twenty days. (The layman who pollutes himself is also to do forty days, we learn in a separate section on fornication.)

> "Who often spills semen through the violence of their thoughts [the subject here is the clergy] twenty days' penance."
>
> "Who spills it in church while asleep, seven days' penance."
>
> "If he/she excites him/herself" — probably masturbation is meant here — "twenty days for the first offense, repeated forty days."

Whether men and women are included in these penances is not clear; the list begins with strictures and penance against monks and sacred virgins fornicating, so the implied subjects include both men and women. But *coinquination*, "defilement," is mostly reserved for men, so we cannot be sure.

These are all comparable to penances imposed for having intercourse during prohibited times or in unnatural positions — entering from the rear, for example, which would elsewhere, unlike masturbation, be much more heavily censured. By contrast, monks and sacred virgins who fornicate will do seven years' penance; a layperson who fornicates with a virgin is to do one year and with a married woman four years.

Masturbation was not innocent. But it also did not matter a great deal. Monks, nuns, and priests constantly struggled to maintain celibacy and remain detached from the worldliness of the flesh; among the laity, the Church battled to prevent incest, maintain the inviolability and sacramental nature of marriage, and condemn carnal pleasure as a reason for demanding the marriage debt. It was engaged in creating a new sort of social order wherever Christianity spread. The haven against concupiscence had to be kept safe from perversions. Kinship had to be bolstered, families maintained, old customs extirpated. In this world, sex alone was a bit player.[87]

Sometime around the middle of the eleventh century, as part of the great reform movement that started to sweep the Church, masturbation finally took on a new and specific meaning. It still had little or no salience for women or for boys and girls, but, first for the clergy and soon for all men, it attained the status of a truly heinous sin. From being a minor and not much noticed vice in a much bigger drama, it experienced a quantum leap into the worst of company.

It made its move, however, on the coattails of a far more pressing issue, one that seemed enormously urgent to reformers, one that far more than solitary sex threatened the community. Masturbation became a sin against nature because it came to be classified with another "criminal wickedness": sodomy.

There were some precedents for this new taxonomy in the early eleventh century. Sodomy had long been understood as anal penetration. Burchard of Worms, writing around 1007, had packaged questions about it, for example, putting one's penis *in masculi terga et in post[e]riora*, "in the hindmost part of a man's backside," so as to commit "fornication as the Sodomites did it," with queries about mutual masturbation, "fornication between the hips or thighs [intra coxas]," and, finally, about garden-variety sex alone: "Did you . . . take your manly member in your hand, and so slide your foreskin, and move it with your own hand so as to delight to eject the seed yourself?" He did not, however, allow his common classification of sins to support a claim for moral equivalency. Sodomy proper — depending on the circumstances — drew severe penances of between ten and fifteen years; inter crural sex merited ninety days on bread and water; masturbation ten days of a similarly restricted diet. Our vice was still a bit player.[88]

It was a generation later, with Peter Damian, the monk, cleric, bishop, and finally cardinal who was both a leading reformer and an important figure in the history of Christian spirituality, that masturbation, on its own, was classified as a species of sodomy, an "unnatural" act. "In an effort to show you the totality of the whole matter in an orderly way," he writes, "four types of this form of criminal wickedness ['the sin against nature'] can be distinguished":

> Some sin with themselves alone; some commit mutual masturbation [literally: with the hands of others]; some commit femoral fornication [literally: sin between the thighs]; and finally, others commit the complete act against nature.[89]

Exactly why, in Damian's view, masturbation was an unnatural, and not simply a filthy, act is not so clear. He cites no biblical precedent or long tradition of interpretation; to the contrary, he complains that not since the fourth-century Council of Ancyra had there been an appropriately resounding condemnation of sodomy in all its horrible glory and variety. For eight centuries, he says, the Church had been dangerously tolerant and made no mention of those who "sin alone." Nor is the problem that masturbation is not procreative. Finally, he makes no mention of the perverse delight the perpetrator might feel by his actions; sexual pleasure is irrelevant. By "nature" he seems to mean something much more literal: "nature" in the sense of "the natural world." "Does a ram leap on a ram, maddened with the heat of sexual union?" he asks. Clearly not. And the stallion stands next to another stallion in his stall without the slightest excitement until a mare comes by, when "lust is immediately unleashed." The desire of man for man thus goes well beyond the sickness of the soul that in the fallen state causes one sex to crave the other. It seems to be explicable, according to Damian, only by a sort of madness: "When a male rushes to a male to commit impurity, this is not the natural impulse of the flesh, but only the goad of diabolical impulse." Not simply the act but the desire itself is mad, which, Damian explains, is why the Council of Ancyra insisted that sodomites pray among the demoniacs and not among Catholic Christians.

However we understand these arguments, they seem to have little to do with solitary sex, since the desire Damian writes about is neither for an object of the imagination nor for oneself but for an inappropriate other person. The "ram desiring a ram" perversion of reason does not seem to fit masturbation. Perhaps the point is that only difference can generate rational desire and that in masturbation there is no difference. But if that is Damian's implicit argument, he never actually makes it, and it would be, on the face of it, implausible. The classical medical and ethical tradition assumed that masturbation was a lesser version of heterosexual fulfillment, and I know of no Christian writer who argued the contrary. Damian's single example of solitary pollution is of a hermit in the desert who at the moment of his death was given over to demons and ruined himself with impurity.[90]

In fact, the *Book of Gomorrah* more or less assumes without justification that masturbation belongs with its more heinous fellow "sins against nature." A cleric does not have to go all the way to commit the filthy act, argued Peter Damian, because the prototypical sodomites — "the inhabitants of Sodom" — did not corrupt "themselves only by the consummated act"; they acted, we should believe, alone as well as with others in a variety of ways. Again, at the bottom of the hierarchy of culpability is the hermit, who "sinned without knowing," thinking "this," presumably sex alone, "was permitted as a right arising from a natural function." Insofar as Damian offers an argument, it is through brief metaphorical allusions. On the vine of sodomical impurity, four offshoots rise from one root. If the cleric picks grapes from any one of these, he "is infected indifferently from the poison," just as he would have been had he picked the grapes from another. Or, with a more zoological twist, the serpent that his disputation has tried to crush has four heads; "it bites with its fangs of any one of its heads and immediately injects its whole poison."[91]

These two sentences and the opening phrase I have quoted are the extent of Damian's explicit references to masturbation in his fifty-five-page-long tract. Most of the disputation is devoted to attacking, clause by clause, what he regards as the laxity of earlier canons that fail to address the foundational evil that homosexual desire poses to the Church in general and to the clergy in particular. Many sections begin with citations from the Council of Ancyra, the only one that, in Damian's view, got it right. Rhetorically, he falls over himself to convey the deep evil of sodomy: "Oh unheard of crime! Oh outrage to be mourned with a whole foundation of tears," he laments. It is a sin born not simply of its abstract "irrationality," a horror that derives not just from its being against nature, although that is the theological foundation of its perversity, but from its being contrary to every possible conception of good order. Sodomy is a defiling of sons by their spiritual father, of those who go to confession by their confessors. If a priest's having sex with a girl who has come to him is sinful, then his having sex with a boy is even more so; sodomy is prostituting those in one's charge; it is like despoiling a virgin but even more disgusting and depraved; it is incest in its highest register of culpability. Monks who seduce males are the most ignominious of the ignominious. Damian's energy, and that of so much subsequent writing against sodomy, is against the erotic culture of the cloister in all its aspects. And it becomes part of the more general mobilization, in the late eleventh century and beyond, against all sorts of lapses in clerical celibacy.

From the modern perspective, the target of Damian's disputation is not solitary sex but sexual harassment, pedophilia, breach of trust, and the profoundly unsettling feeling that the all-male world of the cloister harbors the darkest of sexual threats against social good order. Finally, at the core of the work is a deep horror of incest: father with son or daughter, priest with spiritual son or daughter. Masturbation, however ontologically yoked with sodomy — the great unnatural sin of the clergy — gets barely a mention. In itself, it was not capable of this level of disruption. Only as the first step to something worse — like marijuana as a stage of heroin addiction — did it matter at all.[92]

Damian's text had a checkered history. It was not used, at least not explicitly, by any medieval authors. Pope Leo IX, to whom it was addressed, thanked Damian for his efforts but said that divine mercy should take precedence over apostolic severity, that he would not remove from office any clergy who had committed any of the four sins against nature, and — more important for our history — that there was a big difference between those who had engaged in solitary sex or mutual masturbation or spilled their seed under other circumstances and those who had had anal intercourse. If the former group of sinners confessed and did penance, they could be restored to the office they held before their lapse. Damian's definition of what constituted "a sin against nature" did not make its way into two of the most important canon-law collections of the next century — those of Yves de Chartres and Gratian — which seemed to regard *any* sexual offense as qualifying for membership in that category. If those collections greatly expanded the meaning of the term, then Peter Lombard, the twelfth-century author whose *Sentences* — commentaries on Augustine and other authorities — became a major textbook of Catholic theology in the centuries before the Reformation, shrank it. Somewhat confusedly, Lombard used "sins against nature" to refer to the illicit use of a woman by a man without any mention of masturbation or homosexuality. And somewhere in between is an early-thirteenth-century *Summa of Penance* by Paul of Hungary that enjoyed a great reputation for centuries. Paul held that a sin against nature is "when someone spills seed outside the place specified for it," that is, anywhere other than in a woman's vagina. This, he quickly points out, as had others, is worse than intercourse with one's mother; and the worst species of this ghastly sin was anal intercourse with one's wife. A long discussion of the unspeakable horrors of sodomy ensues.[93]

Somewhere in all this was masturbation, a small part of a theological complex of thinking about sin generally and *luxuria* in particular. Still, by the later thirteenth century, the classification that Damian pioneered had become orthodoxy. In any case, this purported first small step toward full sodomy came to be regarded as "a sin against nature" by the most important theologian of the age, if not for the same reasons that Peter had adduced.

The Angelic Doctor, Saint Thomas Aquinas, declared in his epochal *Summa Theologica* that worst among the sins of lechery (*luxuria*) are the vices "contrary to nature." Like all sin and all forms of lechery in particular, they conflict with right reason, but, in addition, they conflict with nature and specifically with the natural order of venery. They are not procreative; from them generation is impossible.[94]

He specifies four kinds; the first includes masturbation. It is not easy to navigate through the circumlocutions, but the vice whose fortunes we are tracing is, pretty clearly, one of the activities covered: "Outside coitus, when, on account of an orgasm [*delectationis venereae*], an emission [*pollutio*] is procured, this belongs to the sin of uncleanness [*peccatum immunditiae*] which some call unchastity [*mollitiem* again]." The other three vices against nature are more precisely described and are easier for us to translate into our ways of thinking: coition with another species, which is called bestiality (*bestialitas*); coition with the same sex, male with male and female with female, which is called sodomy (*sodomiticum*); and coition where the natural style (*naturalis modos*) is not observed — the use of the improper organ "or other beastly and monstrous practices."

Mollitiem, "unchastity" or "softness," as Aquinas describes it, is too general to refer only to masturbation, but masturbation would certainly count as a sin "contrary to nature," if not as a form of sodomy, in this classification. But despite its elevation,

Aquinas's sin of uncleanness — the *peccatum immunditiae* or *mollitiem* — remained in the shadows in later medieval and Renaissance confessionals and, more generally, in efforts to create a godly sexual order. Perhaps masturbation was so common that the clergy were afraid to speak of it lest it become even more widespread. Once again, we do not know what to make of this silence. But once again, the Church was willing to speak about other sexual sins, which suggests either that it felt they were less likely to be taken up by the laity after hearing them discussed or that these other sins mattered more. I suspect the latter is the case.

Sodomy, as we have already seen, was much noticed, much preached against, and occasionally punished with great brutality after the crackdown of the twelfth century, even if, in many circumstances, it was tacitly tolerated. Marital pleasures, always suspect, went over the brink when they became an end in themselves. Oral sex or any position other than man on top was thus an unnatural act in Aquinas's fourth category, since its purpose was the irrational gratification of lust. Sodomy between men and women — man and wife or client and prostitute — was a particular abomination.

The ramparts being defended here are social, not individual. Sins contrary to nature were a direct assault on the institutions that God had created to allow fallen man to live with his concupiscence: marriage for the laity, celibacy for the clergy. Within matrimony, husbands and wives every day faced temptations in bed that put them in the way of the gravest moral danger. It was the married against whom the authorities preached when they condemned unnatural heterosexual acts — *non in debito vase* (in the wrong orifice) or *non in debitus modus* (in an improper fashion). Albert the Great had classified the postures of sexual intercourse into one natural category — woman on back, man on top — and four unnatural ones that were inimical to the purpose of marriage, that is, to continence and procreation. Sodomy was in all likelihood a much used and effective form of birth control — a sexual act that was *prima facie* a rejection of the one truly acceptable reason for sexual pleasure within marriage — and any position other than the "natural" one was thought to diminish the chances

153

of conception. "*Omnis luxurious attactus* — every erotic stimulation — of the genitals" in which the natural order of procreation was potentially foiled was thus a form of adultery or worse, as Jean de Gerson, teacher, renowned theologian, writer, and chancellor of the University of Paris in the fifteenth century, put it.[95]

The seventh commandment proscribed, it was argued, not only every association and carnal union of man and woman outside matrimony but also every willed and unnecessary pleasure of the marriage bed. Adultery in this sense — the sin of touching for pleasure alone — was worse within marriage than outside it because it flew in the face of the most fundamental purposes of the institution itself. How exactly parish priests were to interpret these wholesale condemnations of almost everything their parishioners might have done in bed is not clear. But the fourth of Aquinas's class of unnatural acts certainly got a great deal of attention, as did the question of where its borders could be drawn. In comparison, the first category, the sins of uncleanness, paled.[96]

An exhaustive survey of French confessional manuals from the fourteenth through the seventeenth century finds that priests were, on occasion, coached to ask questions about masturbation — if that is in fact the sin that is meant by the circuitous language of the queries — but not, it seems, regularly or systematically. And when a penitent had strayed, his solitary sex was regarded as much less serious than the other three kinds of unnatural lecherous acts; serious offenses were sent to higher authorities, whereas masturbation, in all but one case, was left to the parish priest to decide a penance. Moreover, it was almost always treated as far less serious than fornication, a broad category of sins that included everything from intercourse outside marriage to excessively ardent intercourse within. Thus even if Saint Thomas classified "the sin of uncleanness" as the basest form of lechery — "an affront to God" and against "the developed plan of living according to reason" — ordinary men and women, and even their priests, seem to have found rape, incest, seduction, and adultery more culpable than having sex alone. "Unnatural sex" — the general category of mortal sin — meant, in effect, what we would call homosexuality, however many other sins might have been bundled up with it.[97]

Masturbation paled especially in relation to the sin that Damian thought was its telos: sodomy. Beginning in the great age of reform, during the twelfth century, clerical and secular authorities took up, very publicly, the battle against this far worse unnatural act, both between men and between men and women. Solitary sex was once again left in the shadows. "In the whole world there are no two sins more abominable," said the late-fourteenth-century pope Gregory XI, "than those that prevail among the Florentines." The first is their "usury and infidelity"; the second is unspeakable, "so abominable" that he "dare not mention it": sodomy. Whether it was in fact more prevalent in Florence than elsewhere we do not know. Certainly it was more talked about and on occasion prosecuted there, and in Italy generally, than elsewhere. Brothels were municipally licensed, and even maintained, in part, at least, as a defense against sodomy; supposedly, Florentine brothels were established specifically as an alternative. Prosecutions were relatively common throughout the Mediterranean; this may have been a mopping-up operation against the very old homoerotic culture of the ancient world or a response to the particular conditions of the marriage market there. In any case, 100 to 150 men were executed in Madrid, 100 in Palermo, and 100 or so in Seville between the 1580s and the 1650s, and they probably represent only a tiny proportion of those who actually did it. The Florentine numbers are more astounding. The so-called Officers of the Night arrested between 15,000 and 16,000 young men and levied twenty-four hundred fines between 1432 and 1502. Condemned by preachers and harassed by secular authorities, young men nevertheless lived in a material, cultural, and political world in which sodomy was tacitly allowed. And among the clergy, the Church fought a continuing battle against sex between men. Even if Peter Damian's harshest censures were not adopted, the fight against sodomy was relentless and increasingly shrill. On rare occasions, even women came under scrutiny. No one seems to have worried that masturbation led to all this wickedness. The moral energy that after the eighteenth century would be directed so publicly against sex alone was, to some measure, directed against sex between men in the late medieval and early modern period.[98]

Confessors' manuals in the centuries after Saint Thomas seem also to have ignored masturbation in their search for bigger game: *sodomiticum*. The penitents with respect to this question were usually young monks in training. The confessor sneaks up on the masturbation question, whether out of fear of giving his young charges ideas or because, I suspect, it is a ripple in a cascade of offenses: erotic dreams and nocturnal pollutions ("Do you ever experience pollution while sleeping?" "Does dreaming about women cause you to ejaculate?"). Nocturnal emissions, the confessor explains, are a mortal sin if they are habitual and result from evil thoughts. How about erotic fantasies and spontaneous ejaculations while awake, "by yourself with no creature around"? he asks. Then how about masturbation itself, ejaculation caused by the young man's "own touch"? Finally, the confessor moves on to mutual masturbation, rubbing between the thighs, and, in conclusion, the abyss of sodomy. These confessors seem to have been convinced, as Damian had been, that even though the fantasies of their young charges were assumed to be heterosexual, the least of the unnatural sins, sex with oneself, was but the prelude to sex not with a woman but with someone like themselves.[99] Like the Protestant enemies of clerical celibacy after the Reformation, the Church's confessors seem to have imagined a whole category of sexual sins of the cloister, beginning with masturbation and ending somewhere far, far worse.

In the real world of pastoral practice, *mollicies*, the "softness," or the sin of uncleanness (*peccatum immunditiae*) or even that sin of lechery that was "against nature," which we call masturbation, was treated far more circumspectly than other sexual misdeeds and regarded as threatening, especially for young monks, primarily because it would lead to something much worse. For several reasons, producing an orgasm in oneself seems never to have captured the serious attention of those who spoke about such matters, plus the authorities considered other offenses more disruptive and serious.[100]

In the first place, unlike the secular confessors of the eighteenth century — the doctors and pedagogues and philosophers and social visionaries who played coy and were anything but — the

writers of Roman Catholic confessionals and the priests whom
they guided did seem genuinely reluctant, lest they inadvertently
give their parishioners or students ideas, to ask in much detail
about unusual sexual practices. The story is told of a certain priest
in Brabant who began "to dig rashly into the conscience" of a religiously minded girl. By the time he had finished asking her in
detail about the various crimes that she might have, but had not,
committed, or even heard of, she was for the first time tempted.
Troubled, she went to this priest and told him, "You have done me
an ill turn this day by speaking to me of these things." It was with
great difficulty — as she confessed to another priest — that this
pious girl restrained herself from the novel sins.[101]

The "scorpion of lechery," as a thirteenth-century text addressed to three well-bred women in retreat from the world put
it, "has children that it is not fitting for a well bred mouth even to
name." Despite this caveat, some were named: fornication, adultery, the loss of virginity, and incest, as well as foul desires. But
masturbation gets the silent treatment. After warning nuns about
all manner of temptations to lechery — frivolous behavior, wanton
eyes, unchaste touches — the author announces that he "dare not
name the unnatural offspring of this poison-tailed scorpion [lech-
ery]." And indeed, he does not. Instead, he warns that "sorry may
she be who, with or without a companion, has thus nourished
with her lechery the offspring of which" he "may not speak out of
shame, and dare not, for fear anyone should learn more of an evil
than she already knows, and should thereby be tempted." Unlike
eighteenth-century authors who make the same protestations
before going on about the subject endlessly, our thirteenth-century author keeps his peace. On the other hand, what we call sexual fantasy, and particularly masturbatory fantasy, does come in
for censure, if only because it is the prelude to an almost certainly
sinful denouement: "Let her take thought about her accursed inventions in lechery, for in whatever way this is slaked, in a waking
state and voluntarily, to the pleasure of the flesh, except only in
marriage, it is a mortal sin." The silence surrounding masturbation was deep but not complete.[102]

This suggests the second reason, a rhetorical consequence of

157

the fact that other sins mattered more. No one seemed able to stay focused on solitary sex. Occasional references to the unnameable sin in the century after Aquinas always veered onto another track. In one confessional, for example, intended for use with young friars, it is embedded in the spiritual excavation of wet dreams, which has occupied monastic communities since the very beginning. Many, as we have seen, use *mollities* as a segue to *sodomiticum*. In other sources, the masturbatory foibles of penitents seem to provide the fodder for some clerical soft-core titillation with little pretense of extended moral reflection. The chapter on sins against nature by the late-thirteenth-century Dominican Thomas de Cantimpré, for example — *De fuga peccati contra naturam* — has a certain confessional kiss-and-tell, can-you-top-this energy that goes nowhere. He tells four stories about masturbation, each a little more over the top than the one before. One woman who said she did the filthy deed regularly in bed — the first instance I know of in Western civilization of addiction to the solitary vice — told Cantimpré that a devil made loud cries of "fi, fi, fi" and made signs of "indiscrete insertion." She felt sorrowful and ashamed. A second tearfully confessed that she regularly polluted herself because voices told her it would be forgiven. She died shortly after her confession — out of fear, Thomas opines — and so suffers many punishments in purgatory. The third snippet is about a widow living in a convent who is the most abominable (*neffandissima*) of sinners, although Thomas does not specify what she did. It must have been bad, because pigs, presumably with devils inside, dug up her body and scattered its entrails. Finally, in one last anecdote — and the sort of grotesque hyperbole one associates with certain literary forms, the Fabliaux, for example — his readers get rank hearsay: the bishop of Lausanne purportedly knew of a man who reached down between his legs for his accustomed vice and found instead a snake in his hand. Exciting as these stories are, they, and the tiny number of references in confessionals in the centuries after *mollicies* became an unnatural act, constitute the barest trickle in a sea of guilt.[103]

Finally, the solitary unnatural act fit uneasily into the broader jurisprudence and discipline of the Church, which increasingly relied on public sanctions instead of on the private suasion of the confessional to enforce its norms of sexual behavior. "Infamous acts," open wickedness, blatant flouting of increasingly strict standards, not secret vices, got attention. Specifically, changes in the law of evidence and in legal procedures made it easier to bring open violators of standards to account: priests or monks who ostentatiously kept concubines, couples who had intercourse before marriage — a common enough event — adulterers, fornicators, sodomites who sinned in such a way as to draw attention to themselves.

In fact, all this behavior was difficult to regulate; marriage, for example, was made in heaven and depended only on the assent of both members of a couple. It was difficult to prove that a pair of lovers had not made an agreement prior to their tryst and her pregnancy. Trial marriages were commonplace in some areas. Fornication was rife, and even orthodox churchmen conceded that it might well fall within the limits of continence that could be expected from the average believer. Some — heretics — went so far as to hold that it was not a sin at all. In these circumstances, the Church concentrated on bringing the *public* behavior of people whom it had some chance of controlling more in line with precept. Juridical sanctions against sexual deviance, like prosecutions against heretics, were for actions — or views — "publicly avowed and obstinately defended"; what mattered was *infamia*, "being of bad repute," or *notorium* — that is, being egregiously in contempt of standards.[104] In a city as dominated by the Church as York, for example, where the clergy constituted the main clientele for prostitutes, little was said on the subject. Open concubinage — being a "monkwhore" or "friarwhore," essentially a kept woman — and, for her master, keeping such a woman with no pretence of discretion got all the attention.[105]

Even a private denunciation of something done privately needed public proof. And so the secret vice went largely unnoticed. *Onania* might therefore have been right that while "all other actions of uncleanness must have a witness, this [masturbation] needs none," and hence it really did escape much notice before anyone was willing to make the private so fully public.

Perhaps many penitents of the high Middle Ages and the early modern period did not know that this particular "unnatural act" was a mortal sin. There is no way to know. Given the reluctance of priests to ask about it, and the overwhelming weight of worry about both clerical celibacy and the sexual practices of the marriage bed, maybe masturbation simply fell between the cracks. Perhaps cloistered monks managed to separate the casuistry of nocturnal pollution, about which they heard so much, from the practice about which they heard so little. Nuns might not have heard about the problem at all, and children were in all likelihood innocent of knowledge about its sinfulness. There are hints that, even if secret and unspoken, masturbation was not a good thing. A woman in Dijon accused of prostituting a very young girl says by way of mitigation that she caught her masturbating, confronted her with the fact, and kicked her out when she denied it. Both parties seemed to know that masturbation was less than desirable. But since prostitution was not taken terribly seriously, it is hard to know how seriously any of this was meant.[106]

Sometime in the early fifteenth century, however, a distinguished cleric, most likely the famous chancellor of the University of Paris Jean de Gerson, offered more than a casual sentence or two on our vice. Aquinas's new ontology of vice made its way resolutely into the literature of confession in the tract *De confessione mollitiei* (On the confession of masturbation), which for the first time talked about the subject in terms recognizable to us moderns.[107] The strident tone we have come to expect after 1712 is there; so is the confessional insistence that a secret be revealed; and so is the insistence that the sexuality of the young be brought under surveillance. This tract is part of a much larger project to regulate the behavior of children — especially such behavior as might lead to sexual wrongdoing in general and the dreaded sodomy in particular. Gerson is not beyond "pious fraud" to circumvent the defenses of young penitents and make them reveal their most secret vices.[108]

There is in Gerson, too, the insistence that the vice is nearly universal and that it is terribly difficult to discover and put in its proper, terrifying moral perspective. Finally, like *Onania*, "On the

Confession of Masturbation" is anonymous, and it is only *attributed* to Jean de Gerson. It appeared in a manuscript collection, with other works by him and two confessional works by other authors, which was copied in Paris in the 1420s by Nicholas of Clémanges, a humanist churchman who taught at the university and was a member of the College de Navarre. There were perhaps political reasons at first for Nicholas's omitting Gerson's name on any of his works in this collection. Within twenty years, however, when the manuscript was bought for the canons of Saint Victor, Gerson's authorship was established for all of its component parts *except* for the tract on masturbation. It remains in the form of an anonymous report on an informal talk between an unnamed master and students, an "as-told-to confessional": "A certain theology master, according to his rich experience and diligence in his study,... has revealed in Paris the things written below." Transitions are effected through phrases like "The master then counseled."[109]

No one knows who wrote the piece. Perhaps, argues the most careful scholar who has engaged this manuscript, Gerson is the reporter who heard this commentary on masturbation when he was a student and then sent along a copy to his friend in Paris who asked for help in caring for the souls of the young men in his charge. Internal evidence will not help: some scholars think the stridency of this piece is uncharacteristic of Gerson; others think it totally in character. It is not clear why no one in the Abbey of Saint Victor, whose library was famous for its pastoral works, made even a single copy of "On the Confession of Masturbation." Perhaps the manuscript remained so obscure because its author was unknown and it lacked authority, perhaps because the time was not ripe for masturbation to emerge as a sexual practice that was dangerous on its own and not as the prelude to far worse sins of the flesh or as a sign of concupiscence.[110]

For all its similarities to modern texts, Gerson's three-page tract differs enormously in its rhetoric from the much more extensive works of the Enlightenment tradition in an important respect. Those who incorporated *Onania* in the eighteenth century and after assumed that the pursuit of sexual pleasure was right and proper; masturbation for them was a surprising and dangerous deviation from heterosexual bliss. Most modern texts until the twentieth century begin with the "discovery" of how terribly prevalent it was and go on to much hand-wringing about why this should be so. They incorporate it into a perpetual struggle to produce a sexual subject in whom desire is constantly stirred up and modulated; masturbation is part of the making of the secular self. Gerson would have none of this. He assumed that those whose confession he was guiding were mired in concupiscence, that they were children of the Fall. Thus even as Gerson, for the first time in Western history, gives sustained attention to masturbation, he does it in such a way as to make it seem like no great news at all. He evinces no surprise in revealing yet another sign of the soul's estrangement from God, perhaps more insidious than most because it is more private, but still familiar enough. Gerson can relax in a way his modern successors could not; for him, things will be resolved in the hereafter; for us, the problem is endless and very much in the here and now.

The confessor knows exactly what he is after and how to get it. He eases into his interrogation gently: "Do you remember that once in your boyhood, when you were about ten or twelve years old, your rod [*virga*] or private member [*membrum pudendum*] was erect?" Any penitent who denies that this ever happened is to be "firmly reproved for the lie" and assured that this happens to all boys when they get aroused (*calefacti*, "get hot") unless they are defective.

Once he has cleared this up, he is advised to move on to the sin itself by sowing the seeds of guilt. Wasn't it — the erection — ugly? "What did you do to make it go down?" Ask this sincerely and with a calm visage, the confessor is advised, as if honestly seeking a remedy; these conversations were face-to-face. And if no answer is forthcoming, ask more directly, "Did you stroke or rub your member, the way boys do?" If the boy insists that he "never held or rubbed" his erect member, the confessor cannot go further, but he is advised to tell the boy, in a tone of admiration and disbelief, that this is scarcely credible and that the spiritual consequences of this temporary lapse of memory are grave. Lying in the confessional is a serious matter. This is the first time in the historical record that anyone made a claim about the prevalence of masturbation. Like everyone with a subsequent view on the subject, Gerson thought that the practice was more or less universal. But unlike eighteenth-century and later claims that at least purport to be based on observation, Gerson's conclusion is grounded in the fallen nature of the flesh.

However prevalent "the abominable filth of the detestable sin known as masturbation [*mollities*]" might be, it was assumed to be exceptionally resistant to a confessor's queries, in part because it was so secret, and presumably shameful, but also because penitents did not think it wrong. Secrecy is both the sign of the crime's ignominy and the reason why so many people do not know it is a crime. Masturbation is the nearest thing we get to a truly private language whose meaning must be made publicly manifest. And this cannot be easy.

The confessor is warned that if he is not especially skillful and circumspect, he will "rarely and hardly be able to draw out" an admission of vice "from the mouths of the infected [*infectorum*]." (Gerson makes nothing of this medical image—he does not need the authority of the body to underwrite sin—but it will be taken literally in the works of Enlightenment philosophes, doctors, and quacks.) The confessor will face resistance not only from young men, as we have already noted, but also from grown men and women, whom, in slightly different terms, he is also supposed to interrogate. The author says that he knows from "abundant experience" that many infected adults have never confessed to this sin. Some were silent on the subject because they had been ashamed of masturbating and thus forgotten it; others suffered the second-order guilt of having been too ashamed of their action to confess it in the past and too ashamed of that lapse to come clean in the present; and still others claimed that "they had never been asked about it by confessors." So, masturbation was not high on confessional question lists, and penitents were not pressed on the issue.

Presumably, many people also failed to tell their priests about it because they did not think it wrong enough to confess spontaneously. Gerson advises parents and teachers to warn children against stroking or rubbing their private parts, because he knew that later in life many "excused themselves by ignorance, saying that they never heard or knew that this kind of touch is sinful." Many also argued that it kept them from wanting to "know women carnally." In other words, people seem, to some extent, to have bought into the idea that masturbation, like sexual intercourse for some reason other than procreation, was not so bad because it prevented something worse. It would be bad in this way of thinking only if it turned out to be foreplay to fornication or adultery.

Finally, Gerson, like eighteenth-century thinkers, was on to the fact that masturbation was so dangerous because it was so easy to do and so habit-forming. He argues against silence, against the view that young children should be spared warnings because they might learn something bad from them. Even three- or five-year-olds are "inclined to do such things," because they feel an "unknown itch [pruitum] when their member stands erect, and they think they are allowed to rub and stroke and touch that place like they do when they feel itchy in other places." They hardly know what they are doing, but soon they are hooked, and it only gets worse: "The delectation increases with their age," and soon they practice full-scale masturbation or even sodomy, all "out of an act they did not think was forbidden." We are back to the slippery-slope-to-sodomy argument, but not before unprecedented attention to masturbation as a highly specific lapse from chastity.

If we are to judge only by the articulation of ideas, Gerson got there first. Eighteenth-century writers added little to his insights, with the important exception that they thought of the vice as an affront to secular morality and not, as he did, a species of lechery. More than a millennium's assortment of brief, unconvincing condemnations were finally brought to a point in 1427.

But the fact is that Gerson's secret vice remained, quite literally, a secret: secret from confessors, who had to work hard to extract admissions from penitents, reluctant for various reasons to let on that they had done it; secret because confessors were cautioned that, inquire though they must, asking about the practice might stimulate precisely what they hoped to stop, that talking about the secret would make it known and hence more wide-spread; but secret also in the sense that "On the Confession of Masturbation" was almost entirely unknown before twentieth-century historians rediscovered it.

Unlike other pastoral works by, or attributed to, Gerson — works in the same bound manuscript collection and others as well — only two copies are known in addition to the one that made its way first to the Abbey of Saint Victor sometime before 1448 and then, during the French Revolution in 1796 to the Bibliothèque Nationale, where it rests today. By contrast, for example, scholars know of eighty-five copies of his work on nocturnal pollutions; twenty-nine copies of the tract on daytime pollutions. The works by the two other authors in the same manuscript collection were also much copied. Only "On the Confession of Masturbation" was ignored. It was not even listed as an entry to the Saint Victor codex's table of contents; were one to open this bound-together sheaf of variously sized manuscripts, nothing would suggest that the pages on masturbation were anything but the continuation of another work entirely. For half a millennium, the West's first sustained attack on masturbation remained an unpublished, un-noted quasi secret.[III]

But this brings us finally to the question of what this wave of silence means. It certainly does not mean that theologians and preachers had no concept for this vice. Perhaps Gerson's profes-sion of reticence in "On the Confession of Masturbation" was heartfelt and not, as such announcements were in the eighteenth century, an empty rhetorical gesture or a pornographic tease. In other words, the circulation of his little tract was so limited because the vice it exposed was so shameful and dangerous that it could not be written about. Even to announce that there was a secret vice *without* revealing its secret would be subversive to good order. And perhaps once masturbation had been unim-peachably classified among the very worst of sexual sins — sins contrary to nature — it became even more difficult to broach pub-licly than it had been when it was merely one relatively minor way to pollute oneself. Some confessors regarded all sins against nature as such an abomination, such a defilement of the ear, such an embarrassment that even devils were ashamed to mention it, that "the mute sodomite man" — presumably including the masturbator — would confess only to God. Whether even to ask about the secret vice was itself an important and much vexed question, part of a debate in which Gerson played his part.[112]

But reluctance to speak on such topics generally does not explain the relative silence on masturbation in particular. Sodomy, the most wicked form of unnatural vice, produced a continuous uproar, however unpleasant it might have been to hear. It was preached, legislated, and policed against constantly. It was written about and discussed extensively in religious as well as secular literature. Other, lesser sins of the flesh were also much discussed. Prostitution — seen sometimes as a lesser evil that limited the far greater one of sodomy — was a major public-policy question; the sacrilege of sex with nuns, the defloration of a virgin who was not one's wife, adultery, incest, abortion, and living off the wages of a prostitute were all, in various jurisdictions, regarded as serious — even capital — crimes. Pope Sixtus V in 1586 laid down death as the penalty for a long list of sexual crimes. Masturbation in this legal context, if discussed at all, seems to have figured only as a form of homosexuality. Likewise, the profound suspicion of sexuality within marriage and of the impurity of the nude body was, if anything, deepened in the centuries after Gerson. The sustained, endemic embarrassment of the flesh did not engender silence; quite to the contrary.[113]

In a moral universe where sexual transgressions, inside and outside marriage, were diligently pursued, the most likely hypothesis for the almost complete silence that greeted "On the Confession of Masturbation" is that the vice it sought to excavate from the consciences of penitents was not morally or pastorally resonant on its own. Or more precisely, it was not resonant in the form in which "a certain theology master" spoke about. In the perfervid climate of sexual guilt created by the late medieval and early modern Church, impurity threatened to overwhelm the sexual body of the laity at every turn. Sodomy was the much-dreaded sin of the cloister, premarital sexuality of any sort the scourge of the Church after the Council of Trent. "What abomination, what scandal," the touching and kissing of a courting couple; to be amorous was to live in danger, and those who thought impurity a minor matter were said to be seriously mistaken. Masturbation might have been on the preacher's mind, but nothing is said. In a book intended for pastors to the poor, Joseph Lambert suggested that they preach against "secret lewd acts," which included various forms of birth control and not just, or even primarily, masturbation, and — under the same heading — that they attack a long list of sins in the "abyss of horrors": "indecent songs and speeches whether said or heard, shameful insinuations and touches, [and] criminal actions committed with oneself or with different persons of either sex." Historians have found a few other sources, for example, the 1622 Christian pedagogy of Phillippe d'Outremont, which attacks "a most filthy and abhorred sin, whose name horrifies me...the sin of voluntary pollution." Like everyone who has ever commented on masturbation, he regards it as nearly universal because it is so easy to do: "This sin is the most difficult to correct, because one always has the opportunity to commit it; and so widespread that...the greater part of those who go to hell are damned" for it. And always there was sodomy, but not in relation to masturbation. Robert de Sorbon does not even cite Genesis 38.8–10, the verses about Onan, in his condemnation of unnatural vice and starts his list of authorities with chapters 18–19, the story of Sodom and Gomorrah.[114]

Perhaps unpublished works on our vice are waiting to be discovered or further copies of "On the Confession of Masturbation" are hiding in the dusty, long-unread codices that fill Europe's ancient libraries. Undoubtedly, more mentions of masturbation await discovery in the many unpublished late medieval and early modern sermons on other related topics. And the vice did continue to make its appearance in some discussions of sodomy. Still, the silence on the subject of solitary sex is remarkable. By the sixteenth century, the printing presses of Europe were cranking out books and pamphlets on moral education by the thousands, but nothing on this particular unnatural act. And even its subsistence in the queries of some confessionals was little more than a whisper: once a year, maybe one question. Individual sexual sin was not the focus of ordinary Catholics as they learned their way around the new practices of confession and penance.[115] The sexual sins that mattered were, as before, sins with a social consequence, sins that affected the relationship between people, between individuals and society, or between generations: incest, fornication, sodomy, abortion, contraception. Private vice counted for relatively little. In this world, Gerson's now famous tract *De confessione mollitiei* was a dead end until a new kind of problem arose for the desiring, imagining self in the Enlightenment.

Masturbation on the Eve of Onania

Little in seventeenth-century Protestant England would have offered a clue to even the most astute contemporary observer that a new moral and medical concern about masturbation would begin on Grub Street around 1712, make its way into better company within decades, and soon be at the very core of Western thinking about sexuality and the self. Language certainly gave no hints of what was to come.

After Martial in the first century A.D., nothing was heard of *masturbor* or its cognates for almost fifteen hundred years. Supposedly the great sixteenth-century essayist Michel de Montaigne first used a form of the word in French, but I have not been able to find the citation. The first English use comes in 1621 from an unlikely direction. Robert Burton in his *Anatomy of Melancholy* invents a form of "masturbation" to help explain particular cases of women's melancholy, a species, it seemed, of Galen's disease of widows for which genital stimulation was the long-recommended cure. The women of whom Burton writes were sick not because they masturbated too much but because they had intercourse too seldom. Specifically, they, and men as well, were victims of precisely the sexual culture of the cloister that reformers within the Catholic tradition had been attacking for a millennium. The difference in 1621 was that Burton had no interest in making celibacy a reality. His target was the ideal itself, his vehemence born of Protestant hostility toward the "odious and abominable," "the rash and superstitious" popish vows that doomed men and women to lives of unnatural virginity. Tyrannizing "Pseudopolitians," another word Burton invents in this short section to refer to the hypocrites and meddlers who interfered in the lives of others, were the cause of "fearefull maladies, feral diseases, grosse inconveniences," and all manner of sexual depravity to boot. He lays at the feet of Rome and its vaunted commitment to clerical celibacy a dog's breakfast of wickedness, including, just before he gets to sodomy, the English neologism in Latinate form, "mastuprations":

> frequent aborts and murdering of infants in their [popish] Nunneries … their notorious fornications, those *Spintrias, Tribadas, Ambubaias, &c,* [male prostitutes, lesbians — literally, those who rub — and dancing girls], those rapes, incests, adulteries, mastuprations, Sodomies, buggeries of monks and friars.[116]

The first English use of "masturbation" was thus an attack not so much on the practice itself as on something far worse — popery, which encouraged sexual depravity through its immoral and unbiblical insistence on celibacy. Among the many evils that priests and monks loose upon an unsuspecting world is masturbation, condemned less for what it is than as one small sign of a much larger cesspit of corruption. Burton's moral indignation is reserved for the Romish proponents of celibacy, whose misguided views bring nothing but grief and vice to the world. And as for the disease with which he began, the best cure for melancholy lovesickness is marriage and what we would call a healthy sex life. No one would have predicted that "masturbation" would have the future that awaited it.

Nor was there anything in the history of "pollution" or "uncleanness" that would have foretold the new meaning these words took on in connection with the solitary vice in the eighteenth century. Semen out of place — or even where nature supposedly intended it — was regarded as polluting and unclean by both the Jewish and the Christian tradition, albeit for different reasons and under a variety of circumstances. But there is very little evidence that masturbation was regarded as an especially likely, or an especially dangerous, form of pollution or uncleanness on the eve of the *Onania* explosion. A whole treatise on moral dirtiness, for example, written at the turn of the seventeenth century ignored it entirely. "The learned Ostervald" (J.F. Ostervald was a Protestant clergyman in Neuchâtel) in "his *Treatise on Uncleanness in all its branches*" passed over this particular "abominable Sort of Impurity" in silence, as *Onania*'s John Marten points out. He coyly relegated it to some general set of trespasses against cleanliness and failed to "represent the heinousness that it is." Indeed! The phrase "self-pollution or another unnatural and dangerous species of uncleanness," which seems to refer to masturbation, appears only in a preface that had been added to the 1708 English translation, which, in turn, was published by Henry Parker, one of the printers who was also involved with the Anodyne-Necklace empire that later profited from the onanism bonanza.[117] We are already in the ambit of the new world of masturbation.

Ostervald's text in fact offers only the merest hint that masturbation might have been on the learned pastor's mind. Chastity, he says, "governs the Hands and the Body that none may touch themselves, or others, or suffer themselves to be touched in too free and indecent a way." It excludes "the strange effects of sleep and dreams," that is, nocturnal emissions, even if the imagination has some role in causing them, as long as they are not willed. So, some ejaculations do not make a man unchaste but are a sign that the "flesh is not yet brought into subjugation." Fine, but as a semiotics of the wet dream, this view is thoroughly traditional and has little to do with masturbation.[118]

The point, however, is not only that Ostervald is silent about what became so terrible a vice but his silence still echoes in a warren of other, more exigent anxieties about sexual ethics. What mattered to him and to his contemporaries, just as to those in the earlier Christian tradition, were perversions of sexuality as perversions of social life, not as a withdrawal into asocial autarky. He devotes eleven pages to adultery. Unwanted touching was an issue for him, as it must have been for the young men and women of his age; touching oneself was not.

In one of the most remarkably explicit and fulsome confessions of sin that have come down to us from the seventeenth century, the Reverend George Trosse laments that he committed great offenses against God and "*Breaches* of the *Seventh Commandment*": to wit, "*amourous glances, Words and actions*" with the eldest daughter of his master. When Trosse sailed off to new employment, the two connived to have her come on board ship, where they managed to sneak off and behave foolishly and wantonly together. On other occasions, he took advantage of a drunken servant who regularly exposed herself while in her stupor; he repeatedly touched women sinfully. In short, lots of heavy petting, which he construed as violating the injunction against adultery.

Trosse's major self-recrimination, however, is reserved for his out-of-control drinking, which led to the d.t.'s when he stopped and to all sorts of impurity when he didn't. When drunk but not debilitated, he gambled to excess and did almost everything with women except for actual penetration. A "comely but wanton wench" begat in him impure flames that made him do "what led directly to fornication" but never to the "gross complete acts" themselves; during another drinking binge, he and his friends bought wine, with which they plied an old nurse, whom they then "horribly abused." Under his list of offenses against the seventh commandment — separate from reports of earlier dalliances — is that he carried himself wantonly toward everyone and did everything indecent except incest, from which God saved him by "never suffer[ing] him" any "act of fornication" with the particular woman in question. In this repetitive and long list of sexual sins, masturbation comes up only once and then as something that seemed wrong only in post-1712ish retrospective. To wit: "A lewd fellow servant led me to practice a Sin, which too many young men are guilty of, and look upon as harmless."[119] The cultural baggage of "uncleanness" was there to be appropriated by *Onania*, but in the late seventeenth century even as obsessively guilt-ridden a man as Trosse did not find it worth much anguish. He berated himself for social, not solitary, sin.

In the seventeenth or early eighteenth century, being unclean would almost invariably have pricked the conscience for some violation of the ethics of social sexuality: fornication, adultery, incest, petting. "The unclean adulterer" is a standard locution, often followed by an attack on "the uncleanness amongst Christians," which suggests some kind of illegitimate heterosexual intercourse: "A gentleman solicited a citizen's wife to uncleanness" whose husband slew first him and then her; two citizens of London were committing adultery on the Lord's day and "were immediately struck dead with fire from heaven in the very act." There is nothing in this seven-hundred-page book, with its thousands of examples of good and evil, from which these examples are drawn, on masturbation. Jeremy Taylor, one of the best-selling divines on the subjects of the good life and the good death, had no truck with "uncleanness": "of all vices the most shameful." But most kinds involve two souls, he continues, and then proceeds to denounce adultery and fornication. Uncleanness in this heterosexual sense had some of the emotional energy that later coalesced around what became the secret vice; it made one "sneaking, foolish, without courage," as the case of King David's folly with Bathsheba illustrated so well. But masturbation, if that is indeed what he had in mind, merits one sentence against "voluntary pollutions of either sex" in a twenty-page section on chastity.[120]

To seventeenth-century readers, "the sin of uncleanness" would also have suggested prostitution. When Bernard Mandeville, the first great advocate of unfettered commerce, wrote about how virtuous women created the market for prostitution, he asserted that he was far from being an advocate of "the sin of uncleanness" but that he was simply telling it as it was. Prostitution, to be sure, carried many of the associations that masturbation later did: addictive — "how much more difficult to recover from it, than most, if not any other, sin"; seductive — a snare for the unsuspecting that lies hidden in the many other sinful practices of the age; even polluting. But when someone spoke of "polluting oneself," the allusion was to sex with a prostitute, not to sex alone. "I gave the whore two guineas," writes the young Virginia aristocrat William Byrd II in his diary for 1719 about an escapade in Kensington Garden, "and committed uncleanness." On one occasion, he says, he "kissed the maiden 'til I polluted myself"; on another, he kissed the maid "until my seed ran from me." But whatever he did, he seems not to have "polluted himself" or "committed uncleanness" by what came to be called "self-pollution."[121]

"Uncleanness" was a public, social evil. In the sense of "whoring," it follows, for example, "drunkenness" and precedes "swearing, cursing and profanation of the Lord's day" in a list of *public* vices that a group of London gentlemen wished to repress. "Uncleanness" begins with fornication, with lust, with "the criminous conversation of a male and a female," announced a sermon on the subject. But we are not in an ascetic age; the "desires of the flesh are physically good," the preacher went on to say. The moral problem came in choosing the proper object at the proper time.[122] Sex for two and its perversion were at issue.

What so disturbed the vigilantes of the middling sort who founded societies for the reformation of manners was that, with the demise of "bawdy courts," no one enforced decent public behavior. They were interested in creating not a morally autonomous citizen but a new moral police to replace the one that had lost its efficacy. Grotesquely public vices — barely hidden brothels, open sexual coupling in streets and alleys, loud swearing, Sabbath breaking, in short, disorderly, uncivil behavior — seemed, to them, rampant and unopposed. The new moral police was behind the prosecution in Queen's Bench of John Marten's pre-*Onania* work of medical pornography, the first such case in that court. In all this, uncleanness always meant violation of public decency, the sort of thing for which in centuries past churchwardens might have charged parishioners in the archdeacon's court.[123]

In a two-volume exhaustive history, written less than a generation before *Onania*, a learned clergyman surveyed in great detail what he thought the Bible offered as examples of "the most remarkable instances of uncleanness." He comments on Onan but not as the eponymous first masturbator. Whoring, fornication, and perhaps buggery, in all their shameful permutations, are the "uncleanness" that this weighty work most studiously chronicles. Long lists of biblical bad examples fill its pages: Lamech in Genesis 4; Abraham and Jacob because of their polygamy; Esau because of intemperate appetites; the sins of the concubine Zilpah and Bihah — hints of some sodomitic impurity. By the time we get to Er, Onan, and their father, Judah, in Genesis 38, we have been treated to a lot of bad stuff. And more is to come. Er, we are told, was probably guilty of sodomy; Judah, their father, incestuously polluted his own daughter-in-law once his marriageable sons were dead. Onan seems relatively innocent in this bad company; he was struck down by God for "frustrating the End of Nature," that is, for coitus interruptus. Volume 1 ends with Origen, the third-century Church Father who castrated himself.[124]

In 1701, an obscure clergyman writing about the sin of uncleanness did work in a short censure of "mollities" in the course of a full-throated blast against fornication and adultery.[125] But this only makes the point that "uncleanness" was largely a matter of public morality or illicit sexual connection in the minds of those who wrote about sexual ethics on the eve of *Onania*.

The history of "pollution" helped create the moral revulsion to modern masturbation. But before the early eighteenth century, "self-pollution" as a synonym for "masturbation" was extremely rare. One could be polluted by idolatry, by false doctrines, by desecrations of the Sabbath. One could suffer a *pollutio nocturna* or some other emission of seed other than through sexual intercourse, but only rarely was this linked with masturbation and then only in the larger context of ineradicable concupiscence and birth control. Pollution was in its larger sense an inevitable consequence of original sin; the postlapsarian state itself was a defilement of what God had made pure. An individual might "mitigate" pollution, but it was generally not something that one practiced. "*Self*-pollution" before 1712 is rare and difficult to link with what it came to designate.[126]

Likewise, the earlier uses of "abuse" made it ripe for picking around 1712 as part of a new name for masturbation. But before that, it had no such associations. "Abuse" suggested illicit sex but not illicit sex alone. The court at the Bridewell in Tudor London heard cases against a widow at Smithfield and an unidentified man who "abused their bodies together," a woman who confessed that she had twice allowed a man use of her body but that he asked often "to abuse her body," which she refused. Abuse was something akin to our "sexual abuse"; a servant complains against her master that he "attempted to abuse her and hath kissed her."[127] Many other forms of abuse were brought to the public's attention:

the abuse of perfuming tobacco, of curly hair — the deadly mollity that got David's son Absalom into trouble when his wavy locks got caught in a tree and left him hanging. There was abuse of astrology, prerogative, physic, and much more; there was the "abuse of the boundless power of Cupid"; and there was self-repugnancy made manifest in the abuse of Scripture. I found "self-abuse" — or at least a variant on it — only once in connection with a sexual act. However, not masturbation but "homosexual-ity" or, to be more precise, the "abusers of themselves with mankind" — was at issue. These "liers with mankind," they who practice "the filthiness of the Greeks," will not enter the kingdom of heaven, says Calvin in his commentary on 1 Corinthians 6.9.[128] "Self-abuse" thus has a history but was seldom uttered before around 1712 in connection with solitary sex.

Clearly words like "uncleanness" and "pollution" and "abuse" that were not specifically connected to masturbation offered the weight of the past to the new "trouble and agony of a wounded conscience" when it appeared in the early eighteenth century. Unlike "homosexuality" and "homosexual," however, which as terms may well have come into use only when the thing to which they refer came sharply into focus — a particular sort of person or state defined, at first by doctors, as having a constellation of fixed desires — or "sodomy" and "sodomite," which covered a variety of acts and ways of being, "self-abuse" or "self-pollution" or "mas-turbation" or "the sin of Onan" referred after 1712 to something that had been perfectly well understood since Antiquity, even if it was variously classified and named. There had been masturbation by its own name and by unambiguous circumlocutions well be-fore "self-abuse," "self-pollution," or "onanism." The authors of major seventeenth-century works of English pedagogical and normative literature were clear on what it was. They simply had almost nothing to say on the subject: I could find less than three pages of print, *in toto*, before the eighteenth century compared with the avalanche of the centuries that followed and with the constant stream of books on sin, child rearing, and pedagogy.[129] And even when someone wrote about masturbation, he did it in a broad context of sin and guilt relevant only to adult men; there

175

was no discussion at all about women, children, or adolescents.

The Puritan divine Richard Capel, for example, embeds his censure of "selfe pollutions" — a rare use of the term but one that clearly includes masturbation — within a cascade of moral theology that, like the great tradition of Christian thinking on the subject, has as its object concupiscence and the sins of lust. First, Capel lectures, there is the "sinfulness of sin itself," which is most evident in the fact that it hides itself and, once discovered, seeks extenuation: "Sinne and shifting came into the world together." In other words, all sin, and not specifically masturbation, is in an important sense secret and can be countered only through exposure and watchfulness. Second, he gives a general account of lust, which, he argues, works both through temptations, which "entic[e] and bait the heart of man as men do fishes," and through our original sin — through concupiscence — which provides a constant forest of tinder: "Fire burns not where is no matter for it to worke upon." The fundamental problem is the absence of singleness of heart, of estrangement from God. Third, Capel spends ten pages discussing how "all our tentations, if they may be let runne, will become unnatural." Indeed, the more natural a sin, the "more headlong our lust for it." Nothing in this section is recognizable as masturbation, although there are references to what the Sodomites and the daughters of Lot did; pollutions against nature get a mention but nothing more specific. The point seems to be that lust in general knows no bounds. Uncleanness — all sex outside marriage — presses especially upon the conscience because it is so very sensual and brutish that it deprives men of their reason. Many instances of uncleanness are committed with a second person, which makes them even worse, and many have terrible consequences in the world. Adultery, for example, results in bastardy and allows "strange birds to inherit the nest": "the sin is great, the consequence is greater." On page 210 of a 687-page treatise, we come to a chapter on "unnatural uncleanness" and specifically to section 1, titled "Of selfe pollutions." It finally takes on masturbation but ever so briefly. "Unnatural uncleannesses," Capel argues, are worse when practiced alone than with someone else because sin is worse when it offends most aggressively against the order of love; love of other begins with self-love; one cannot love one's neighbor's chastity if one does not love one's own. Therefore, the worst wrong one can do is that done to oneself, and uncleanness alone is worse than uncleanness with others. This is the opposite of the modern argument, articulated most clearly by Havelock Ellis and Freud in the twentieth century but present already in eighteenth-century discussions, that the big moral problem with masturbation was that it was the result of rampant narcissism, too much, not too little, self-love. Capel has no interest in such psychological arguments.

In fact, after these brief observations on the gradations of uncleanness, the discussion turns to self-pollution as "spilling seed" in the most obvious sense of Onan's sin: coitus interruptus. It is a very bad thing, a kind of murder, in fact, even if "this is not the intention of the doer"; "he that feeds the Ravens will provide," readers are assured; people should marry on the poorest of terms rather than "fall into such illicit, darke and abominable practices." But all of this has little if anything to do with masturbation. Capel is warning against sins that a man and a woman commit together.

However bad as a class of sins "self-pollution" might be, it remains a bit player even among the temptations of "unnatural uncleannesses" more generally. Capel devotes less than two pages to it, a few more lines to "beastiality," and then over twenty pages to "sodomy." All sins have a voice, this one, sodomy, "hath a loud and a crying voice." The dangers of servants in corrupting families, the dangers of religious men and women — monks and nuns corrupting each other — are adumbrated in great detail with respect to the third, and most prominent, unnatural uncleanness. The whole category of "unnatural uncleannesses," in turn, gets much less attention than uncleanness generally, that is, adultery and fornication. And finally, if we look at the promising section on "tentations that come from our selves," we find it silent on masturbation. So, "self-pollution" does make the briefest of appearances in the seventeenth century, but it is scarcely recognizable in the company it keeps. There it subsisted, in quite another moral universe, until the eighteenth century.[130]

Of course, there is nothing magical about the dates I have used so often: "in or around 1712." The material was there from which the new vice would spring; the social world that gave it resonance had existed probably from the 1680s or 1690s. Daniel Defoe in 1705 replied to a question in his *Review* that, yes, self-pollution was a mortal sin but that the problem ought no more to be discussed in public "than to be acted in private." He was not about to make a bid for the share of the literary market place that John Marten would claim. There were other would-be *Onanias* that might have made it. In 1698, for example, a man named Hadriaan Beverland published, in England, a Latin tract on fornication that went on for thirty pages about masturbation. Nothing came of it; the book languished unknown and unnoted, never translated, never cited in any of the eighteenth- or nineteenth-century literature. Not even the learned Tissot, always on the lookout for predecessors, seems to have heard of it. But had Beverland's tract taken off, the story of how modern masturbation started in the gutters of Grub Street would not have been very different. It and *Onania* shared a common world.

Beverland, like John Marten, who started it all, was a shady character. Born in Zeeland (now part of the Netherlands) in 1652, he became a student at the University of Leiden in the early 1670s and immediately got into trouble for publishing a book in praise of pederasty. When he was twenty-six, he was kicked out of the university and fined for publishing a book on original sin which claimed that Adam and Eve's only failure had been their "carnal conversation." Off young Beverland went to the University of Utrecht, from which he was also expelled, this time, it was said, for writing a satire on the *magisters* of his former alma mater. He then went to Oxford, where he continued his studies in law and philology but fared little better, supposedly because he wrote satires of various English bishops that did not sit well with his hosts.

Our troublesome Dutchman finally earned his J.D. while at Oxford, but *De fornicatione*, which he had started in 1689, went rapidly off track. Beverland may have drafted it with a serious intent: getting back to Holland. But when it was published, it was pretty clearly a satire. He had a well-developed taste for classical erotica and it shows. In any case, the tract did not earn him a reprieve at home or much else either. The author of the first sustained treatment of masturbation went mad; Beverland died in exile and insane. Perhaps his views had no resonance because, unlike John Marten, he had no medical tie-ins — no nostrums — which gave onanism as Marten conceived it entry into the commercial mainstream of eighteenth-century London. But had Beverland beaten his much more successful would-be rival to the punch, neither the beginning nor the early history of modern masturbation would have been very different.[131]

I have occasionally used as the date for that beginning 1712. This is cheating. "Early eighteenth century" or "around 1712," as I usually say, is more honest. We do not know the actual date. There may have been an edition of *Onania* in 1710, the year given in the British Library catalog for a now-lost copy; the first mention we have of it in a reliable contemporary catalog of pamphlets is 1716. Some scholars have suggested that it appeared as early as 1708.[132] "Around 1712" splits the difference.

Whenever the book first appeared, John Marten is basically right to claim that this is the first work to bring masturbation to the world's attention. Of course, it came with a legacy: a medical tradition that held that excess of any kind was harmful; a link to the abject, the silly, the derisive from classical culture; an association with Christianity's and Judaism's revulsion toward birth control; a family tie, in some Jewish and many Christian texts, to sodomy and unnatural vice; a solid foundation in the long Christian tradition of suspicion of the flesh and its pleasure from which the Protestants and liberal Catholics who created modern masturbation wanted to distance themselves. But masturbation made its own history even if it did not make it entirely as it pleased. It did it by explicitly jettisoning the moral problem of sex with oneself as it had been conceived by almost two millennia of Christianity, by creating for it a new ethical centrality and by inventing a disease about which classical medicine and its heirs knew nothing.

We do not know if *Onania* is right in claiming that a new guilt was born when it made the world aware of the heinousness of self-abuse. One can well imagine that a boy — and certainly a girl — coming of age before the early eighteenth century grew up thinking that there was nothing terribly wrong about masturbating. Only one of the many prescriptive books published in England during the seventeenth century would have warned him; none in other countries as far as I can tell. Perhaps somewhere in Catholic Europe, a confessor nervously brought up the topic in his once-a-year encounter with a young parishioner. But basically there was silence, and it is against this silence that *Onania* and its successors struggled for the next centuries.

About the history of the guilt of real people we know little. Whether it ebbs and flows with the rise and fall of proscriptions and whether the guilt of the many can be gauged from the confessions of the few — or the absence of confession by the great majority — remain open questions. Based on the evidence we have, we can say that masturbation seemed remarkably innocent in the decades before it became the locus of primal sexual guilt.

Every so often we can catch a glimpse of someone's conscience in this regard, a kind of before-and-after-1712 comparison. Samuel Pepys, the first great English diarist and the father of modern naval administration, masturbated regularly, in public and in private. He conjured up the object of his desire in his inner fantasy theater even if she was present in the flesh. With his eyes closed, his body responded to the imagination's erotic stimuli, and he made himself come, sometimes with his hand, sometimes just by thinking hard. Sometimes, especially during the first year of his diary, when he is guilt-ridden about his compulsive play attendance and visits to pubs, he seems to feel a twinge of conscience about masturbating: June 29, 1663 — "Never again to make bad use of my fancy with whatever woman I have a mind to," very much the same vow he made repeatedly about staying out of the playhouse and the public house. Within two weeks, he was at it again, twice, these times without self-reproach. He continued to feel bad about succumbing to the theatergoing or boozing habit and promised to put money in the poor box each time he fell off either wagon; he did not fine himself for masturbating.[133]

Over the years, it was only doing it in inappropriate places that pricked his conscience, and then not always. On Sunday, November 11, 1666, he did it in church, his mind on a friend's teenage daughter. "God forgive." At High Mass on Christmas Eve that year, the queen and her ladies so aroused him that he did it with his eyes open, "which I never did before — and God forgive me for it, it being in chapel." (It is not clear whether the offense as he understood it was masturbating in church — which he had done before, although not in a Catholic church — or masturbating with his eyes open, which he had not previously reported.) Perhaps for a vehement anti-Catholic like Pepys, just being there and finding all the pageantry exciting were enough to induce guilt. In any case, the next year he reports doing it again in church, this time with his lids closed and with a merchant's daughter sitting in the balcony providing the excitement in his mind's eye. No guilt. And when he managed to bring himself to orgasm by the force of his imagination alone — no hands — as he was lying in the bottom of a boat that was ferrying him up the Thames, he was positively proud of himself. He had passed his self-imposed "trial of my strength of fancy" and "had it complete avec la fille que I did see aujor-duy in Westminster Hall. So to my office and wrote letters." In fact, he seems to have been perfectly, guiltlessly, cheerful about reliving the erotic pleasures of his daily rounds among the court ladies in his bed at night: "to bed — before I sleep, fancying myself to sport with Mrs Steward with great pleasure"; "to bed, sporting in my fancy with the Queen." He also seems to have been unfazed by masturbating with his sleepover guest and was positively rapturous about the wet dream he had one night while in exile from plague-infested London. "The best that ever was dreamed," he said of the nightlong romp of his unconscious with the king's mistress, the Lady Castlemaine, who in his reveries had allowed him every possible liberty. If in the grave one could have such dreams, he wrote, one would not be so fearful of death as one was during this time of pestilence.[134]

In the famous episode in which he took a copy of the new French pornographic rage *L'Ecole des filles* to bed, his anxiety was about having so inappropriate a work found amongst his library treasures. He burned the book but did not comment on how he felt about masturbating. In short, Pepys enjoyed with himself the sort of self-absorbed sexual life, founded in the imagination, that doctors, philosophers, and moralists came to regard as the fundamental evil of masturbation. He was caught up in the round of seemingly endless and unlimited pleasure that made self-abuse so threatening. But except when he was already in a high state of worry about his theatrical obsessions and sometimes when he did it in church, Pepys did not find making "bad use" of his "fancy with whatever woman" he had in mind a big burden on his conscience. One might argue that he secretly knew that masturbation kept him out of even more trouble than his carousing already produced. The danger of rejection, failure, or raising the ire of Mrs. Pepys, always there when he tried to cop a feel, or get someone to play with his penis, or have a quickie, was absent when he had sex with himself. (He never seems to have worried about getting caught masturbating.) Nothing here of the anxieties of the cloister or sins against nature; but also nothing of the secular guilt that enveloped masturbation in the next century.

We have one other case study from before the eighteenth century. John Cannon, a schoolmaster and an officer of the excise, tells us in an unpublished manuscript memoir how, in 1696 at the age of eleven, he learned to masturbate. He begs us not to judge him by the standards of the 1730s and 1740s, when he was writing, but to reflect on how we readers had passed our own "adolescencious years." "After some Aquarian diversions," the oldest boy at a swimming party "took an occasion to show ye the rest what he could do if he had a female in place, and withall took his privy member in his hand rubbing it up and down till it was erected and in short measure followed Emission." Cannon and the other boys were told that this would be a good way to prevent "lustful venereal thoughts."[135]

Even as an adult writing his memoirs, Cannon was not sure what to make of his youthful exercises. "This I am of opinion sounds much of self pollution or ONANISM." But when he reflected on what he had done, he reminded himself — and his readers, whomever he imagined them to be — that "wise men or

Kingdoms" may be surprised and be "guilty of doing foolish things." Only habitual foolishness is reprehensible.

There is in all of this the air of an old person excusing the moral insensitivities of his youth. One could not know back then. Perhaps one ought only to be taxed with "inadvertency at the first commencement of folly." It would be the work of *Onania* and its successors to make sure that such inadvertency was erased and that guilt about solitary sex was as firmly and as early implanted as possible. A new guilt was soon to be released upon Europe.

We will take up the questions of what masturbation was and why it became a problem in the next chapters. In this one, the point has been that in every age and tradition there is guilt sufficient unto the hour. A connection exists, argues the French historian of sin Jean Delumeau, "among guilt, anxiety and creativity." The medieval and Renaissance regime of sin and fear produced enormous guilt but also intense introspection and self-scrutiny; a particular version of the bad conscience developed, he suggests, at the same time as the portrait, the sonnet, the essay, and much that we take to be characteristic of the early modern world.[136] Freud had it right when he said that nothing focuses one so intensely upon oneself as the moral queasiness of having done something bad. The history of the new modern regime of guilt is thus part of a larger history of the self, of creativity, of limits, and of excess. It is a guilt born of a newly problematic relationship between the individual and society.

CHAPTER FOUR

The Problem with Masturbation

By now two things should be clear: solitary sex was not much of an issue for several millennia, and beginning in the early eighteenth century it swept the Western world. The next question would seem to be why this should be the case. But before taking it on, we need to know *what* was suddenly so disturbing about masturbation: What was, and is, the problem? I ask the question in this general form because there is a general answer beyond the specific answers that were generated as solitary sex took on ever more meanings — mostly negative, more recently positive. That is, I think a constellation of features came to be associated with solitary sex around 1700 and has remained associated with it ever since. Anxiety about these features led almost the entire medical profession to believe that masturbation could cause spinal tuberculosis, epilepsy, pimples, madness and other mental infirmities, general wasting, and hundreds of other diseases. It continued to unsettle those who were unsure whether masturbation caused disease or not, as well as those, after about 1880, who were sure it did not but thought it was nevertheless abominable. The problem of masturbation also grabbed those who did not care about the disease question one way or the other but identified sex with oneself as a sign of something terribly amiss about a person, an institution, or a whole culture. Finally, in the twentieth century, and more prominently in the 1960s and after, some began to think that solitary sex is healthful and much more besides: the way to individual autonomy, spiritual self-realization, and liberation from a repressive heterosexist regime. They too derived energy from

185

that essential "*what*" even if the question is no longer "What is the problem?" but "What is the solution?"

After some ground clearing, I will begin with doctors and quack doctors to ask first *what* it was — in nontechnical, and then technical, terms — that they found so dangerous about masturbation. I start with medicine not because it offers all the answers. The birth of new anxieties, fears, opportunities, fatal and not-so-fatal attractions, and freedoms that gave new meaning to masturbation is part of a far bigger story. But medicine is an important part of the answer for two reasons. First, physicians of the body, in their various ranks and strata from the eighteenth through the twentieth century, increasingly took on the mantle of earlier physicians of the soul; they welcomed every opportunity to become arbiters of morality and good order. As the authority of divine revelation became less convincing and that of nature ever more so, doctors became its voice. Masturbation went from being just another instance of a great complex of divinely condemned impurities or non-procreative sexual practices to being a subject for enlightenment, a moral question refracted in nature whose violation was empirically discoverable. Second, and related to this point, is the fact that there is one indisputable novelty in or around 1712: the claim that masturbation per se makes those who do it sick unto death. Its fundamental evil was visited, first and foremost, in the body, and anything that wreaked such havoc in the flesh had to be very bad indeed. A new, secular morality was thus forged, articulated, amplified, and legitimated in the language of medicine.

From what doctors said was wrong with masturbation we will work backward to excavate the moral underpinning of their pathophysiology — to answer why guilt, shame, and danger came to be so sharply focused on what had been a relatively unnoticed kind of sexuality. The medical question will thus turn into another, larger one: What is it about solitary sex in western European culture since the eighteenth century that makes it a problem in an ethics of the self? Or more specifically: What is it about solitary sex since the Enlightenment that makes it exemplary of something to be feared and — later — welcomed? What makes masturbation so protean as a way of thinking about ourselves and our sexuality in modernity? Only with these questions answered will we be in a position to ask "why?" A causal explanation depends on understanding *what*, precisely, is to be explained.

Ground Clearing

More Masturbation?
One answer to the question of what the fuss was about might be, simply put, a boom in the practice itself. Masturbation had not been a terribly important moral or medical question, in this view, because there was not very much of it before the eighteenth century. Or conversely, an increase in the incidence of solitary sex created the problem, and doctors addressed it; like the plague or cholera, it came to medical and more general public attention only when it reached epidemic proportions.

To put this view more subtly: new circumstances made masturbation more attractive, thus more prevalent, and thus more attention grabbing. Freedom from old constraints is one explanation. C.F. Lallemand, the nineteenth-century medical high priest of seminal loss, and Edward Shorter, the modern historian of the supposedly liberatory qualities of the Industrial Revolution for the masses, both argue that the relative silence of ancient and early modern doctors on the subject is due to the fact that people did not masturbate very much and that something about modern society freed them to do it.[1] Given the chance provided by more privacy and more stimulation, they did it, and medicine responded accordingly.

Alternatively, there was more solitary sex because other kinds became scarcer, what economists might call a sexual substitution effect: a sort of hydraulic system in which energy pushes the system in one direction proportional to pressures from another. One of the most learned contemporary historians of sexuality and the family argues, for example, that "solitary practices ... appear to have increased in proportion to the repression of other forms of sexual behavior."[2] A fixed amount of libidinal energy will make itself felt in another direction if its original destination is blocked.

187

So, the Church's successful efforts to impose premarital celibacy — the culmination of centuries of efforts that found their fullest expression in the Council of Trent — and economic pressures that resulted in both a higher proportion of celibates in the population and an increase in the marriage age forced sexual energies from heterosexual into solitary sexual channels. (The seemingly successful repression of wholesale sodomy would have had a similar effect.) Masturbation, in other words, rises and falls inversely with the availability of something better; it is a cheap, readily available alternative in hard times.

Both versions of this story might, to some extent, be true. Modern civilization may well have increased the incidence of masturbation, and the absence of heterosexual — or homosexual — opportunities may well increase interest in other outlets. Certainly, the idea that masturbation is a cheap alternative form of sexual release goes back to Diogenes and beyond, and there is a great deal of anecdotal evidence for what the German sexologists of the late nineteenth century called *Notsonanie*, "masturbation of necessity."[3]

But there are problems with this story as an account of what it was about masturbation that so disturbed the eighteenth century. In the first place, contemporaries had no way of knowing that the incidence of masturbation had gone up, if indeed it had. Jean de Gerson in the 1420s assumed that everyone — or at least every male — had done it and that any boy who denied he had ever rubbed his penis in response to an erection was not credible. More to the point, no one in the eighteenth century claimed that the problem was *more* masturbation; every commentator says simply that wherever one looks there it is: shockingly endemic. They thought that masturbation was everywhere and especially dangerous because it was so easy to do and so difficult to detect. The novelty seems to have been not the act itself but the remarkable attention it suddenly garnered.

Finally, even if someone did think solitary sex was on the rise — and even if it really was — these putative facts would not explain why it became so dramatically exigent. It takes little cultural mediation to account for why plague, cholera, and ague demanded a response; they kill people. Masturbation, on the other hand, does not, and no one before the eighteenth century thought it did. So, the "what" we are looking for cannot be simply numbers. It has to be a much bigger issue that these numbers represent.

The strongest empirical evidence against the increase of masturbation because of a substitution effect — solitary in place of social sex — comes from England, the birthplace of the new anti-masturbatory literature, and from its American colonies, where sexual intercourse seems to have become more, not less, available than it had been before. Repression, if that is what one wants to call it, collapsed all around. Lower marriage age meant that young couples entered into regular sexual relations earlier; higher rates of prenuptial conception and of illegitimacy suggest that they had more sex before marriage and that it was harder to make them get married if the girl became pregnant; and a decline in the percentage of the population never married means that fewer people remained outside the game entirely. In short, the barriers to heterosexual intercourse had seldom been lower. Perhaps there was more masturbation in France because marriage age there was higher and the Catholic Church in the countryside enforced strictures against premarital sex more successfully than elsewhere, but there is nothing to suggest that the circumscribed conditions of the peasantry were what disturbed those who wrote about masturbation. Their prototypical masturbator was the schoolboy, schoolgirl, or apprentice of the middling sort, not a sex-deprived peasant. For them, venery — excessive venery — seemed rampant in the cities of Europe no less than in the proto-industrial villages of Switzerland.[4]

Sexual Pleasure

The attack on masturbation was not an attack on sexual pleasure as something good and worthwhile outside the narrow categories in which it had been considered acceptable in Catholic moral theology. Nor was it part of a latter-day neo-asceticism.[5] Neither medical doctors in the Enlightenment nor the pedagogues and moralists who took up the cause shared the Church's long and deep suspicion of the pleasures of the flesh. In fact, one striking

189

aspect of the post-1712 discussion of masturbation is its indifference — active hostility in many cases — to the moral universe in which solitary sex subsisted after the rise of Christianity. The Protestants who led the modern medical assault against masturbation were generally hostile to the celibate life as an ideal; they did not regard marriage as a second-best option, nor did they regard sexual intercourse as a threat to health or to salvation. Indeed, the Calvinist tradition in England produced the novel idea that the constant heat of sexual love between man and wife mirrored the constancy of the saints' commitment to God. Enlightenment anticlericalism lived off the sexual exploits of supposedly celibate priests, monks, and nuns. One of the things that was so bad about masturbation, according to Voltaire, was precisely that it was the vice of the cloister and the choir, a perversion of desire that the Church tried, stupidly in his view, to repress.[6]

Radically new valuations of sexual pleasure were on the front lines of medical-theological contestation: enlightened support of virtuous enjoyment versus the clerical opposition to pleasure for its own sake. Doctors were allies of the novelists and moralists who made the world safe for sexual love; they certified it as beautiful, virtuous, entertaining, and healthy. The philosophes who articulated a medico-moral attack on masturbation extolled the virtues of married sexual love. Indeed, sexual love outside marriage did not seem so bad either; there was no binding, universal, divine, or natural truth in the matter. Diderot's *Supplement to the Voyage of the Bougainville* famously painted the sexual freedoms of a South Seas culture as an attractive alternative to repressive European mores.

The problem with masturbation was not that it was a species of sexual pleasure but that it wasn't. At best, it was false pleasure, a perversion of the real. In general, medical naturalism and speculative anthropology supported the rightness and moral innocence of heterosexual bliss.[7] Even unmarried love was not so bad in certain medical circles; some doctors went so far as to recommend prostitution as a cure for the habit of solitary sex. And of course libertines existed for sexual pleasures of almost any sort. But both they and the doctors found masturbation detestable. (There is an exception. A well-documented, avowedly libertine club — The Beggar's Benison — was started in Fife in 1732 and soon had branches in Edinburgh and Glasgow. Precisely because it was so outrageous and unconventional — a parody almost of the club's devotion to breaking with sexual norms — masturbating in front of the membership became the central feature of its initiation ritual.)[8]

The popular quack tradition lived for a century off the idea that masturbation was so bad because it ruined sexual pleasures. Men who masturbated faced mortification, apprehension, and suppressed rage in the nuptial bed, which ought to be "teeming with hallowed, ecstatic, and indefinable delight." Women addicted to masturbation were said to eschew the "legitimate rapturous enjoyments" of sexual intercourse in favor of the agonies, punishments, and remorse of self-abuse.[9]

Eighteenth-century doctors also had almost no interest in the Christian taxonomy of sexual sin. They certainly understood masturbation as "unnatural" but only in the sense that a physiological process had more dire effects if carried out under unnatural rather than natural circumstances: "Too great a quantity of semen being lost in the natural course produces direful effects; but they are still more dreadful when the same quantity has been dissipated in an unnatural way." "Unnatural" here means not non-reproductive but artificial, out of the course of nature in the same way that a weir alters the course of a river with possible ill effects. As one of the many popular rehearsals of the views of Sanctorious, the seventeenth-century savant of physiological mechanism, put it: "Coition upon natural provocations is good." Even excessive coition is not so bad if care is taken. But "upon the Incitations of the Mind, it is injurious."[10]

We will have to tease out exactly what this means to figure out why doctors and others thought that one sexual practice, one way of having an orgasm, was so much more dangerous than another. But for the time being, all we need to say is that the distinction is *not* between sex for the purpose of generation and sex for any other purpose. Aquinas's classification of permissible sexual acts, (within marriage for the purpose of reproduction), those that are offenses against reason (incest, fornication, adultery), and those that are offenses against nature (nonreproductive practices like sodomy, bestiality, masturbation, positions and practices within the marriage bed that prevent conception and reproduction) is not operating here. Modern worries about the very young — three-, four-, five-year-olds, well below the age of reason — who learn to abuse themselves from nurses are outside the world of penitentials and of Thomist moral theology, as is the solitary sex of women. New questions about the uses of pleasure are put on the agenda as sexual pleasure itself goes from being suspect to being sublime.[11]

Medicine and the Morality of Masturbation
One might better look to medicine as a discipline to discover what was suddenly so bad about masturbation. In one sense, it might seem that Enlightenment doctors were simply taking up the cudgel of priests: vice kills and its consequences are dire in this world, not just for eternity. But they were doing so in new terms; they so radically revalued solitary sex as to make it something genuinely novel. Nature, not God, vouchsafed its wickedness. Masturbatory disease was not understood as providential; Tissot goes out of his way to disassociate himself from those who think that it is "the special will of God to punish this crime." Everything, he says, can be explained by "the mechanical laws of the body, and those that unite it to the soul."[12] He allies himself with Hippocrates and with the materialist medical tradition more generally in a search for natural causes of natural consequences. Moreover, nowhere in Tissot or in any other eighteenth-century medical authority do we get the idea that the evil of masturbation resided primarily in its being nonreproductive or ritually polluting. It certainly did not produce children, and spilled semen was certainly thought to be nasty, but these were not its root horrors. The historical problem is therefore to discover what about masturbation made it unnatural in new, materialist ways.

There are no new medical observations or discoveries or even hypotheses that would account for what came to be regarded as so dangerous about masturbation, nothing that would link solitary sex to death. In fact, the remarkable continuity over several millennia of views about the physical consequences of sexual engagement and of orgasm makes the sudden explosion of medical writing about masturbation all the more puzzling. The connections between epileptic seizures and masturbation, for example, have their origins in the classical medical notion that orgasm produces a corporeal tremor, a shaking of the system, that mimics and might actually initiate a fit. Deeply steeped in this tradition, Tissot cites case after exemplary case from contemporary physicians in which sexual excitement was said to have induced horrible racking seizures. One colleague "knew a merchant in Montpellier who never made any sacrifices to Venus, without having immediately after a fit of epilepsy"; another knew a woman who "usually had a fit after every act of venery"; a third offers the most spectacular case, that of a man "who in the midst of the act was seized with a spasm and the disorder continued twelve years."[13] Finally, Tissot appropriates Galen to give these contemporary observations a good pedigree.

Two things to be said about these cases: they are not, on the face of it, ridiculous; but also, they offer no hint as to why masturbatory orgasm all of a sudden came to be regarded in the eighteenth century as an especially dangerous version of this admittedly jarring experience. A violent orgasm might look like an epileptic or other seizure in some people, and there *are* "brain phenomena" during sexual orgasm that give this very old observation some credence. While in normal people there probably is no link between ordinary, garden-variety masturbation and paroxysmal activity, in some people there clearly is an association. A perfectly respectable late twentieth-century neurologist with no moral ax to grind reports the following case: a forty-one-year-old man with generalized epilepsy but no history of sexual deviancy masturbated uncontrollably during seizures accompanied by staring and rapid eye movement. There are other cases of young children who are brought to a teaching hospital because they have what appears to be an epileptic or some other kind of paroxysmal event. The attending pediatrician suggests that before more expensive tests are undertaken, one ought to consider another possibility in the differential diagnosis: the violent, sometimes painful tremors of benign masturbatory orgasms. Some people get sharp shooting pains in the back from masturbatory as well as other sorts of orgasm.[14]

But if the orgasm-and-seizure story is old and not entirely implausible, the *masturbatory*-orgasm-and-seizure twist is new. Before the eighteenth century, no one connected it specifically with what we would call neurological symptoms, and even Tissot produced no cases in which a seizure was occasioned by masturbation. The argument is by indirection: if heterosexual excess is bad and may result in seizures, solitary sexual excess is worse and will result in more severe ones. When the moral argument against masturbation became largely independent of medicine in the early twentieth century, the claim that it was linked to epilepsy disappeared as well. Although onanism is certainly common "among epileptics of low moral gauge," concluded a major Anglo-American reference work in 1901, "it can hardly be considered in light of a cause," whatever some Continental writers might think.[15] So the question remains, "*What* about masturbatory orgasm" — about the tremors of solitary pleasure — marked it out for particular scrutiny and danger?

The moral physiology of semen gets us closer to an answer but only after a very long detour that takes us far from the quotidian fluid that we might recognize. If, as a number of eighteenth-century observers and modern historians have suggested, the "what" that is so threatening about masturbation is the loss of precious bodily fluids, we are well on our way to resolving both of our remaining questions. Loss of semen might then be linked metaphorically with worries about other sorts of loss, and we would be close to a general explanation for the advent of modern masturbation. The argument might work as follows: semen, money, and energy are all in short supply and are profligately expended at the wastrel's peril. Just as in the world of trade and commerce one must discipline one's use of scarce resources, so in the spermatic economy men need to save and to husband their precious bodily fluid. Anxieties about not enough time, not enough money, not enough security are assuaged by imagining an autarkic body safe from leaks of all sorts and threatened by the willful

194

expenditure of its most highly elaborated fluid: semen. The economic realm maps nicely onto the corporeal one.[16]

In the eighteenth century, as in the millennia before, semen was regarded as bearing "the vivifying fire" that enlivened the fetus and more generally was "the torch-bearer of vitality," a "balmy-spirituous-vivifying essence," a "luminous principle," in the words of the quack sex-therapist James Graham, whose rental bed was guaranteed to kindle a man's fire. Testimonies to its wonders are everywhere and of long standing: it is the froth of the blood by which "man is animated, is sustained and lives," reports the seventh-century encyclopedist Isidore of Seville; the Promethean spark "leaping with so much spirit" that triggers new life, thought William Harvey, discoverer of the blood's circulation. Clearly important stuff.[17]

In Galenic medicine and still in the eighteenth century, despite the inroads of mechanism, chemistry, and much else, semen was regarded as the most thoroughly worked over, the most energy intensive, of the body's fluids: the very finest distillation of the entire digestive process. The body expends varying amounts of effort to extract its vital materials from food; male semen requires more than female semen, semen more than milk, milk more than blood. "In a word," said Tissot, "it appears by the many testimonies" he had assembled, and by a variety of others that would only gild the lily, that semen is "the most important liquor, which may be called the Essential Oil of the animal liquors... the rectified spirit"; "concentrated life force"; "the source and substance of life." It is, as the *Encyclopédie* put it, "that most precious humor in whose production the body lavishes more care and energy than on any other." Its loss is extremely debilitating, writes the famous and much-read Friedrich Hoffmann, "just as if it were the flow of blood and nervous liquid," and hence must be carefully moderated; immoderate excretion "offends against health."[18]

In this context, Tissot's long-lived, endlessly cited, and completely spurious pseudo-quantitative dictum that one part of semen was worth forty of blood made perfect sense. It was still trotted out 150 years after he said it as if it were the latest word from Science: a Leipzig-trained M.D./Ph.D. who wrote one of the standard early-twentieth-century physiology books claimed it as indisputable that "there is a far greater loss from masturbatory orgasm than from equivalent loss of blood."[19] And it had been around for at least seven hundred years before Tissot appropriated it to nail home the dangers of masturbation. In his popular early-seventeenth-century health guide for students, Thomas Cogan told his readers: "If seed pass us above nature's measure, it does hurt us more than if forty times as much blood were avoided." Cogan at least cited his source: the early-eleventh-century Arabic Prince of Physicians, Avicenna. Tissot may have been embarrassed to acknowledge that he took his famous observation from a work that his master Albrecht von Haller had labeled "methodic inanity." Still, everyday observations could be adduced to make it seem plausible: a wet nurse can give pints of milk and not feel tired, whereas one small ejaculation is exhausting. Men especially are much more tired after orgasm than after other activities of comparable duration. Extirpation of the testicles produces the flabby, malformed body of the eunuch; the advent of semen in a normal boy is coterminous with the vigor of youth.[20]

Clearly, losing this remarkable fluid faster than it could be replenished would have disastrous effects on the corporeal economy. Conversely, if everything was in good order, semen, like blood, circulated and nourished the body's most critical elements first, especially the nerves and the spinal fluid, with which it was intimately connected. Loss of semen thus had its most deleterious effects on the brain, which could literally shrivel up in the skull, reported Tissot, from loss of seminal life force. Indeed, he explained, the testicles were so much in sympathy with the whole body that the brain of one man given to sexual excess "was heard to rattle in the pericranium." And finally spermatorrhea — the leakage of sperm that was regarded as both a consequence of and an important stage in the pathophysiology of masturbatory disease — was considered dangerous enough to become a little medical realm of its own. The early-nineteenth-century French doctor Lallemand was its king, thought contemporaries; to return to him is progress, proclaimed a German successor in 1869.[21]

But this does not get us very far in accounting for *what* it was

196

about masturbation, in particular, that brought it to prominence in the eighteenth century as the cause of a specifically new version of a very old disease. Seminal loss as a key step in the pathophysiology of excessive venery was not news in 1712. In fact, a long clinical tradition from Antiquity to his own time offered Tissot scores of cases to prove that losing semen kills. But the striking thing is that *all* the cases he cites from before the eighteenth century and the majority of contemporary ones involved severe illness and death that were the purported result not of masturbation but of that very old problem — excessive heterosexual intercourse.

New discoveries about semen from the late seventeenth through the nineteenth century had, as far as I can tell, no impact on the discussion of masturbation and seminal loss. Certain thinkers in what we might call philosophical medicine, terribly important to the elaboration of a naturalistic secular ethics, did hypothesize that semen constituted the fundamental, basically electrical fluid that was the spark of life. This was a novel view, but it had little to do with the visible stuff that was ejaculated or with the old physiology of concoction and humors that still informed the horror stories Tissot gathered from eminent colleagues. None of their victims was said to have masturbated: not Hoffmann's wounded patients for whom "the danger of amorous pleasures" was especially acute nor those with fevers; not Fabricius of Hilden's patient who had connection with a woman on the tenth day of pleurisy, got a fever, experienced immoderate trembling, and finally died on the thirteenth day; not Bartholin's young bridegroom who got a fever as a result of his "conjugal excesses"; not Chesneau's young married couple who during the first week after their nuptials were stricken with fevers and flushed faces and died after a few days; not Tissot's two young men, "strong, healthy and vigorous," one of whom was seized on the morn of his nuptials and the other a day later, in 1761 and 1762, respectively. In fact, Tissot's one on-point case is of a man who died of smallpox; masturbation, he said, rendered the "disorder mortal." All these men died from other diseases made worse by the exhaustion of garden-variety sexual intercourse.[22]

It is a big leap from all this sickness and death laid at the feet

197

of "excessive venery" to the new view that masturbation was a specifically and uniquely dangerous practice. It is an especially big leap in the context of contemporary standards of "excess." Nicolas Venette, an authority much admired by Tissot and much in favor with a broad European public for the better part of a century, thought that a twenty-five-year-old man on the plains of Barbary could safely engage *five times a night* in the summer whereas a forty-year-old in the dead of the Swedish winter could do it once or twice a night. Presumably, men more prosaically situated could gauge their limits by interpolating from these exemplary cases. Women, Venette thought, "truly do not feel themselves exhausted," no matter how often they couple. If these levels are compatible with good health, it is hard to see why even daily masturbation would pose a threat to fit young men; young women should be able to indulge freely. Or conversely, as an early attack on *Onania* joked, if a man were capable of abusing himself eight times in an hour, as the book claimed, the news would make a very bad impression on lascivious wenches, who might demand this level of performance from their husbands. Any man should in fact be able to keep a woman satisfied unless some disease intervened, and the medicines *Onania* peddled wouldn't help for that. In short, the expenditure of a prodigious amount of sexual energy was thought compatible with health.[23]

The key, of course, was to distinguish masturbatory orgasm from other kinds, but this undermined the idea that seminal loss per se was what mattered. In fact, the problem of making a plausible and robust distinction would haunt the enemies of masturbation to the very end of its days as a medical question; here is where the serious cultural work lies. "Prominent and preliminary in the study of the effects [of solitary sex]," wrote the eminent American educator and psychologist G. Stanley Hall in 1904, "is the problem whether self-abuse is more pernicious than excess in the natural way, and how they differ." Some people in the past decades have argued that the effects are the same, he continued, but now — at the beginning of the twentieth century — there is "no competent authority who does not assert that abuse is far more injurious, and that in many ways."[24]

Tissot would have agreed: onanism is "more pernicious than excesses with women," he declared. And the generations who followed him chimed in: "Excess of venery is a dreadful and common cause of dangerous diseases," writes an early-nineteenth-century American doctor, but self-pollution is "tenfold more destructive." Onanism is much worse than coition, wrote a prominent English forensic expert, because "it is more vivid and violent."[25] So, in the absence of relevant new ideas about semen, something about masturbatory orgasm in particular suddenly became a threat in the century of the Enlightenment.

Whatever this might be, it had little to do with neo-humoralism — the physiology of fluid balance — or with a seminal economy in particular. It did not express a longing for the ideal of an autarkic body or the dangers of loss in a world of shortage. Masturbation is born as a medical and a moral problem at a moment when plenty seems poised to replace paucity and when the last thing anyone advocated was autarky. But more to the point, seminal loss is simply too narrow a category to capture what really bothered those who put onanism on the agenda.

To begin with, there was the problem of children from infancy to puberty. Classical medicine had had almost nothing to say about the sexual lives of this whole class of people: they were not prone to excessive venery; they produced no semen; indeed, this is why they were not pubescent. What Freud would call infantile masturbation or masturbation during latency was raised as an issue for the first time in the eighteenth century; its importance, then, makes it abundantly clear that losing semen was, at most, only part of the problem. Tissot and his successors thought that onanism was manifestly dangerous to children well before they had anything to lose but their lives. A leading German pedagogical reformer notes that among twenty well brought up children between the ages of six and ten at most two were not caught in the snares of self pollution totally innocent of its horrible consequences. Worse, the epidemic seemed to grow by a sort of spontaneous combustion; fully half had discovered the vice on their own. Parents and educators were thus duty bound to warn their children — beginning no later than age eight — of the body- and soul-destroying consequences of their actions. Here, then, is a whole world of supposed victims who were entirely outside a putative seminal economy. Looking back on a century and a half of carnage, Larousse's *Grand Dictionnaire* in 1875 announced to its lay audience, "We find in the annals of medicine plenty of cases of five-, six-, and eight-year-old children dead as a result of masturbation." Obsession — a more generalized dissipation of energy, or more complexly, moral collapse — not loss of precious bodily fluids, destroyed their immature nervous systems and their constitutions, but that is another story.[26]

Finally, and much more telling, there is the question of women. With the advent of the modern version of onanism, the old crime of pollution was suddenly open to everyone; solitary sex broke the gender barrier. There were almost no references to female autoeroticism in classical Antiquity except for the occasional quip about dildos when the real thing was unavailable. There was not much more, as we saw, about male masturbation: mostly rude jokes and other vulgar allusions. In the new Christian ethics, sodomy and bestiality were male offenses even if they were possible for women; and the whole complex of sexual dangers associated with the spilling of seed — through nocturnal emissions with or without erotic dreams and pleasures, through inadvertent rubbing, through an unexpected daytime erection, through handling the penis during more innocent acts — threatened men alone. Pollutions in all of their niceties were, with very minor exceptions, a male problem, the worry of monks and celibate priests that made its way into confessionals for the laity.

Onanism, on the other hand, was democratic; after 1712, the hands and the genitals and, more important, the imagination and the will of women were as likely to offend as those of men. The fifteenth edition of *Onania* (1730) perhaps sensed a lack of conviction in earlier editions and promised still more girls' letters to prove not only that they engaged in masturbation but also that they harmed themselves by it. Stories of the fall of girls through self-exploration or through experimentation with friends were an advertised feature of the *Supplement*. The most respectable of medical encyclopedias, published under royal privilege, leaves no ambiguity in its entry on voluntary pollution: "Persons of both sexes suffer equally when they unhappily give themselves over to these pleasures." Tissot cited the confessions in *Onania* of women masturbators — "that cannot be read without horror and compassion" — and concluded, "The disorder seems even to make greater progress with women than with men." On a more clinical note — and with almost no corroborative cases in his own book — he argued that women no less than men "often perish the victims of this detestable lewdness" and that "if anything the malignity of the disorders occasioned by it" seems to have "a superior degree of activity among them." His friend Zimmermann thought likewise; twenty-five years of experience had taught him that, dangerous as self-pollution was for boys, it was worse for girls. Various French doctors of the early nineteenth century cite both their contemporaries and many German authorities to establish definitively that girls masturbate and that the practice is even more dangerous to them, morally and physically, than to men.[27]

This would continue to be an important theme in the Enlightenment tradition of thinking about sexuality right up through Freud and beyond. Freud, like Tissot, thought that in general women "tolerated" masturbation worse than men: they fought against it more; they were more restrained than men in finding the circumstances to engage in it; and, most important, it was more unnatural among them. There were exceptions, but it appeared to Freud that

> masturbation was further removed from the nature of women than of men.... Masturbation, at all events of the clitoris, is a masculine activity and that the elimination of cliteroidal sexuality is a necessary precondition to the development of femininity.[28]

In other words, more cultural weight needs to be brought to bear on the sexuality of women to channel it into its normative course, more guilt needs to be generated, and hence their psyches — if not also their bodies — bear heavier scars of the confrontation with the work of civilization than do the bodies and psyches of men. Whether the views of Freud, or of Tissot, and their colleagues are right or not is irrelevant here. The dangers of masturbation were thought to be real and present even though women admittedly produced either no semen or a very weakly elaborated, lesser version whose loss could not amount to much.[29]

Clearly something else is at work, something that would continue to kill, maim, or psychologically damage well after anyone believed in female semen. O.S. Fowler, the immensely popular and widely read guru of phrenology — the nineteenth century's version of materialist psychology — quoted unimpeachable medical authority to back up his claim that while girls *may* be less infected by masturbation than boys, they were still dying by the thousands from consumption caused by it. Another American writer of the mid-nineteenth century quotes "the highest medical authorities" (he is referring to Copland's *Dictionary of Practical Medicine*) to the effect that masturbation, the "solitary indulgence of amativeness," is "fully as common — perhaps more common — with girls than boys." Whether they were diagnosed as sick more often is difficult to say. Wasting diseases seem to have been thought to strike females as much as, or even more than, males; men, however, were diagnosed with masturbatory madness more frequently than women. At one asylum in early-nineteenth-century Germany that has received careful recent study, *Selbstbefleckung* — self-pollution — was consistently near the top of the diagnostic charts for male inmates and not used at all for females. Late in the century, Krafft-Ebing diagnosed twelve cases of male masturbatory insanity, only three of the female variety. On the other hand, a well-informed American author on health matters writing in the 1840s thought that masturbation was second only to alcoholism in causing insanity and said she "had it on good authority, that, among the insane admitted into the lunatic hospitals from this cause, the proportion of females is nearly as large as that of males."[30] Whatever the proportion, women from the beginning of the worry about masturbation until its end as a medical problem were thought to suffer its ill effects quite independently of semen but not independently of the social context of solitary vice.

Among women, the secret vice was at its most secret. Zimmermann could not believe that people were so "unbelievably indifferent" to female masturbation just because they knew less about it. He therefore made a point of warning of the danger, especially in very young girls, who might be thought least vulnerable. The internationally translated educator Christian Salzmann thought that "even more girls" than boys had fallen prey to solitary sex; in fact, he, like almost every commentator on the subject, declares himself shocked and surprised that the practice seemed universal wherever he looked. But he declined to say much about girls, because he did not know enough about them; clearly, no girl would write a man the sort of self-revelatory, guilt-ridden letters he received from schoolboys. The women who taught adolescent girls, it appears, did not share their experiences with the reading public, and, of course, there were far fewer schoolgirls than schoolboys. It was harder, in short, to find out about what girls did and how they learned to do it. That said, everyone thought they did it as much as boys. The two sexes vie with each other in making their "hands serve as criminal instruments" — with equally grave consequences — claimed the *Encyclopédie*.[31] And whenever over the centuries we catch a glimpse of real experiences, this seems to be borne out.

Anastasia Verbitskaia, the turn-of-the-century Russian novelist and notorious proponent of gender liberation for women, wrote about her experiences at boarding school, and her reminiscences testify to the agonies of adolescent-girl longing and to the place of masturbation in withstanding them. Crazy longings tormented her and her fellow students; they were ordered to sleep with their hands outside their blankets, and some girls who could not fight their desires walked around exhausted, whether from masturbating or from resisting is not clear.[32]

In fact, masturbating women made the most perfect of onanistic tropes because they literally produced desire and only desire in their solitary reveries. Loss of substance is simply irrelevant. The ineffable, not the material, constitutes danger and attraction. In the vast pornographic explosion of the eighteenth century, which both served masturbatory purposes and took masturbation as a major theme, women masturbating were an especial turn-on: in one survey of erotic fiction, 75 percent of the books surveyed play on the subject, and 73 percent of the masturbators were women. (In at least some areas of popular culture today, the proportions have been reversed. One Web site that offers a learned summary of masturbation in film found 172 movies that featured male masturbation and only 96 that featured women.)[33] That said, in the eighteenth century, there was clearly a whole imaginative world of masturbating women that was well outside a seminal economy. And the existence of such a world should suggest to us that the danger of masturbation was not dearth — not running out of something — but excess. Onanism stands at the center of a sexual economy threatening to whirl out of control from its sheer energy, an economy in which the restraints of the ordinary world, the restraints of nature, did not seem to operate.

The medical world in which onanism took root in the eighteenth century certainly talked about semen a great deal. But medicine did not become the voice of morality by sticking with the old saws about precious fluids and their effect on vigor. It claimed, much more grandly, expertise in the natural limits of permissible human behavior. Morality was far more deeply embedded in physiology than could be represented by the loss of even the most precious of liquors. Tissot was one of a distinguished group of doctors and philosophes — almost all of them Protestant — who articulated a new ethics grounded in nature and reason, not in divine authority or otherworldly metaphysical authority. Onanism was the child of the same parents who produced sensibility — "the mother of humanity" — which linked the physical and the mental, nature and the soul across the spectrum of human activity.[34] More important than blood or semen, nerves and nervous fluids were at the physiological core of this worldview. Whether a soul emerged from their elaboration or not, the senses, which stimulated nerves, were thought to provide the most direct access possible for the outside world into the innermost reaches of our being. Excitements, joys, sorrows, desires, frights — the whole gamut of human emotions, whatever their source — soothed or racked the body. We are creatures open to endless stimulation, material and psychological.

This was the century in which the pain and suffering of others

204

were thought to translate directly into sympathy, in which the feelings aroused by literature were said to have an immediate effect on the bodies of readers. Readers wrote to Rousseau's publisher, for example, about tears and sighs, heart palpitations, weeping, seizures, and convulsive sharp pains induced by reading *La Nouvelle Héloïse*. And yet they read on. "All things fatigue us at last," says Tissot in his book on the diseases of literary people, and "above all great pleasure." The philosopher Malebranche is said to have had the most dreadful palpitations while reading Descartes; a professor of rhetoric in Paris — still living, we are told — fainted while "pursuing some of the sublime passages of Homer."[35]

This was also the century in which an empiricist, associationist psychology held that the mind was entirely stocked by what it took in from the outside world. A more or less blank slate at birth, it was literally constituted by the proper flow and organization of sensations. And even the faculties with which it was endowed — the imagination and memory, for example — were vulnerable to environmental distortions. Without resorting to theology or to providence, doctors and moralists — and doctors as moralists — could thus easily translate a wrong or inappropriately modulated set of stimuli, whether physical or mental, into madness, wasting, and death.

And, finally, this was the world in which luxury and material excess were ever more widely available and potentially ever more corrupting. Boys and girls, men and women were thought to feel what we call the commercial revolution in their flesh and bones. Modern civilization was jarring, stimulating, and dangerous, and, worse still, it led to precocious unnatural desire, to self-stimulation. But we will return to this later.

Tissot's version of the philosophical physiology that supported the idea of masturbatory disease came from his Swiss Protestant compatriot Albrecht von Haller, one of the most read and most influential of eighteenth-century doctors and moralists. When a young man, Tissot had taken charge of seeing his older colleague's work into print. He wrote the preface to the various vernacular translations from the original Latin and could not have been more enthusiastic. Haller's discovery of irritability was the "key to nature," he proclaimed; the man was the successor to Bacon, the great proponent of experimental and rational philosophy, a worthy star in the firmament of a period in human history that had witnessed the discovery of the circulation of blood, the properties of airs, and so much more. Tissot, in short, held Haller in the highest regard.[36]

Like the clinician and theorist Hermann Boerhaave — another Calvinist — and other famous doctors we could point to, Haller regarded nerves as the essential building blocks of the body. But wary of the Dutchman's unrepentant materialism, he distinguished the property of mere muscles — the intestines in peristalsis, the contracting gastrocnemius of a frog — a property he called "irritability," from the property of nerves and ultimately the brain, a property he called "sensibility." The soul finally emerges at the top of this physiological ladder. The two properties of living things — the merely biological and the biological that ultimately produced consciousness, morality, and the finer qualities of humanity — were intimately connected; what affects the one affects the other to moderate or exacerbate reactions to stimuli. One important implication of this for our story is that the travails and excitements of the body could thus make their way directly into the soul, while derangements of the soul — or, in any case, of the inner reaches of the self — could damage the tubes, tissues, and nerves of the body. Haller, in short, provided the framework for moral physiology, and his pupil Tissot filled in its details. So, for example, in his introduction to Haller, Tissot points out that some people cannot have the slightest unusual impression, the least alarm or shock, without suffering extraordinary symptoms — vapors, hysterics, all manner of nervous complaints. Too great "an irritability of the parts" — a heightened jangling of muscles — "combined with sensibility" accounts for disorders of all kinds and eventually death from a sort of corporeal overload.[37]

Nerves, in short, lie close to the root of what was so bad about masturbation. In no bodily function are the high and the low — the mind and the genitals — more dangerously linked than in the throes of sexual excitement and orgasm. Nowhere else is the body more thoroughly aroused; nothing is more thoroughly mediated by the imagination and the emotions. The phenomenology and physiology of orgasm — quite apart from ejaculation — its affinity to its near neighbor, the seizure, and more generally its manifest turmoil are beyond question: the body of whatever age or gender is in high dudgeon. Such a state is potentially dangerous to all those parts that transmit its frenzy. "Convulsions" "wear out the constitution by destroying the Strength and Elasticity of the solid parts," because during coition — and by extension in self-pollution — the fibers are "intensely drawn up"; "overstraining Apoplexies compress the brain," writes an expert on the passions, and are a prime example of how "every faculty of the mind depends on the nervous system." "The body," announces an eighteenth-century doctor who is agnostic about such niceties as whether nerves are fibers for conveying "aetherial fluid" or solid matter for conveying mechanistic vibrations, is made up of "flexible pipes and yielding fluids."[38]

This account might seem so mechanistic as to leave no room for mind. And there is a sense that the danger of masturbation was too much friction too violently applied. This was John Marten's view at its simplest before he elaborated it in *Onania*; Aristotle had long ago suggested that excessive rubbing might be dangerous. But even in the most wildly materialist physiology, masturbation is more than a simple jangling of nerves or chafing of parts. The *Statics* of Sanctorius, for example, in which the mechanistic message could not be clearer, still leaves a lot of room for state of mind especially when it comes to sex. Intercourse provoked by "natural provocations," it argues, is far healthier than intercourse to which a man has aroused himself. "Unnatural intercourse" is understood here not as a violation of the telos of generation but as confusion about its driving force: it is intercourse to which one is aroused by the "Incitations of the Mind." The discussion, like those of Antiquity, is entirely in terms of male physiology, but women had been incorporated by the eighteenth century. The point is that when something incorporeal, something not quite real, created excitement, it was more dangerous than if the body were responding to something more real, something present there and then.

"State of mind" seems to have been understood not as the condition of the soul or some mental substance but as a sign of the body's ability to sustain the rigors of sex. When one exerted oneself in sexual acts beyond one's needs, the equilibrium of nature was thrown off, rather like a chemical reaction that refuses to come into equilibrium. It is almost as if there were an algebra of orgasm and masturbation left one with equations that would not balance.

Intercourse with "one [whom one] hath been desirous before to enjoy" is both a sign of health and a guarantee that damage from even immoderate venery would be limited, because the pleasure of the occasion "assists the perspiration of the heart, and gives it Vigour"; "what is wasted is soon recouped." Tissot, who was generally not sympathetic to so mechanistic a view, nevertheless borrowed its language without explicitly aligning himself with its metaphysics. He cites a number of cases in which doctors advised debilitated patients to lie with their nurses so that they might "inspire" the healthy stuff perspired by these robust young women. In one case, the young man was advised to stop sleeping with his nurse once it became clear that he was about to lose his new vigor by abusing whatever strength he gained thereby; the revival of King David in the arms of a virgin provides another example. In coition, people perspire more than at any other time and thus might enfeeble themselves were it not for the fact that one person's loss is the other's gain, and vice versa: "The one inhales what the other exhales." The masturbator "receives nothing."[39]

This has the beauty of offering a thermodynamic account of the masturbatory disease, an explanation of why it might be ten times more healthy to have intercourse with a prostitute than to masturbate once, why it would be healthy to fornicate with one's nurse but not to have sex alone. And it had some appeal. For example, the 1805 catalog of a museum of medical curiosities that displayed in Paris — among other horrors — full-scale models of the visages and bent backs of masturbators compared the relative dangers of good old-fashioned coition and "the vicious action." In sociable sex, the losses of bodily fluids and energies are mitigated by "une jouissance RÉELLE" — the sexual ecstasy of real presence

— and by "an invisible blush" that escapes in abundance from the pores of one's beloved. But for the solitary orgast, it is "pure loss," made "all the more prodigal in that the *imagination* goes well beyond reality."[40] But we are getting ahead of the story.

Several things should by now be clear about what doctors thought was the problem with masturbation. They said it was seminal loss, but they had to scramble to distinguish one kind of orgasm from another and to bring women and children under the general umbrella of the solitary vice. A new interest in nerves and in the physiology of irritability offered a less hydraulic model; the problem was not so much fluid loss as nervous exhaustion, always a danger with sexual gratification and all the more so in the unbalanced act of sex alone. And then there were the mechanistic views derived from Sanctorius and his followers, who thought that venery was healthy only if practiced ecologically and that the energies lost by one partner were taken up by the other and vice versa. But whatever it was that became so threatening about masturbation in the early eighteenth century, it was not primarily losing highly elaborated bodily fluids, or uncompensated gas leaks — more perspiration in than out — or irritation of the nerves, although that comes closest. All of these were novel ways, in this case, of speaking about something more fundamental: the relationship between the mind, the soul, the feeling human being, on the one hand, and "nature," on the other.

No single medical philosophy provides the precise answer to "what" was wrong with masturbation. In fact, even proponents of rigorously classifying diseases based on their nervous origins debated how masturbatory disease should be categorized.[41] Doctors and moralists quoted authority eclectically. But everyone shared — and continued to share even after the physiology of sensibility was passé — the sense that masturbation constituted an unnatural state of desire.

What Was So Unnatural About Solitary Sex?
One of the great doctors of the Enlightenment believed that masturbation was "much the more to be dreaded" than smallpox. And he ought to know: Tissot, who made the comparison, was an

209

expert on both. Something was so terrifyingly unnatural about sex alone that in the early twentieth century, long after the foundations of eighteenth-century medicine had crumbled, otherwise reasonable people still regarded masturbation as "the most inevitable and most fatal peril of all." (And so it was for Frederick Arthur Sibly. After a long career of prying confessions of self-abuse out of his pupils at Wycliffe, he was accused by one especially pretty boy of fondling his penis, allegedly to relieve the lad of semen and prevent self-abuse. Sibly lost his job.)[42]

Three things made solitary sex unnatural. First, it was motivated not by a real object of desire but by a phantasm; masturbation threatened to overwhelm the most protean and potentially creative of the mind's faculties — the imagination — and drive it over a cliff. Second, while all other sex was social, masturbation was private, or, when it was not done alone, it was social in all the wrong ways: wicked servants taught it to children; wicked older boys taught it to innocent younger ones; girls and boys in schools taught it to each other away from adult supervision. Sex was naturally done *with* someone; solitary sex was not. And third, unlike other appetites, the urge to masturbate could be neither sated nor moderated. Done alone, driven only by the mind's own creations, it was a primal, irremediable, and seductively, even addictively, easy transgression. Every man, woman, and child suddenly seemed to have access to the boundless excesses of gratification that had once been the privilege of Roman emperors.

Masturbation thus became the vice of individuation for a world in which the old ramparts against desire had crumbled; it pointed to an abyss of solipsism, anomie, and socially meaningless freedom that seemed to belie the ideal of moral autonomy. It was the vice born of an age that valued desire, pleasure, and privacy but was fundamentally worried about how, or if, society could mobilize them. It is the sexuality of the modern self.

Nature, Artifice, and the Dangers of the Imagination

"Masturbation," said that son of the Enlightenment, Sigmund Freud, "contributes to the substitution of fantasy objects for reality."[43] It would be the middle of the eighteenth century before this core horror of solitary sex was fully articulated, but its elements were already there in *Onania*, which consolidated what had before been the stray anxieties, not focused specifically on masturbation, which we surveyed in Chapter 3. The rabbis of the Talmud, as the reader will recall, had worried about the dangers of a man touching his penis and specifically about the man "who brings his bone [penis] to the hands of impure fantasy [or heated imagination]," the man whose offense is, in at least some measure, that he "incites his evil inclination himself." Solitary sex was not this particular rabbi's concern, but fantasy in all its idolatrous potential very much was.

In *Onania* and all its successors, the "impure ... imagination" became crucial to explaining what made solitary sex so dangerous. The very definition of the vice that John Marten was putting on the West's moral agenda pointed resolutely to both mental and societal depravity. The solitary vice is, readers will recall, as already noted,

> that unnatural Practice by which persons of either sex may defile their own bodies, without the Assistance of others. Whilst yielding to filthy imagination, they endeavor to imitate and procure for themselves that Sensation ...

Elsewhere, while supposedly responding to critics in the *Supplement*, Marten says that he, too, thought that the biggest part of the sin was "an impure imagination." One simply could not commit it "free of mental impurity"; purely medical masturbation — *pace* Diogenes the Cynic — was not possible.

This theme bounced around the popular and learned literature for forty years. Masturbation was the most common crime of impurity and that to which there was "more and stronger incitement" than to any other because the incitement was "always WITHIN ourselves," announced one of the many, many variants of *Eronania*, the *Onania* rip-off; it is carnal pleasure that people "*imitate* within themselves."[44] Chambers's *Cyclopaedia* in 1728 distinguished "Self-pollution" from pollution more generally by its resort to artifice: "defiling of one's own body by means of lascivious frictions and titillations, *raised by Art*." Nocturnal pollution, in other words, happened because of a natural surfeit of material that was relieved with the attendant natural pleasure; both the excitement and the means for self-pollution were artificial.

When Tissot and the *Encyclopédie* pronounced on the subject, they located the evil genius of masturbation not in the lusts of the flesh but in a generally benign faculty of the mind. Both distanced themselves from theological condemnations based on violation of the telos of sex or the triumph of concupiscence. Tissot announced that sin was not within his expertise. Menuret de Chambaud, writing for the *Encyclopédie*, was more straightforward. Leaving theology aside, as he clearly wanted to do, masturbation would not be so bad if — and here comes the big "if" — it were not in the thrall of an unmoored psyche: "Masturbation which is not so frequent, which is not excited by a fiery and voluptuous imagination, which is, in a word, spurred only by one's need," is not harmful at all. Diderot, the general editor, is even more explicit on the point. He never quite endorses masturbation and is clearly on the side of normal heterosexual relations, but Dr. Bordeu in *D'Alembert's Dream* makes a persuasive case that it is better than the alternatives. The stern Roman Cato the Elder might not today, Diderot suggests, offer a young man visiting a prostitute to relieve himself the same advice he did in his day: "Have courage." Catching the boy "alone, *in flagrante delicto*," that is, masturbating, these days, he might have told him that "he was doing better than corrupting someone else's wife or risking health and reputation." And as for the view that lots of strenuous exercise might get rid of the surplus, the answer is, "Why deprive yourself of a little pleasure?"[45]

In other words, if masturbation were natural — that is, the result of real sexual need — it would be fine; Menuret de Chambaud clearly has no interest in the problem of its being "unnatural," as that term was used by Saint Thomas, or in the bigger issue of sexual pleasure and concupiscence that had for long exercised theologians. His point in the *Encyclopédie* article is that it is not so easy to maintain moderate masturbation simply as an alternative way of satisfying ordinary, sociable sexual desire when other outlets were not available. It was almost by its nature immoderate, because the imagination was not easily restrained. It had "the greatest part of the crime," and thus the seat of the imagination — the mind and all that is connected to it — was most severely punished for doing it. This is almost a direct quotation from *Onania*, specifically from a letter in which an onanist confesses, "I look upon the Imagination which often goes along with, and always facilitates the Operation, to contain the greatest part of its Sinfulness."[46] A central problem with solitary sex as understood by the canonical text of the high Enlightenment was that it was generally driven from within, driven by a "voluptuous, a fiery imagination" that had only the most tenuous connections with all those charms, tricks, arrangements — and physiological natural processes — that drive a more social passion.

Tissot makes the same point even more clearly. Masturbation, he says, stands outside the natural economy not because it is unnatural in the traditional Christian sense of going against the natural purpose of a sexual act but because the desire that motivates it is quite literally the opposite of natural. It is artificial, made-up, chimerical, the figment of unbalanced minds. The masturbator constitutes an economy of one, an unregulated cottage industry of desire that produces both the urge and its perverse satisfaction: "Men subject themselves to false wants, and such is the case of those addicted to self-pollution. It is imagination and habit that subject them; it is not nature."

Masturbation in this formulation is like a metastatic wet dream to which every man, woman, and child was susceptible. In old-fashioned nocturnal pollution, "ideas relative to amorous pleasures, . . . objects which are painted to the fancy," affect the organs in sleep just as they would during the day. Then if "the act is consummated in the imagination," it is also physically consummated. That is, dreaming about orgasm produces a real orgasm. This in turn weakens the organs that weaken the imagination, because bad thoughts are rewarded with pleasure. So, in a vicious cycle, the nocturnal polluter has more dreams of orgasms and more real orgasms. In solitary sex, this sad process is even more completely out of control because the onanist wills the seductive chimera into existence repeatedly. Pleasure is at his beck and call; every

213

act reinforces fantasy. Almost every word of Tissot's account continued to have resonance from the eighteenth century to the present. "Men subject *themselves*"; they have "*false wants*"; they are "addicted" to "the imagination and [the] habit that subject[s] them." The enemies and — in the past forty years — the friends of masturbation who want to rehabilitate it agree on at least that.[47]

The work of solitary sex is done consciously in the mind, and from this follows its moral and medical evil. There was no question, as there had been with respect to nocturnal emissions, whether or not lascivious thoughts, or unconscious traces of such thoughts, might deepen the blame. Such willful thoughts were of its essence. Nor did concupiscence — a craving in the soul estranged from God — drive the onanist; not even temptation, although that might have started it all, is to blame. The wickedness of masturbation arose from the fact that those who do it purposely stride into trouble; they conjure up the whole enormous emotional, psychological, historical weight of sexual pleasure in the vacuum of solitude. Kant zeroed in on this: the moral insanity of masturbation, what made it worse than suicide, was that the masturbator "himself creates its [desire's] object. For in this way the imagination brings forth an appetite contrary to nature's purpose." Fictions and phantasms — the made-up, imagined, self-fashioned products of the mind — always at the ready, were the real villains of the piece.

This was widely understood in the best of circles. Goethe's, Schiller's and Herder's physician in their Weimar days, Christoph Wilhelm Hufeland, for example, articulated fantasy's danger cogently but without feeling the need to justify himself very much. Here once again the connection between masturbation and advanced Enlightenment thought is clear; Hufeland was one of the progressive giants of his era. In addition to treating the cultural heroes of his day, he was at the forefront of what became modern medicine: one of the great proponents of smallpox vaccination on the Continent, an enemy of what he took to be pseudosciences — phrenology, mesmerism, and such — the longtime editor of a major medical journal that ran for decades. His book on long life continued to be translated into English and other languages well

214

after his death in 1836. And on the subject of masturbation he could not have been clearer.

In general, Hufeland thought that modern youth engaged in sex at too early an age, *tout court*; in the Teutonic forests, he noted, warriors husbanded their strength and stayed away from women until they were twenty-five. But of all the varieties of sex, onanism was the worst because it was forced and hence "unnatural"; it responded to inner, not to real, needs: in both sexes, "it is endlessly more damaging than any natural act." And "moral Onanism" is its constant companion: "the expansion and inflaming of fantasy with all sorts of indecent and unworthy pictures." Indeed, it is the habit of such excitation through which "fantasy is armed and takes over the whole being." More and more excited by fictions, the young seem to stand on the brink of mortally dangerous art.[48]

Many less famous doctors and moralists made the same point for lay readers, male and female. "Imagination is the artisan," announced D.T. de Bienville, for "the fatal rage of Masturbation." Obscure in his day, Bienville did invent the putative disease that takes its name from the book in which this and other thoughts about solitary sex abound: nymphomania.[49] "The imagination, having without cease occupied itself in *dissembling* those things which will more and more excite the organs of generation," acquires thereby dominion over them, claimed a major 1771 French medical reference work. More than a hundred years later, the biggest of all nineteenth-century medical encyclopedias made the same point: natural discharges are good; those caused by the imagination weaken it. And on the eve of a new century, a year before the publication of Freud's *The Interpretation of Dreams*, the internationally successful author of a sex-education guide for girls informed them, in the section on the solitary vice, that feelings awakened by the imagination were by their nature morally wrong and more dangerous physically than actual deeds.[50]

The problem was not that masturbation created sexual pleasure outside of reproduction; it was not lumped with transgressions involving inappropriate partners or inappropriate ways of engaging with appropriate ones. The problem was that it lacked any partner at all except those in the mind's eye. The "pollution" part of "self-pollution" had lost most of its literal connotations when it branched off from its relative "nocturnal pollution." That which sullied, that which transgressed, was no longer semen in all its sticky specificity but rather the imagination reveling in desires of its own, unnatural creation.

A.P. Buchan, an English doctor, scion of a popular medical tradition, and a serious professional in his own right, captured the essence of what Rousseau had found so dangerous in his own masturbation: "the *absence* of the proper object of sexual intercourse," the absence, in fact, of any object or thing. This lack, in turn, is filled by "the imagination actively excited and the attention actively engaged in forming an image to supply the place of the legitimate object of desire." Fantasy provides where reality fails. The "exertions of the imagination" endeavor, by "an effort of will," to keep "in the mind's eye the form of some, perhaps favorite, female" and thus to provide a phantasm in place of the missing real thing. Herein lay the problem. The "improper interference" in the normal "indulgence of sexual appetite," the "interference of the will with an action wholly instinctive," was the chief cause of the "evil consequences of this vicious habit."[51]

Thomas Beddoes, the radical physician and father of the poet and physiologist Thomas Lowell Beddoes, makes the same sort of connection between onanism and the imagination — again, hostility to masturbation in the most progressive of circles and especially among people otherwise devoted to the Romantic project of self-realization. In the first place, he would agree with Rousseau that the vice, "which shame and timidity find so convenient, has a particular attraction for lively imaginations." But he is more specific in his pathophysiological speculations. Masturbation can begin with some chance stimulation: "Voluptuous ideas will arise in girls from any accidental irritation." But then, in those of considerable sensibility, these "ideas get possession of the imagination," causing them "to seek pleasure without any bodily irritation," that is, to indulge in the act he could not call "by the offensive name." In other words, stimulation and irritation are not enough to account for the dangers of the unnameable act. The mediation of the most protean of the mental faculties is required.[52]

This is, of course, the opposite view of the hygienic, if not the moral, valuation of masturbation that would have been given in classical medicine. Diogenes the Cynic was so often cited in ancient sources — a sort of exemplary masturbator — because they held that rubbing oneself to get sexual satisfaction was even less engaging, and hence less depleting, than sex with an anonymous prostitute, the most minimally engaging form of intercourse they could imagine. For them, masturbation was the most efficient, if not the most dignified, way to relieve oneself. One famous eighteenth-century surgeon tried to revive this view and met with universal condemnation. But the contretemps does show, once again, that a deranged mobilization of the imagination stood very near the heart of the newly articulated problem of solitary sex.

John Hunter was a lion of eighteenth-century medicine: a well-known surgeon, anatomist, medical writer, and public figure, he more than anyone else would probably have come to the mind of an educated British person if asked to name a famous homegrown public medical figure. In general, Hunter was unimpressed with the evidence that masturbation did much harm. Yes, many patients were all too eager to believe what they had read in books; among the men who consulted him, many were "ready to suppose this cause" for their impotence. But it seemed to him that this problem was "far too rare to originate from a practice so general." More likely, given how "the imagination acts . . . to make men believe they are really weakened," they suffered from what they read, not from what they did, and they were made doubly miserable because they supposed that youthful indiscretion had caused their adult debility. If there was an objection to "this selfish enjoyment," it was the probability that it would be "repeated too often." But Hunter's heart was not in even this mild rebuke. To these perfectly sensible clinical judgments, Hunter appended, in the first edition of the treatise, a theoretical justification for why he thought masturbation generally benign. His was one of the few medical voices that spoke out against the dominant view that solitary sex killed; it was crying into the wilderness — the only eighteenth-century version of the standard Stoic medico-sexual ethics to have survived in print. Diogenes lived on here.[53]

217

Masturbation, Hunter argued — just once because his editors suppressed such subversive views — "does less harm to the constitution" than the "natural [act]," and intercourse with a prostitute or a woman to whom a man feels indifferent is less debilitating than intercourse "where the affections for the woman are also concerned," because the mind and the passions are less engaged in the former two cases than in the latter. Contrary to what everyone else since *Onania* had said, orgasm from solitary friction is thus the most purely "constitutional act" of the three. It is "simple"; only "one action takes place." Next comes intercourse with a prostitute — a bit more involvement. And most threatening to health is sex with someone who engages the mind. The mind

> becomes interested, it is worked up to a degree of enthusiasm, increasing the sensitivity of the body. . . . [W]hen the complete action takes place it is with proportional violence; and in proportion to the violence is the degree of debility produced or injury done to the constitution.[54]

No one agreed with Hunter in his ordering of the "actions" in question, in his assessment of what kind of sex engaged the mind the most. But everyone would have agreed with the underlying dictum that the more affected the mind, the more danger to the body. And except in Hunter's account, masturbation from the early eighteenth century to the present has been understood as the paradigmatic sex of the mind, specifically of fantasy, of its capacity to imagine something other than the here and now; therein lay its pleasure and creative possibilities but also its dangers.

Freud's colleague the Hungarian psychoanalyst Sándor Ferenczi offers a wonderfully precise modern inversion of Hunter's order. In onanism, he argues, the sense organs are silent, and conscious fantasy, along with the genital organs, has to provide all the excitement. The sheer effort of all this mental work — "the forcible retaining of a picture often imagined with hallucinatory sharpness" — causes the fatigue and debility, short-term if not repeated too often, of solitary sex. By extension, men who have sex with their wives frequently, "in spite of a diminution of sexual interest," manage to do it only by replacing, in the imagination, the wife with someone else. This, of course, is just onanism by another name — *per vaginam* — and has the same physical and psychic consequences as the solitary kind. But — the clinching argument — if such men occasionally have sex with someone who provides complete satisfaction, that is, with whom they do not have to do the heavy lifting demanded by fantasy, "they are invigorated by the act."[55]

Perhaps because Hunter's views in the post-1712 climate were so out of sync with his contemporaries' — or perhaps because they were soon suppressed — rebuttal seemed pointless. Only one pamphlet straightforwardly announced itself as against Hunter's treatise "in favor of onanism or masturbation." It was mostly a pastiche of plagiarisms from Tissot — pages on end — with occasional evidence drawn from other, long-dead authorities. The author says he could quote a thousand more on the dangers of solitary as opposed to other kinds of sex but that he will limit himself to a few choice quotes and ripostes: Nicolas Venette, who wrote the standard and long-lived late-seventeenth-century sex manual much attests, for example, to the apparently well-known fact that immoderate venery with a beautiful, engaging woman was far less exhausting than similar extravaganzas with an ugly one because it had "charms which dilate our hearts, and multiply its spirits." The lover did not have to fantasize to find pleasure; reality supplied all he needed. Social, aesthetic, and emotional circumstances thus redeemed even the wildest excess. Furthermore, Hunter's views were said to be counterintuitive. If it were true that the less alluring one's sexual partner, the healthier the act, because the imagination was less engaged, then we would only couple with the old and deformed, and that would stop procreation in its tracks. We should, the author concluded, be much more indulgent of the rake or libertine, whose only crime is overindulgence in an "inclination which nature has engraved in all our hearts," than of the masturbator, who furtively indulges in a passion of his own creation. Kant would agree with that.[56]

But Duncan Gordon, the author of this pamphlet, need not have been so worked up. Hunter's analysis of the sexual imagination —

so commonplace in Antiquity — was not long for this world. It disappeared from the second edition, leaving only his clinical skepticism about masturbation as a cause of impotence. And by the time his son-in-law, himself a famous surgeon and scientist, issued a third edition, there was nothing left but an apology from the editor saying that onanism was more harmful than the author had imagined and that venereal acts with women, when the passions are strongly excited, can be repeated more often without debilitating results because the body compensated for such fervor.[57]

One answer to the question of *what* made masturbation so threatening is the following: it entailed the willful mobilization of the imagination engaged in the endless creation of desire — fictive desire — that had at most a tangential relation to its real counterpart. Why this happened in terms of a history of the imagination and society is another question that we will take up in the next chapter. For now, the point is that masturbation was threatening not because solitary orgasm felt any different from the pleasure of permissible orgasm, or because, on any given occasion, it rattled the body more. Masturbatory pleasure was dangerous because it was a sham version of real pleasure: virtual-reality orgasm we might say. It partook of the wickedness of subterfuge, fraud, fakery, the very opposite of natural transparency.

"Deceitful" and "counterfeit" were the adjectives that came to Rousseau's mind when he wrote about the teacher's worry in *Emile* over the collapse of his whole educational project should his pupil succumb to the secret vice. This is the idea in another of the *Encyclopédie*'s articles that takes up the topic: "Manustrapratio" suggests that we see further "Pollution nocturne." Here we learn that masturbatory emissions were "sacrifices" to a "false Venus." They had no origins in the real world; they were born, as we already know from the masturbation entry, in a "fiery and voluptuous imagination." Perhaps this particular image, so suggestive of classical paganism, was an allusion to the oft-repeated story in Pliny about the man so taken with Praxiteles's naked Cnidian Aphrodite that he hid himself at night so that he could embrace the image, the representation, the simulacrum (*simulacro cohai-*

sisse) we might say. A stain on the marble betrayed what he did then. (The people of Cos had bought the clothed version of this statue for the same price and apparently did not have trouble with this sort of vandalism.) Renaissance retellings of the tale have a reclining Venus being "of such beauty that men [in Antiquity, when the pieces were first presented] burned with sacrilegious lust, violating the statue by masturbating on it." "Deceitful" was the adjective that made its way into authoritative nineteenth-century medical texts to describe the nature of masturbatory passion — the lust for the object of fantasy.[58] And there is, of course, the more general sense in which representations were thought to encourage eros, however it might be satisfied.

In this context, solitary sex was the perversion of one of the mind's most protean and admirable faculties. The onanist mobilized the imagination not to produce art or poetry or compassion; in fact, he or she produced nothing at all or, worse, nothing but bottomless self-absorption at the expense of any possible social good. If the sleep of reason produced monsters, the triumph of fantasy produced them twice over.

One did not have to read the philosophes to get the idea. The most self-serving bit of eighteenth-century commercial doggerel, written to sell quack nostrums, paints the masturbator as an artist gone mad:

> But what more base, more noxious to the body
> Than by the power of fancy to excite,
> Such lewd ideas of an absent object,
> As rouse the organs formed for noble end
> To rush into th' embraces of a phantom,
> And so do the deed of personal enjoyment.[59]

These lines do not scan, but their meaning is clear enough. The "power of fancy" is where the interior peril of solitary sex resided after 1712 or thereabout. The power of the mind to create images, whether mirroring the real world or combing it in new and fanciful ways, still captivated Freud and his colleagues when they held their contentious meetings about masturbation two centuries

221

later. One of the few things they all could agree on was the importance of the fantasies that accompany masturbation. And more recently psychology has recognized — yet again — their centrality. But this time science seems to have shown that masturbatory daydreaming might be a good thing. Modern survey techniques and personality measurements suggest that elaborate story-like fantasies correlate with a positive approach to daydreaming, which in turn correlates with a rich erotic life and positive attitudes toward life generally.[60]

But before such a rosy prospect came into view, more than two hundred years passed during which masturbation was associated with a bad conscience. Guilt arose from doing something that would not survive the light of day, and masturbation was paradigmatically such an act. In the eighteenth century, it became the *secret* vice and all the more dangerous because it was understood to be so essentially an act of the shadows.

Solitary and Secret

The perceived threat of masturbation to the social and moral order is almost self-evident from the names by which it came to be known: the *solitary* vice, *self*-pollution, the *secret* vice. The adjectives are decisive. No other antisocial act, not even other antisocial sexual acts that captured the attention of doctors and moralists, occasioned the chorus of revulsion that met any mention of masturbation. This vice's solitariness and secrecy went beyond the merely antisocial or morally reprehensible; the act was outside the pale of not just this or that but any possible moral order. Onanism represented the deepest sort of secret: not like the secrets of conspirators or Freemasons, known to an inner circle that was bound together by holding it in common; not like the shared secret of illegitimate lovers hidden from a disapproving world but there to be discovered if one were to betray the other or if a child were forthcoming; not like the secrecy of all sin that stained the soul and made itself known only to God in prayer or to a confessor, however much its outward signs might be visible; not like the secrecy that interpretation seeks to penetrate or the opacity that religious texts acquire to separate an in- from an out-group.[61]

222

The secrecy of masturbation went beyond the general reticence that accompanied talk of sin, especially sexual sin. Moral and confessional literature had for centuries made full disclaimers: the author, almost as a matter of form, was reluctant to speak of this or that topic lest public condemnation were to plant the idea of some new transgression in the minds of innocent readers or hearers. It even went beyond the secrecy that seems so deeply embedded in the language of sex: the privates, organs not for public view; the German *scham* (from the same root as "shame"); the pudenda, from the Latin *pudendus*, meaning "of which one ought to be ashamed." This sense of secrecy transferred to the language of sexual disease — secret diseases for those of venereal origin. All this is old.

But to those who invested masturbation with its peculiar modern significance and then maintained its status in the pantheon of perversions for the next centuries, the secrecy of the new vice had something fresh about it. This vice was uniquely, fundamentally secret, like no other. All other sins, *Onania* announced, had to have witnesses except for this one. All other sins were to some measure restrained by law or custom; not this one, deceptively free as it was from outside detection and danger: no problem of disadvantageous marriage, no problem of virtue lost, no risk of rejection or of being thought too forward, no need to confess, because the sinner herself did not know she had sinned and who was to tell her. Women who would "rather die than betray their weakness to any man living" have "by reason of [its] SECRECY been unhappily betrayed" into onanism. "Secrecy" also beguiles many otherwise sober boys. "Using THEMSELVES, separately and alone," they subvert nature as nowhere else.[62] Like the tree falling without witnesses in the forest, this sin threatened to vanish in the absence of a beholder and, with it, all shame and all restraint.

"Secret" modifies "venery" in the subtitle of Tissot's wildly popular and much-quoted book; secrecy is what distinguished onanism from all other kinds of venery; secrecy is what made it worse than smallpox, more to be dreaded because, "by its working in the shades of mystery," "it secretly undermines without

those who are its victims thinking of its malignancy." "It undermines without noise," stealthily, free from outside scrutiny and
alarm. Here is a sin one can, in principle, commit in complete
ignorance that one is sinning, rather like speaking prose without
knowing it but with far worse consequences.[63] It is not *a* but *the*
solitary vice, not *a* but *the* secret sin.

Solitariness was regarded as a necessary condition for the
secrecy that constituted masturbation's fatal attraction but in a
sense that went beyond the fact that one usually did it alone as one
might practice a musical instrument alone or study alone. In fact,
one worry of teachers was that students did it together. But the
fact remained that solitary sex was autarkic sex. The masturbator
was free from the prying eyes of authority and the restraints of
good company but, more important, from the need for anything
or anybody. The whole apparatus of desire — creation, elaboration, fulfillment — was self-contained, an old-fashioned mercan-
tilist's dream and a moralist's nightmare. "Nothing can be more
ensnaring," said *Onania* in what became the standard refrain, than
a "Satisfaction that can be procured without any Body's Assistance, Leave or Knowledge . . . any hour, one day as well as another,
up or in bed." All one needs is to be alone and "hardly that when it
is dark."[64] The solitary vice stands wholly divorced from everything that might bind a man or woman, girl or boy to the social
order.

Even Richard Carlile, one of the most impassioned of nineteenth-century sexual radicals, recoiled in horror from the secret
vice. He envisioned a utopian regime of social sexuality, a regime
of cheerful relationships in which "sexual intercourse with affection" and without the danger of conception would replace the
perversions of the cloister, the joylessness of marriage without
passion, and the miseries of trying to support more children than
one could afford. In the sad old world he was struggling against,
"self-excitations and unnatural gratification," specifically "Onanism, pederasty and other substitutions," thrived at the expense
of "natural and healthy commerce between the sexes." He recommended "chaste and proper commerce" with its exchange, sociability, and mutuality in preference to the disgraceful, disease-

224

producing, and painful "artificial and unnatural means," to subdue temporarily the passions of love. And Carlile, like all eighteenth-century commentators, brought the social question back around to the question of fiction, to masturbation as the demon of fantasy: "We encourage reality and decry artifice," he announced. Birth control, in his view, meant that one was not tempted to perversion and could enjoy healthy heterosexuality without fear of children or childbirth.[65]

The meaning of the adjectives "solitary" and "secret" would seem to be simple enough to describe a vice. But both carry a lot of cultural baggage. Not every activity we do alone is solitary or private; not everything we choose not to share with another is a secret. Certainly neither word generally carries a negative connotation. "Solitary" and "private" might be opposite, complementary, or supplementary to "communal," "public," or "social" or some combination of these. "Secret" or "secret something," like "private" or "something private," covers a great variety of cases. It might describe something we have been forbidden to share or something that would be dangerous, embarrassing, unfair, or inappropriate were it known. It might be something that is kept as a sign of trust, love, or religious devotion: private prayer, the secret, or prayer, closet. "Private" and "secret," in other words, do not just describe the inner as opposed to the outer self, that which is not available to others as opposed to that which is. They help create this distinction; they are a part of the modern process of self-fashioning and developed alongside it.[66]

There is, of course, a history of this, secular and religious. Private — as opposed to public — confession, instituted by the Council of Trent, asks each penitent to delve deeper and deeper into his or her soul, to probe not only misdeeds but also mis-thoughts, mis-desires. The English Protestant tradition made the prayer closet, the place of solitary prayer, into a venue for the most intense interior self-scrutiny, a place where the private self stood in sharp contrast to public acts and expressions. If it was a theater of the self, it was a theater before God. "For man is that certainly, that he is secretly," announced *The Privie Key of Heaven*; a prayer closet is "a closed or secret chamber, a retiring place, where a person is not seen or heard."[67] The century and a half before *Onania* witnessed an enormous elaboration of the private — the secret — in the religious sphere as a space for self-articulation, a space not only of physical retreat but of self-absorption in its positive senses.

And in the secular world, too, the private came to be regarded as much more than just an alternative to something else. The private arena was where each individual could seek his own advantage, as opposed to the public arena, in which he worked for the general good. On the other hand, somehow the two were thought to mesh. Some private vices were said to translate to public goods; this was the basis of one of the earliest and greatest defenses of the marketplace. Some private reading was a road to self-knowledge and also to the knowledge of others. The rich interior realms that had been the province of saints were democratized; this is the century in which Rousseau wrote his *Confessions* as a secular monument to Augustine's *Confessions*. This was the world that witnessed the creation and burgeoning of the modern autobiography. The realm of the private was the basis for civil society in which individual interests negotiated and contained each other. In other words, privacy and secrecy also had all sorts of positive associations as sites of truth and as foundations of a real self.

It was in contrast to this affirmation that *the* private vice assumed such importance. It was the negative of all this, the paradigmatic emblem of solipsistic privacy or secrecy of the wrong sort. Masturbation represented socially inappropriate and uncontrolled privacy. Prayer closets were the privilege of the rich, as were the other modern venues of privacy; they belonged to adults who might be expected not to abuse them. But adolescents out of sight, prey to the teaching of some older, loutish, perhaps lower-class, sexually knowledgeable boy, or children of the middling sorts at the mercy of unsupervised servants were ready victims of a private vice that escaped the gaze of civilization. The battle against masturbation was one of the main engagements in the long war fought to ensure the right kind and just measure of bourgeois privacy.

However private the sin, however solitary the act, those who wrote about it thought that its origins were social, that it was on

226

occasion practiced in groups, and that the young often did not know that what they were doing was "secret" — something to be ashamed of. In other words, they did not know they were meant to feel guilty about some kinds of privacy and social isolation. (I have found no sources that suggested that adolescent boys masturbated in groups as an act of rebellion precisely because they knew that adults considered it to be outrageous.) A few nineteenth-century doctors suggested that infants and children might discover masturbation inadvertently, on their own, by scratching their genitals to relieve an itch and finding pleasure thereby. But no one before Freud formulated the notion of poly-morphously perverse sexuality — basic equipment with which the human organism comes into the world and which it is the work of civilization to channel into its proper course. (No one, of course, imagined that a thirty-two-week-old female fetus in the womb, who had not had the opportunity to learn anything, would one day be observed caressing the region of its clitoris, giving all the signs of pleasure.[68]) Masturbation, in other words, had to be learned, and it had to be learned from someone. Artifice entailed an artificer, and even a perverse craft seemed to need a teacher. "In my experience," writes Johann Georg Zimmermann, calling on twenty-five years of medical practice in many countries, "only a very few young people discover this vice for themselves."[69] Thus the existence of solitary sex in itself bore witness to failure, specifically to the failure of society to inculcate the right kind of bad conscience.

Sexual intercourse, by contrast, was thought to require no "art," because "nature" taught it to each of us when the time came. Thus learning to masturbate came to be represented as a secular reprise of the Fall as each innocent new generation of the young stood to be corrupted. In the role of the serpent were either vicious servants — nurses who played with the genitals of their charges to keep them quiet, others who taught their young masters to masturbate out of simple perversity or for their own pleasure — or vicious friends such as school chums or neighbor-hood mates. In any case, the sin came from the outside; it was learned.

227

This contrast persisted despite evidence that heterosexual attraction and intercourse were not all that natural either. The well-publicized case of the "wild boy of Aveyron," who had grown up outside society and was seen as a purely "natural man," suggested precisely that. Jean-Marc-Gaspard Itard in his studies thought that the most astonishing aspect of the boy's emotional world was that he was indifferent "to women in the midst of the violent changes attendant upon a very pronounced puberty." "Beyond all explanation." Despite what seem like blind furies of passion and adolescent mood swings — "passing suddenly from sadness to anxiety," tears, pulse racing, face apoplectic — the boy did not seem to realize the nature of his passion or that a woman might satisfy it. And Itard was reluctant to teach him lest he gratify this need like he did all his others, in public, which in this case would be intolerable. Cold showers did not help. Itard concluded that having never been taught the difference between men and women, something other adolescents learn before puberty, he could not imagine what one might do with the opposite sex. Itard does not mention masturbation, but his finding belied the distinction that one was born to heterosexual intercourse but one learned the evil art of masturbation. His subject seems to have discovered neither on his own.[70]

The insistence that the adjective "secret" differentiated solitary sex from all other sexual vice also flew in the face of evidence, horrifying evidence, to the contrary. Tissot, ever the magpie who cannot resist picking up another good story, tells about a college of students who, according to a reputable journal, "sometimes diverted the tediousness of metaphysical scholastic exercises...delivered by a drowsy old professor" by masturbating. It helped them stay awake. He admits, "This story does not so much evince the truth of what I advance, as the scandalous dissolution into which youth may be led." He thinks masturbation is contagious, spreading from student to student, from wicked servant to helpless charge, like smallpox or fever. So, this anecdote ought to be a warning: boring lectures can produce a masturbation epidemic. Indeed, the most common advice to teachers and parents is never to leave groups of children unsupervised lest the vice leap from one infected party and take hold more generally: "As far as is possible never let the children under your care work or play without being watched," advises the pedagogue C.G. Salzmann, on the grounds that someone will teach them about self-pollution and ruin the lot of them. "A father needs to know what is done in the darkest recesses of his house — use that vigilance which discovers the coppice where the deer has taken shelter, when it has escaped all other eyes" — in an effort to protect his children, advises Tissot. In this story of the etiology of vice, the problem is that young people take it up before they learn it is secret, solitary, or wrong. The problem was to enlighten them in this regard. This was a wicked secret; it was done in the wrong sort of private place; it ought thus to produce shame and guilt, which, alas, were not inborn. If they were, there would be no need for so huge an apparatus to make the private vice public.[71]

Children thus had to *discover* masturbation was wrong; they had to be taught, so the story went, not only the act itself but also that what they might regard as innocent pleasures were, in fact, something horribly shameful called self-pollution. This is where books came in. Letter after letter, Zimmermann attested, offered evidence that Tissot's book, more than any other source, was what first informed his patients that masturbation was wrong. Half a century later playwright August Strindberg reported that he learned to masturbate in his early teens through a game — while swimming, an older boy taught it to the younger children; no one, he says, made a secret of it; there was no shame as they played, out in the open, on a steamship dock. But he "soon gave up the habit when a book of sex horrors fell into his hands." (This was probably the widely translated and long-lived *Warnung eines Jugendfreundes vor dem gefährlichsten Jugendfeind; oder, Belehrung über geheime Sünden, ihre Folgen, Heilung und Verhütung* by the German bishop Sixt Karl Kapff. The title, at the same time coyly insinuating and threatening, says it all: "The warning of a friend to youth of youth's dangerous enemy; or, Instruction about secret sins, their consequences, cure, and prevention.") The young Strindberg, in other words, learned that he was publicly practicing a *secret* sin and with this knowledge began what he says was a struggle with instincts that he could never fully conquer and that lasted until he began having intercourse at age eighteen. His efforts to abstain from a secret vice became the arena for self-mastery, a constant test of his will to resist, an inescapable contest with himself. Strindberg's most thorough recent biographer claims that his subject and thousands of other Swedish children were much relieved when a Board of Education inquiry showed that they were not, contrary to what they might have believed, alone in their private vice. Most boys and girls did it. Having the report published in newspapers and widely discussed seems to have assured at least Strindberg that the subject was "a necessary part of normal human experience." We do not have enough evidence to know how general these inner battles were among nineteenth-century men and women or how much having them discussed in public might have assuaged their guilt. We do know that, looking back through the lens of Freud, the guilt seems common enough and that sharing it with others did not help much. Nor do we know how, if at all, Strindberg's confrontation with masturbation shaped his well-known misogyny and the hopelessness of sexual relations in his plays. We do know, from him, that he did not have a restful night of sleep during these years of overt guilt and temptation and that the repressed images of his waking hours returned to haunt him in his dreams for years, whatever he might have thought about the normalcy of his not-so-solitary private vice.[72]

From the eighteenth to the early twentieth century, a great deal of literature was addressed not to masturbators but to their mothers and fathers, whose job it was to let their offspring know there was no such thing as innocent masturbation. By the late nineteenth century, parents, especially mothers, had moved to the front line of instilling into their offspring the appropriate sense of secrecy, shame, and guilt. They in turn were also made to feel guilt for the inevitable failures of surveillance. "Perfect Womanhood" meant that a mother who saw her little boy handling himself would not let it pass, thinking "he will outgrow it." She might not "realize what a strong hold it has on him"! "I say to you who love your sons," Dr. Mary Ries Melendy warns, "watch." The message differed little from what eighteenth-century parents were taught about keeping their eyes open for secret acts in secret places.[73]

Masturbation, in short, was private in a way that was deeper and more sinister than other activities, even sexual activities, which one would not do in public and about which one might be ashamed or embarrassed. It was regarded as solitary even though children seemed to learn it from other children or from servants in all sorts of social contexts; and it was singled out as the private vice from among other vices that were themselves not so terribly public either. This was sex in a truly private place, private as it emerged in the late seventeenth and the eighteenth century: the private as the venue within each of us where our innermost feelings, responses, and sensibilities, as well as the whole structure of self-government, dwelled. More than the thinking self of Descartes's "Cogito ergo sum," the authentic individual dwelled in this private place. It was the place of truth, the place of revelation; to sin here came to be regarded as a terrible violation, while at the same time that violation helped to define its boundaries.

To those charged with the process of civilization, solitary sex held out the disturbing possibility of the impossible: a private language of the body in which only the masturbator knows what the signs mean, a totally self-contained system of fetish and arousal that nowhere touches down in social reality. Less epistemologically radical but still an enormous threat was this truth: there existed a purely private realm of pleasures and of commerce in which communication took place that deprived those outside it of their roles as interlocutors. This world could not be socially regulated because it was, by definition, hidden from view. A whole paranoid style developed among pedagogues, doctors, parents, priests, and clergymen as they contemplated among the young an epidemic of vice that at no point articulated with the visible and manageable world. One could teach children that nakedness was shameful by wearing clothes and chastising them for not doing so; one could preach against fornication with plenty of examples. Shame had to be mobilized to make young people, especially girls, behave chastely and modestly. But how was one to preach against something that children did without their knowing that they were

231

doing anything, without their thinking there were any consequences, and without their doing it in view so that they might be
rebuked? Shame was almost by definition public; one was shamed
in the eyes of someone else. Masturbation escaped all this.

Onania captured this fear of primitive privacy — masturbation
as private language — at the beginning of the eighteenth century,
and the theme never went away: people of both sexes, it seems,
continued to masturbate, believing they would not do themselves
any harm thereby, without any sense of immodesty, without restraint. And critics continued to worry about it in these terms.
"That trick of childhood," the "first darling sin . . . which infects
with strong habits of impurity" in *Onania*, became, in Freud, "the
foundations for the future primacy over sexual activity exercised
by this erotogenic zone." Freud means that censoring genital masturbation marks the organs for the great future they have before
them; girls, of course, will have to readjust, but that is a story for
later. Failure to get a cultural hook into infantile masturbation
would, Freud says, "constitute the first great deviation from the
course of development laid down for civilized man." Over the
years, masturbation — or, more specifically, the sublimation of
masturbation and the resulting guilt — loomed ever larger in his
thought. In 1915, he commented in a new edition of *Three Essays
on Sexuality* that the question of why neurotics' sense of guilt is
attached to the memory of some masturbatory activity, usually at
puberty, still awaits an exhaustive analysis, though the truth of the
observation is beyond question. In 1920, he added that masturbation represents the executive agency of the whole infantile
sexuality and therefore takes over all the guilt attached to it. The
curious thing is that masturbation comes to represent a guilt
about secret pleasure, pleasure with no redeeming social function, that seems to be almost primal — the original guilt — and yet
at the same time the work of so much cultural effort.[74]

I am not simply reading Freud backward. Beginning with *Onania*, the moral desperation of two centuries of literature on the
solitary sin was rooted in the sense that there might be a realm of
privacy into which the civilizing process could not reach. One
could curb violence and aggression by banning knives and stop-

232

ping fights; one could bolster the boundaries of bodily integrity by teaching table manners, encouraging polite people to make their toilets in private, and discouraging spitting and farting in public; one could enforce discipline in schools and in the army. All of this was about creating in public spaces the sort of people who could control their bodies themselves whether in public or in private. Masturbation outside of public view seemed capable of escaping all this. It became a particularly horrible transgression not because it *was* private and solitary but because it was made to be exemplary of the private and solitary in their negative registers. It represented the dark side of a much-admired state, the threat of independence and autonomy. Guilt about endless, asocial pleasure, and shame at one's delights being discovered, were the creations of the age that created both the realm of the private and its perverted doppelgänger. In other words, as the virtues of privacy, solitude, and autonomy were being created, their vice was being shaped as well. Freud once claimed that it was easy to commit a crime but difficult to remove its traces; finding the signs of inner transgression is precisely what *Onania* and its successors set out to do.[75]

But contemporaries seemed to recognize that these signs were not a natural consequence of the act even if they did not recognize the ironies of their analysis. It was not inevitable that masturbation was, or ought to be, secret because it was manifestly shameful. Its shamefulness had to be taught and its supposed consequences — guilt at repeatedly succumbing to a shameful pleasure, averted glances, melancholy, and dejection — could not be simply assumed. Yes, they were evident but only after culture had done its work. Yes, much of the injury of masturbation arose from the tortures of secrecy but secrecy was clearly not inherent in the act. Undisturbed "solitary lewdness meets no obstacle"; one has to watch a child carefully — here Tissot cites Rousseau — to intervene, to teach the child that his or her seemingly innocent entertainment was, in fact, both deadly and profoundly demoralizing. But still, Tissot and many others also believed that the unnaturalness of solitary sex — its interiority — somehow produced a poisonous secrecy quite on its own. Those who are "seduced by

natural sex are to be forgiven," argued Tissot; they had simply
succumbed to the excessive gratification of "what nature engraved in our breast." But the masturbator "is tortured by secrecy,
by how horrible he must appear to society when discovered"
because of the unnatural sources of his or her desire. Tissot quotes
a letter — almost certainly genuine — of a patient who thinks that
everyone can read on his face that he is a masturbator, which
"makes all company insupportable" and turns him to solitude,
which brings on melancholy, which then leads to all manner of
other symptoms.[76]

An early-nineteenth-century doctor — one among many —
criticized Tissot for creating so much anxiety that patients thought
they had symptoms caused by masturbation which in fact had
other origins — scurvy, for example. Tissot himself thought he
might have gone too far as he was deluged with letter after hypochondriacal letter from folks claiming to be sick because they had
masturbated as children. He very soon stopped responding and
announced that he had said his piece on the subject and was moving on. But such criticism, such awareness of the origins of anxiety
did not keep the same nineteenth-century doctor from suggesting, as if it were a fact of nature, that solitary sexual gratification
in either sex was "so foreign to human dignity" that people who
yield to it had the usual physical side effects of excessive venery
aggravated by an "anxious state of repentance." One of the most
virulent of the late-nineteenth-century anti-masturbation tracts
announced as a commonplace that "the most constant and invari-
able," as well as the earliest, indication that someone was a masturbator was the "downcast, averted glance, and the disposition
to solitude."[77]

Right up to the present, masturbation has sustained the sense
that it is pathologically, transgressively secret even though no one
believes anymore that it causes horrible diseases and few would
place it above sodomy, adultery, or premarital intercourse in their
list of wrongs. It is the most prevalent sexual activity, and yet it is
still the one that people are most reluctant to speak about, one of
the very few truly discomforting things to air in public. Hardened
interviewers in a recent large-scale, thoroughly professional study

234

were unembarrassed to ask viva voce questions about anal sex and same-sex relations; they balked at inquiring about whether their interviewees masturbated. Only questions about personal income occasioned similar reticence, which says something about what is regarded as personal in our society. A self-administered questionnaire had to be used in place of the usual protocol. But not just interviewers' sensibilities were at work here. Government officials willing to find out about so much else insisted that questions about masturbation be excluded from the survey. Men who were judged "unresponsive" to various research instruments and who had to be revisited five or more times to ensure the statistical reliability of the study were also especially reluctant to let on that they had masturbated.[78] Other studies, too, have found that no aspect of sexual behavior is more sensitive — more hidden from the probing eye of social science — than masturbation. It is about as secret a kind of sexuality as exists today, the legacy of almost three centuries' efforts and the heir to *Onania*'s original formulation.

The great moral question of the modern period would be how the private self, with all its desires, fantasies, and infinite wants, could be made to articulate with the world outside itself. And more particularly, how was it to be mobilized for the public good. An autonomous, private being was not — could not be — autarkic if society was to exist. But masturbation suggested that maybe this truth was not a fact of nature but a construct of culture. It came to represent the dangers of solipsistic collapse, of sinister privacy at a time when the private was being extolled by philosophers, economists, writers, and artists as the repository of so much good. In the battles against private vice, the war to civilize and socialize the endlessly desiring self was fought.

The Threat of Excess
Rousseau, always ready with the psychologically astute reflection, always poised to transform a personal anxiety into a general truth, got it right when he considered masturbation in his *Confessions*. It was, he famously said, "the dangerous supplement": there was always something more, something unbounded, something

235

that could not be satisfied and laid to rest. When he masturbated, the greatest and most original of the philosophes tells us, he would conjure up a sexually exciting image or story, become excited, and satisfy his desire, all without recourse to anyone. There was nothing to stop him from doing it again and again, "with" whomever he wanted, whenever he wanted, and without any natural satiety. Therein lay its fatal attraction and the seeds of ruin. Masturbators were able

> to dispose, so to speak, of the female sex at their will, and to make any beauty who tempts them serve their pleasure without the need of first obtaining her consent. Seduced by this fatal advantage, I set about destroying the sturdy constitution that Nature had restored to me.

In heterosexual intercourse — to which onanism was "the dangerous supplement" — there was always some external restraint: he might be refused; he might lose interest in the woman at hand.[79]

Masturbation, however, was outside not just this or that form of restraint but all bounds whatsoever. There was no stopping it because it was so terribly easy, because it was so alluringly free, because it seemed to escape from any and all consequences, because it was so perfectly outside civilization. *Onania* was already onto this: some men were constrained from visiting prostitutes by their stinginess or poverty; others abstained from fornication for fear of disease; some women feared having children; and lascivious widows feared that they would lose their fortunes, their liberties, or their reputations if they had intercourse with a man. But masturbation stood outside custom, economics, and law; no statutes forbade it, as they did sodomy. No punishment was its consequence.[80]

The father of British utilitarianism, the eighteenth-century legal reformer Jeremy Bentham, uses this legal otherworldliness of masturbation as a sort of *reductio ad absurdum* argument against criminal sanctions for other sexual acts. "Of all the irregularities of the venereal appetites," the "most incontestably pernicious," the one that is "incomparably more enervating than any single act of those kinds" that the law does proscribe — bestiality, sodomy, and perhaps "lesbianism" — the one more enervating than "any single other exertion of the venereal faculty," the one most harmful to the welfare of society, remains beyond the reach of the police powers of the state. If masturbation can go scot-free, then so should sodomy.[81] Bentham thought that the hostility toward sodomy was due to an irrational antipathy to pleasure — the foundation of his utilitarian calculus — and an exaggeration of its social costs. Even the century's most pro-pleasure theorist could not find a place for solitary sex in his philosophy.

Other sins might be avoided by exercising caution and avoiding trouble: "Lead us not into temptation," Jesus taught his followers to pray. But one could not be delivered from this evil. It is so attractive, as the *Eronania* family of pamphlets observes, because of the "great Ease there is in engaging" in it; it is so common because, once started, "escape is difficult because the Incitements to it are always within ourselves." "The fuel and treacherous enticements to it always accompany us," and it is not a crime that can be stopped or at least moderated like any other because it is private. "Once started it is near impossible to stop"; once the masturbator is aflame with desire, nothing out there seems to quench the "inner fires."[82]

Thirty years later, Tissot offers many more learned accounts of why this should be so, but they amount to the same thing: masturbation *is* excess. The onanist is never satisfied but wants to do it more and more; the urge to masturbate always exceeds any natural urge; it is always the supplement, always out of control. Sociologically, the story is as it was in *Onania* and would be in more or less every other treatment of the subject for centuries: "There are no obstacles to a solitary debauch, which is unlimited." Physiologically, Tissot explains the excess in terms of other bodily functions. The part of the brain occupied by thinking about masturbation is like a muscle that has been extended or worked over a long period of time. It either learns this wickedness so deeply that it is permanently imprinted on the body — "the attendant motion in the part cannot be stopped" — or goes on so long that the muscle is exhausted "by perpetual fatigue" beyond revival.

237

Alternatively, he suggests, the masturbator is like someone who has ruined his elimination of waste by "bad habit," rather like the abuser of laxatives or some other unnatural intervention in the working of our bowels or bladders. Normally, he points out, the necessity to void stool or urine is "signified by certain conditions." One really needs to get rid of something and one does. But this natural economy can be "so far pervert[ed]" that evacuations no longer depend on the "quantity of matter to be evacuated." Then the body goes beyond what it needs into a realm where the reality principle is seemingly in abeyance. Nothing now governs what it does. "We subject ourselves," he says, summing up this analogy, "*to want without being in want; and such is the case of masturbators.*" Driven by imagination and not nature, masturbators come unmoored from social and even physiological necessity, unencumbered and autarkic: masturbation is, by its nature, excessive and abusive. "It is all the more dangerous because one has incessantly the possibility of giving oneself over to it," the standard nineteenth-century French medical dictionary tells us.[83]

In the eighteenth century, masturbation seemed more and more to look like what we would call addiction; it enslaved just like alcohol, drugs, or some other object of unquenchable desire. Its intellectual heritage had roots not so much in old-fashioned concupiscence as in the Platonic trope of the ever-emptying jars — "of the souls of fools where their appetites are located." Like the masturbator's appetite, these souls could not be sated; the more they were indulged, the more they demanded indulgence. *Onania* is full of letters from those who tried to stop but found it impossible to "keep the mind free from sinful, or at least from vain and foolish imagination"; others report masturbating eight times in one hour, which, far from quenching the fire, "blew it into a flame." An autopsy report purported to show that a girl died from "insuperable" desire and titillation, made evident on her dead body by the state of her clitoris. "Nothing can be more ensnaring," we are told.[84]

With only slight changes, Tissot's accounts of masturbation could have come from a modern twelve-step program: "Many efforts are necessary to conquer a habit which every moment

recalls to the imagination . . . The sight of any female object creates desire in me . . . My filthy soul is but too much disposed to
represent incessantly to my fancy objects of concupiscence . . . I
combat [it] — but the conflict exhausts me . . . If I could find some
way of diverting my thoughts . . . I believe my cure would be at
hand." Tissot remembered a fellow student at Geneva who had
arrived at such a "pitch in the practice of these abominations, that
he was incapable of abstaining from them." A watchmaker reported that his soul was a slave to masturbation despite the weakness he felt with every repetition; he says he "was incapable of
forming any other idea, and the repetition of the crime became
every day more frequent." A piteous lad of six or seven had been
taught the vice by a servant; his "rage for the act" was so great
that "he could not be restrained from it the very last days of his
life," but when, as he lay dying, he was told that masturbation
would hasten his death, he was consoled by the thought that he
would all the sooner meet his dead father in heaven. Eighteenth-
and nineteenth-century observers talked about masturbation with
the same combination of moral repulsion and grudging sympathy
with which we view drug addiction. Their point is that there were
no natural limits to this vice; unlike other desires — for food, for
drink, even for heterosexual intercourse — this one produced only
more desire, not its fulfillment.[85]

The language of addiction and of masturbation quickly came
together. Tissot had talked about a young man who "had given
way to masturbation" when he was fifteen and by the time he
was twenty-three "was in a kind of intoxication." Thomas Trotter,
credited with the classic account of alcoholism, regarded the
addiction on which his fame rests very much in Tissot's terms. It
results in "sudden death, apoplexy, palsy, dropsy, madness and
a hideous list of mental disquietudes and nervous failings." It is
born of the same cultural milieu: "the present state of society
where human kind is almost taken out of the hands of nature . . .
[where] fashion now rules everything." Artifice, in short, sets up a
slippery slope to addiction, and the alcoholic, like the masturbator, "forsakes his former friends, [and] seems to shun his honorable acquaintances."[86]

239

But addiction to masturbation seemed even more insidious than addiction to spirits because its stimulant was always available in the sensual hothouse of the mind. Licensing, control of hours, economic cost that regulated the supply of opium and drink were of no avail. Each bout encouraged the next, one arousal made the next more likely, and a feedback loop to the genitals made a fall into addiction almost inevitable: "A soul ceaselessly caught up in voluptuous thoughts causes the animal spirits to be carried to the genitals, which by repeated touches become more labile [*mobile*] and more obedient to the dissolutions of the imagination." This, says the *Encylopédie*'s entry on masturbation, results in more erections, orgasms, spasms, and convulsions in a cascade of excess. Sixty years later, a considerably less elevated source spoke in the same terms: the genitals "become so familiarized to the dictates of the imagination that they are ever more readily excited into action by this morbid and vitiated influence." The solitary vice produces "that kind of lust or appetite which grows with what it feeds on," warns an early-nineteenth-century self-help tract. "You who are addicted to the solitary vice," intones another, should realize that it is a well-known fact among physiologists that masturbation excites and agitates the system much more than sexual intercourse: "In consequence of the facilities to repeat the crime, and the delusion it causes, [it] makes rapid inroads on the constitution."[87]

By the nineteenth century, this language had made its way out of medicine into the reflections of sensitive souls. When I first mentioned the fact that the Russian critic Vissarian Belinsky had started to masturbate as an over-stimulated university student suddenly exposed to Schiller and Byron (see p. 62), I did not give the rest of the story. It began when the anarchist Mikhail Bakunin confessed to him at the beginning of the two young men's friendship that he had recently triumphed in a major psychic struggle and was now ready for a full spiritual life. He had been an onanist, he announced as a gesture of intimacy and openness, and was finally cured. Not to be outdone in this duel of mutual revelation, Belinsky reported that he, too, had masturbated, that he had begun in just that stage of life when Bakunin had freed himself from the habit. When Belinsky was nineteen and a student at university, poetry had done him in. This was serious one-upmanship of suffering and moral turpitude. Belinsky's imagination had been unbearably pricked, he told his new friend, his whole body had shaken with fever and heat, and his only escape from the "disgusting dream" into which literature had thrust him had been the even more disgusting reality of masturbation. Finally he weaned himself, slowly and methodically, like an addict in a self-help group: first he limited himself to two times a week, then once a month, then once a year. His excuse was straight out of *Onania*: Belinsky said that he acquired the habit because he was too shy to take up with girls and that he had continued it because he could not stop once he had started. After these revelations, the two men became "eternal friends" because they had been so honest and open about their struggles, so revealing in their blushes and downcast looks. There is, of course, a heavy air of homoeroticism about all this, but the explicit context is the romantic notion that friendship is grounded on the baring of souls. There is nothing, however, in the tone of their exchange to suggest the ironic comedy of the *Seinfeld* episode — about which more later — in which the main characters make a bet as to who can keep from masturbating the longest. The nineteenth century's horror had become the late twentieth century's joke.[88]

Alcoholism and onanism were linked at many levels in the eighteenth and nineteenth centuries. The Wellcome Library's copy of Tissot, for example, was bound with another work on masturbation and once belonged to the Society for the Study of Addiction, formerly the Church Temperance Society. A French medical dictionary in 1826 defined *abus* as the improper use of something, as, for example, "abus des liqueurs alcooliques" or "de soi même," the abuse of alcoholic drinks or self-abuse. In fact, this notion of masturbation as by nature excessive, compulsive, unstoppable carries right through the nineteenth century into the twentieth. Masturbation is "in the same proportion more dangerous, as one can engage in it incessantly," said another French dictionary published in the period when Freud was a medical student in Paris.[89]

241

The young Sigmund Freud could draw on an almost two-century-long tradition when he wrote in a letter to his best friend, Wilhelm Fliess, that masturbation was the primary — meaning, I think, the prototypical or model — addiction, for which later addictions like those to tobacco, to alcohol, to morphine, or, in Dostoyevsky's case, to gambling were a substitute. Onanism sets the self and the body on this dangerous track, just as marijuana supposedly sets its users on the road to heroin. Indeed, "moderate masturbation," writes a twentieth-century French doctor active in a variety of socialist and other causes, "is an illusion in the same way that moderate opium addiction or moderate cocaine addiction are illusions." The alcoholic, le morphinomane, and the masturbator are on the same road to ruin, thought this doctor, a self-consciously progressive man on sexual matters, in 1926.[90]

The cry of the addict suffuses the most intimate, private agonies of the early-twentieth-century masturbators whose voices we hear in the letters to Marie Stopes, the proponent of sexual happiness in marriage, asking her what they might do. "During the past year I have been making frantic efforts to pull myself together," writes one man; in a bad month, it happens every six days or so. "Is there anything I can do apart from constant efforts at self-control?" he pleads. "Impossible for me now to shake off the vice," writes another. Would circumcision help? "I have it more or less under control," says another; "at last practically succeeded in breaking the habit," but not before he was a physical wreck. Sometimes Stopes got cheerier news; like an alcoholic at an AA meeting announcing how long he has been free from drink, one reformed masturbator writes triumphantly in 1929 that there has "not been a single instance where I've had recourse to masturbation since the end of 1915." Another thanks her for her books, the thoughts of which "often help [him] overcome a terrible craving to give way to self-abuse."[91]

Psychological and physiological accounts for why substance abusers and self-abusers found it so difficult to kick the habit have coexisted for centuries. As late as 1923, a major English reference book offered an account that did not differ too much from that in the Encyclopédie. First the imagination fires up the system. In men, masturbation initially has the same effect as coition, but when it is frequently repeated, it causes prostatic congestion, which sends signals to the brain, which sends signals back, resulting in "*hyperesthesia* such that a vicious cycle is formed." In women, it seems to work the same way, although it is not clear what, in the absence of a prostate, sends up the signal. And as for "psychic masturbation" — here we are firmly back on eighteenth-century turf — the higher parts of the brain send signals to the "sexual centers," which send signals to the genitals, just as in regular coition; but because the act is repeated so often, these higher centers become hyper-irritated. So, it "takes stronger and stronger mental images to arouse them to activity." "The nervous drain upon the higher centers can be easily imagined."[92] From the eighteenth to the twentieth century, moderate masturbation, like moderate heroin use, seemed impossible. To masturbate was to masturbate excessively, to be in the throes of unquenchable desire.

This view was inherent in the logic of solitary sex, driven as it was by the imagination, practiced outside social restraints, standing at the beginnings of a modern sense of secrecy. And empirical observations seemed to confirm it. Or rather, genuinely compulsive masturbation, for which there was, and is, good evidence, was construed as a version of ordinary masturbation. The most egregious, florid cases, which we would regard as the result of an independent, radical collapse of inhibition, were generally interpreted in the eighteenth and nineteenth centuries as a consequence of the act itself. We have already seen this way of thinking at work: the dying six-year-old boy Tissot recorded who could not stop masturbating; his fellow student who masturbated compulsively. The tradition continued. Of all the horrors encountered by a nineteenth-century medical student who wrote his thesis on masturbation, a shepherdess who was so much the "victim of her imagination" that the mere sight of a man sent her into "voluptuous spasms" made him most aghast. She would even engage in self-pollution while he was trying to take her pulse! The modern reader might think that there could scarcely be a better way for her to show anger and hostility toward her doctor and the hospital. Patients today seem to follow in her footsteps. Or maybe, a

modern clinician would guess, she had the neurochemical im-
balances associated with OCD, obsessive-compulsive disorder. But
the nineteenth-century medical student interpreted the girl's behavior as ordinary masturbation's predictable next stage, in which
the imagination had become a bit further unhinged from reality.[93]

The notorious, sad, but mercifully tiny number of nineteenth-
century cases in which girls who masturbated obsessively were
subjected to clitoridectomy or clitoral cauterization also seemed
to support the equation of self-stimulation with excess and its
near-total triumph over the psyche. Inflamed by the imagination,
the girls had fallen so far that even the guilt and shame born
of secrecy no longer restrained them from the most desperate
means to gain satisfaction. They represented the far limits, and
modern commentators have made too much of them as typical of
the ways in which nineteenth-century doctors dealt with masturbation. Tissot and his successors were normally more gentle in
their treatment. But the abyss of psychic anarchy loomed before
those who thought about even ordinary solitary sex. Or rather,
the private vice always hinted at its extremes.[94]

Doctors were not making up cases of spectacular excess.
Whether people compulsively masturbated in public before masturbation assumed its place on the frontiers of civilization we do
not know, just as we do not know what people with Tourette's
syndrome shouted in periods and places where explicit sexual
language was not as transgressive as it is today. But we do know
that compulsive and very public masturbation exists in our age.
A thirty-six-year-old man at a hospital in Israel was successfully
treated with serotonergic drugs when he asked doctors to castrate
him because, he said, he was consumed with thoughts of masturbating in public and could not stop himself from masturbating
despite feeling both guilt and anxiety about his fantasies. He low-
ered his trousers and masturbated outside the doctor's office. A
mildly disabled woman stopped compulsive public masturbation
after she started taking lithium carbonate. Children are sometimes subjected to all manner of tests for organic problems when
in fact their flushing, pallor, and short-term weakness are due to
masturbation.[95]

In other words, Tissot and his colleagues probably saw what they reported seeing. But they interpreted the exceptional cases that came to their attention as representative of solitary sex in all its many ordinary contexts. Secret and outside the constraints of both nature and culture, masturbation could not, in their eyes, be anything but excessive, out of control, addictive: a debilitating habit. Exceptional instances of truly compulsive, unstoppable masturbation that did, in fact, fly in the face of civilized behavior only proved the rule. In the crazed person of the obsessive public masturbator they saw everyone who had ever given in to the secret vice.

Masturbation was a peculiar vice born of three paradoxes that weave their way through each of my sections on what specifically so disturbed those who created modern masturbation. It was not just a solitary vice but *the* solitary vice, and yet it supposedly reached pandemic proportions because it circulated endlessly and freely from one masturbator to the next. We are not born into solitary sex; we learn it from others, and there seemed to be no resistance, no immunity to its diffusion because it was so easy: nothing more was needed than the imagination and a hand. Second, it was not just a secret vice but *the* secret vice, and yet those guilty of it were not at all secretive about their crime until they learned it was shameful and deserved the most severe punishment from an avenging nature. Unlike other vices, it seemed harmless enough and socially inconsequential until someone in authority pointed out that precisely the opposite was the case. And, finally, it was thought to be antisocial in the sense that it hindered the enjoyment of normal, healthy heterosexual pleasure, and yet it was all too social in that it encouraged perverse and libertine sexuality and was fostered in communities beyond the control of the authorities.

The problems with masturbation fed off those psychological, social, and moral virtues that created the modern self. It was a vice of paradox. Now the question is, finally, why all this happened: Why did the age of reason and enlightenment create so peculiar and novel a vice?

245

CHAPTER FIVE

Why Masturbation Became a Problem

We are finally ready to account for why masturbation burst so spectacularly onto the scene in the early eighteenth century. But even now I ask readers, once more, to be patient. For every explanation a more fundamental, tantalizingly more satisfying one always lies just one layer down. If we can account for why the guiltiness of some action or thought was widely broadcast by those who created guilt in our culture, we are still left to account at a psychological level for why people actually came, or ceased, to *feel* guilty: perhaps the consequence of repressed infantile sex, as Freud suggests. But this and other psychological theories have broadly cultural explanations. There is always one more question: "Why all the interest in sexuality or in the body to begin with?"[1] Let me therefore be clear about what I want to explain, about the parameters of my explanation, and about how many elephants standing on turtles, as the old story of what holds up the earth goes, I plan to expose.

First, I want to account specifically for those things about masturbation that became so disturbing after 1712. My question in this chapter might be reframed as follows: Why was masturbation reconfigured from its amorphous, varied, and not terribly pressing earlier construals — as a species of unnatural sex, as one among many possible signs of concupiscence, one among many ways to rid the body of a surplus fluid, a relatively minor infringement on chastity, a lapse in the sumptuary laws of sexual propriety, a non-reproductive sexual act, an embarrassing joke — into the paradigmatically fraught mix of fantasy and the imagination, secrecy and

247

solitude, addiction and excess writ upon the body that we saw it become? The old associations did not go away, but I will not account for the many instances in which they resurfaced. This is because, as I argued in Chapter 3, there is such a thing as "modern masturbation," because I have already explained why solitary sex was problematic as an element of more important problems within other earlier sexual regimes; and because some of the old explanations are still relevant today. Masturbation jokes at the expense of hapless characters in contemporary films are not so very different from Aristophanes's, Juvenal's, or Martial's.

My explanation will therefore be framed in terms of the three features of masturbation — its claim on the imagination and fancy, its secrecy and solitude, its tendency to excess and addiction — that came to be regarded as threatening in the eighteenth century and have remained exigent ever after. With only slight modifications, they became the foundation for a new, redemptive masturbation in the late twentieth century. I will therefore not dwell on lots of other local explanations that account for why a particular writer or group took on the problem at some time over two hundred years: why seminal loss or the nonreproductive qualities of masturbation became especially problematic in nineteenth-century American or French contexts or how the introduction of the notion of irritability and sensibility in medicine helped create new anxieties about solitary sex. I regard the association of other deviant forms of sexuality like homosexuality with masturbation not as a cause but as an example of how the new vice came to represent almost every conceivable form of illicit sexual pleasures and desires. All these explanations of the evils of masturbation stem, I suggest, from more fundamental ethical issues.

Second, my explanation will proceed by reversing the terms of the pre-Enlightenment history of masturbation, where other questions in the ethics of the body were far more pressing. The Jewish tradition, classical Antiquity, and Christian teaching all regarded sexuality as a deeply social phenomenon, one that had to be understood in terms of the human relationship to a transcendental order. What mattered was with whom one had sex, how, and when. Then, sometime around 1712, the question of autoeroticism became exigent because the relationship between the individual and a newly emerging social order became deeply problematic. Masturbation is a moral problem of the modern self, a reflection of the very deepest problems of modern life. Conversely, modernity in certain of its critical aspects, through the social world it created, invented — one might even say needed — the problem of solitary sex.

The next steps are to argue that fiction and the imagination, secrecy and solitude, excess and addiction became so clamorously important because they were important in the making of a new cultural landscape and finally to explain the connection. Near the very beginning of this book, I said that it was not an accident that *Onania* was published in the same decade as Defoe's first novels and the first stock-market crashes. I might have added that it was published within two decades of the foundation of the Bank of England in 1694, in the same age as the vast expansion of coffeehouses and newspapers, in the decades that saw Mandeville and Hume defend luxuries, within a lifetime of the tulip mania. If I were pressed to come up with one sentence to explain why masturbation became a problem, it would be, "Because it represented, in the body, some of the deepest tensions in a new culture of the marketplace; solitary sex was to civil society what concupiscence had been in the Christian order." If I were allowed to add a sentence, it would be, "Masturbation hijacked some of the central virtues of civil society and transformed them into evils; it was the dark underbelly of a new social and cultural order that seemed to threaten its very core."

This is as far down as the turtles and the elephants go.

Some Ground Clearing, Major and Minor
I begin with the claim that there is no explanation, then turn briefly to explanations that are simply wrong, and finally address those that do explain, at certain times, some aspects of the new centrality of masturbation but that need to be put within a more general framework. (Readers who want to skip these engagements with other views and go straight to my own should turn to p. 276.)

First of all, there is an explanation in history. Endemic paranoia, the eternal need for a scapegoat, another round of the
return of the repressed will not do. Nor can the question be
fobbed off as some ill-understood, slightly mysterious social phenomenon more akin to an act of nature than to the work of
culture. We are not dealing here with a "great fear," seemingly
irrational, disproportionate to immediate provocation, virulent
while it lasts, and then gone. The advent of modern masturbation;
in other words, is not like a peasant revolt sparked by a bad
harvest or a new tax; in fact, peasant revolts were not all that irrational or lacking deeper causes either. If there had been no
Onania, there would still have been a worry about masturbation;
although once the book existed, its views were reinforced by the
social mechanisms through which any belief might be sustained.
Every doctor who supported the view added "evidence"; every
patient who believed a doctor added more. And then, just as mysteriously, the process is reversed, without a deeper explanation.
This is a more elaborated version of the view that the rise and
purported fall of the masturbation problem is akin to that of hem-
lines: a question of fashion. It "probably came and went with a
tide of lay belief...it was invented in the eighteenth century by
the sensationalistic *Onania* and died at the beginning of the twentieth century for no better reason."[2] Fashions are sustained by all
sorts of things, but nothing very important accounts for why one
style succeeds another except for novelty itself.[3] But, if the problem is that of modernity, it did not mysteriously appear or dis-
appear, and its causes go beyond this or that contingency or
supposed correlation of masturbation with something else.

There is the claim, for example, that the incidence of venereal
disease rose in the early eighteenth century and that there was an
increase in masturbation to avoid getting sick. We have already
argued that greater incidence of the practice was not what disturbed contemporaries. But also, we have no evidence that its
incidence rose at all, though it might have, and we certainly have
no evidence that such a purported rise was due to a new worry
about venereal disease. If anything, VD was less virulent in 1700
than it had been a century earlier. And even if there were more

masturbation as a substitute for dangerous heterosexual intercourse, such an increase would not elevate solitary satisfaction
into a major moral problem. Nor does the decline in witchcraft
as a cause of madness and a new interest in its physical causes
account for new medical interest in masturbation as an alternative
cause. Western medicine since Hippocrates has almost always
looked for natural causes for disease, mental illnesses included,
and, in any case, no sources offer even a hint that masturbation
replaced witchcraft or magic as an explanation. Nor was the reason for the collapse of the "masturbatory hypothesis" in the late
nineteenth and the early twentieth century due to the realization
of how common the practice was and thus how unlikely that it
could be the cause of so many ills. On the contrary, the unimag-
ined, undreamed-of prevalence of onanism is part of the structure
of the whole phenomenon: a universal secret waiting to be discovered and tamed. It was thought to be universal in 1712, still so
regarded in 1900, and still centuries later in 2002.[4]

Similarly, there is the view that masturbation rose as a purported cause of disease because of the paucity of other explanations, and then fell because other explanations became more
plausible. Of course, the new masturbatory etiology thrived in the
absence of better explanations for lassitude, tuberculosis, fevers,
acne, irregular heart rhythms, madness, and much else. But these
complaints were nothing new, and they had existed without
masturbation as their cause for millennia; none became suddenly
problematic in the Age of Reason. At the modern end of the story,
new explanations for some diseases — bacteria as the cause of consumption, for example — made masturbation a less attractive one.
But there were, and are, plenty of mysterious ailments of a general sort that lack specific explanations: chronic fatigue syndrome,
headaches and muscle aches, depression, and obsessive behavior,
for example. Under the right cultural conditions, they could as
well be attributed to solitary sex as to a type A personality, mysterious unidentified viruses, anxiety, or radiation from high-tension
electric lines. Nothing in the history of medicine accounts for the
shift of focus in the early twentieth century away from masturbation as a major cause of unexplained ailments. If what now seems

so manifestly organic and florid a disease as schizophrenia could still be attributed to certain patterns of family behavior or inadequate mothering in the 1970s, there is, in principle, plenty of room for masturbatory madness today.[5]

I do not deny that medicine helped sustain the seemingly endless conversation about masturbation. Once a constellation of behaviors and attitudes came to be regarded as wicked, threatening, or antisocial and once such deviance was thought to have recognizable signs and symptoms — jangled nerves, obsession, seminal loss, and lethargy, for example — it was not difficult to link suspect acts and moral failure with real or putative diseases. This is especially true because the lines between pathophysiology and politics were — and to some extent still are — blurred: slaves who tried to escape were said to have an "obtuse sensibility of the body" that produced "rascality"; the working classes in the late nineteenth century were thought prone to alcoholism, drug addiction, and crime because of measurable "degenerative" traits. Other anxieties, too — the very real danger of bankruptcy or social collapse in the unpredictable, raw capitalist culture of late-nineteenth-century America, for example — were translated into threats to the body. A seminal economy seemed to mirror that of shops and markets; the importance of careful husbandry of resources in one realm was reflected in the other. So, waste of money and waste of semen did not seem so terribly different, and losses in both realms could be disastrous.[6] In short, a moral vision translated into the body undoubtedly produced a self-verifying, ever-lengthening list of complexly interrelated ills.

Each "successful" exposure of these kinds of diseases sustained the moral vision that was the foundation of the diagnostic process. Syndromes make signs and symptoms cohere. Once established as an entity, the syndrome sustains its premises. Each case of a lethargic, depressed, ill-nourished, hostile, or consumptive teenager who had masturbated demonstrated yet again the danger of the solitary vice. Diagnoses of madness from masturbation in German asylums made the same diagnosis in Canada or Philadelphia seem reasonable. Everywhere the incarcerated insane masturbated; everywhere adolescent sufferers from many com-

plaints admitted to doctors and parents that they had masturbated; everywhere tired men and women confessed that they had
done it too. *Post hoc, ergo propter hoc* has great appeal, and the
occasional skeptical comment directed against the whole idea of
masturbatory disease fell on deaf ears until well into the twentieth century.[7]

But neither physiological theories nor the sociology of belief
and of diagnosis explains why medicine took up the cause of a
heretofore-obscure form of sexual gratification in the first place.
They also do not account for the philosophical, and more broadly
cultural, attention to solitary sex that began in the Enlightenment
and continues to our day. It is not difficult to understand why,
once the masturbatory hypothesis was in place, doctors and lay-
people continued to believe that the secret vice was debilitating,
if not deadly. It is more difficult to plumb the reservoirs of anxiety
that sustained the centuries-long intense interest in the subject.

There are other historical explanations that offer us very little
but that do take us away from medicine and its foibles: for example, the Protestant Reformation or various of its children —
like Puritanism or evangelicalism — raised the level of anxiety and
guilt about sexuality generally, which then made itself felt in various practices, including masturbation. This view has one great
merit in that it points to the fact that the anxiety about masturbation was almost entirely the creation of Protestants: John Marten
and his *Onania*, the Genevans Tissot and Rousseau, Kant, Campe,
and the German reforming pedagogues. Alternatively, the worry
about masturbation might be regarded as a kind of Protestant
counterphobic reaction: or it comes up as an aspect of the attack
on Catholics and their views of celibacy and chastity. Masturbation and worse are the practices of a religion that proscribes
healthy sex. This was Voltaire's entry into the subject. But the
association between masturbation and Protestantism had very
little if anything to do with the question of sexual guilt generally
nor, as Lawrence Stone suggested, with evangelicalism in particular. The resistance to solitary pleasure stands in sharp contrast to
a much wider acceptance of secular heterosexual pleasure that
came to be regarded not just as a defense against concupiscence

but as a good thing for its own sake or for the sake of marital harmony and good feeling. Progressive thinking, whether Protestant or Catholic, stood on the side of reforming traditional sexual morality, not reinforcing it. Anyway, evangelicalism came on the scene too late to explain how things started. The striking thing about the extraordinary new attention to masturbation is that it was the product *not* of old guilts and anxieties about sexuality but of their collapse in some circles. Protestantism may be connected to the masturbation problem through its deep and much-debated links to individualism and to the freeing of desire, but that is taking us into a whole other aspect of the history of modernity. As an explanation for the rise and fall of worry about masturbation, Protestantism will not do.[8]

A more historically precise account links a new anxiety about homosexuality in the early eighteenth century — "a failure to engage in appropriate heterosexual" relations would be more precise — with the new problem of solitary sex. The argument goes as follows. There were vigorous persecutions of male homosexuals and even occasionally of women across Protestant northern Europe, the territory of the new masturbation. Coming in batches — 1730–1732, 1764, 1776–1777, 1795–1798 — the number of prosecutions for sodomy in the eighteenth-century Netherlands, for example, was four times the number in the previous centuries. There are no good comparable figures for England, but it appears that new ways of prosecuting sodomites gained favor in the eighteenth century and produced more convictions: prosecutions for "assault with intent" were more than double the number of the older kind of prosecution of sodomy as a felony, which was much harder to prove, and this allowed the authorities to bring offenders within their reach.[9] (One ought not to make too much of this, however; no one has examined systematically the incidence of prosecution for other sorts of "unnatural sex" that were proscribed by law. In Sweden, for example, only twenty cases of homosexuality were tried in the courts between 1630 and 1734, but more than fifteen hundred cases of bestiality were tried in roughly the same period, 1630–1750, with 470 death sentences. Homosexual prosecutions in Holland or England may or may not be correlated with bestiality prosecutions, and if they are, this would suggest that normative heterosexuality was not the, or not the only, driving force behind the former. Sweden quietly dropped homosexuality from its criminal code in 1734 because to include it might, reformers argued, have given people ideas. Silence was the wiser policy.) In short, roughly coincident with the rise of sodomy trials in some places was an intense new interest in masturbation.

Putting these two observations together, we get the claim that "straight and narrow heterosexuality was bounded on one side by the avoidance of sodomy, the avoidance of masturbation lay on the other." When James Boswell felt pangs of guilt at having masturbated, he swore not only to stop doing it but also to "never pleasure but with a woman's aid." In other contemporary sources, masturbation was construed as precisely this sort of deviation for both men and women; it kept men and women from the appropriate venue of pleasure that was the marriage bed, or at the very least the bed of heterosexual union. For men, though not for women, the solitary vice also made its appearance precisely when a major reconfiguration of masculinity was in full swing. The old sorts of male friendships — eroticized, physically intimate, perhaps even consummated — had become suspect or worse. The secret vice thus seemed to track new anxieties about the collapse of decent heterosexuality; or, more accurate, it became a matter for serious concern at the same time that new standards of heterosexual masculinity appeared. Masturbation in this story is a special case of a more general revolution in what was considered right and proper for men and *perhaps* by extension for women.[10] The explanation for a new heterosexuality — not in itself a trivial matter — will account for our vice as one of its defining boundaries.

There is considerable evidence for the linkage itself. To begin with, masturbation shared the closet in the eighteenth century with men's love for other men. "What is this secret; this untold tale?" asks one monk of another in Horace Walpole's tragedy *The Mysterious Mother*, referring directly to murder and sexual transgression but in a wider context to the secret loves of its author. Erotic male friendship and the private vice shared the sexual secrecy that became so important a part of modern consciousness.

Masturbation and homosexuality will share coming out of the closet in the late twentieth century.[11]

There is more. Eighteenth-century jokes at the expense of the sodomite veer off easily into digs at onanism. "Of Crimes and the Man I sing" starts a satire of the unfortunate Mr. Foote, who was tried for buggering his servant:

> Sodomy old, see at the van appear
> Polluting Onan fly, brings up the rear.

or

> He tampers in subordinate degree
> And Onan introduces sodomy.[12]

Perhaps the writers of this attack on a prominent man of the theater knew of rabbinic commentaries that identified Onan's sin with Tamar as penetrating her ground, that is, anus, or as more vaguely linked to the sins of Sodom. In any case, Onan stands well outside the gates of normal heterosexuality. The sense that masturbation was the foul, guilty alternative to taking one's pleasure as one should became explicit in much eighteenth-century writing on the subject. "An abominable and *unmanly* practice," Robert James's *Medicinal Dictionary* labels "*manustrapratio*" in 1745, after having announced that it constitutes a vice, very near the words of Oscar Wilde on homosexuality, "not decent to name."[13] "Of this crime in WOMAN HATERS," reads a section heading of *Eronania*; "Of those wicked Clubs and Societies of Women Haters," "Of ABUSERS OF THEMSELVES WITH MANKIND — MOLLES," the table of contents promises, although nothing further is said on the subject. *The Crime of Onan* promises to explain the meaning of "MOLLES — an ugly word enough" — by then used in the English form "mollies" to refer to cross-dressing homosexuals — in connection with self-defilement, but again, this is a tease. One masturbator whose letter is quoted in *Onania* reports that when he finally did get a girl to his room, he panicked; he "did not so much as salute her" and instead once more gave himself over to self-pollution. A father writes that his son's "one passion" is self-pollution and that in consequence he has recently refused marriage to a woman with £17,000. (This is odd in many respects: the crazy decision, the fact that the boy apparently also whores around. But still the theme of failed masculinity is there.)

By the nineteenth century, these associations had become canonical. Larousse's *Grand Dictionnaire* took as two exemplary uses of the word *onanisme* the following: (1) "Love for love's sake leads to pederasty, Onanism, and prostitution"; and (2) "*Onanism* has as its corollary bestiality*." Both are from Pierre-Joseph Proudhon, the anarchist who coined the phrase "Property is theft," exerted an enormous influence on modern French working-class radicalism, and was a well-known misogynist besides.[14] Of course, these examples cover much more than homosexuality or even deviance from heterosexuality; Proudhon's views on what counted as acceptable were circumscribed to say the least. But the neighborhood is marked out. Connection, of course, does not make causality, but we are closer to explaining the modern discovery of the secret vice if we can place it as part of the broader phenomenon of failed heterosexuality with elaborate genealogies of its own.

Women fit much less well onto this sodomy/masturbation axis, but they, too, seemed seduced from the paths of heterosexual satisfaction by taking their pleasures alone. *Onania* offers many examples. Doing it alone, reported an inveterate masturbator who had begun at age eleven, was better than lying with her husband; "we shamefully pleasured one another," says a girl about herself and her servant. Tissot thinks the problem is greater for women than for men: "A common symptom in both sexes... more frequent among women is the indifference which this infamous practice leaves for the lawful pleasures of Hymen." That said, the case in point is a man who was taught to masturbate by his preceptor and then developed an aversion toward the marriage bed. More generally, Tissot thought, the debility caused by the secret sin made boys and girls mutually unattractive: dull eyes, rickety body, the end of a youthful complexion and plumpness, without which even beauty led only to "cold admiration."

257

These are the Uriah Heeps of the next century, the sallow-skinned, weak creatures — epicene at best — who are useless in normal heterosexual life. "Woman has no real charms for the miserable being who no longer controls his passions"; The polluted imagination destroys all.[15] Conversely, women come to prefer the "odious practice" to the "legitimate and rapturous enjoyments which are followed neither by agony, nor remorse, nor punishment, nor peril." The, to us, implausible claim that the consequences of the "fashionable vice of young women" were more dangerous and painful than the likely results of heterosexual intercourse — pregnancy and childbirth — is less important here than the anxiety that masturbation leads, at best, to female celibacy.[16] We are on a track now that leads with various twists and turns to the eve of the twentieth century. Krafft-Ebing explicitly regarded masturbation as a cause of that complex of *feelings* that constituted "inversion." (Only rarely were there physical signs of inversion or putative brain pathology.)[17] Other well-known physicians offer case after case in which homosexuality — uranism in their terms — and masturbation were linked. One young man consumed with guilt about his play with his genitals confessed to an older classmate who "enlightened me, reassured me, and formed a connection with me" that led to mutual masturbation. Another "congenital invert" reported that he had never been interested in girls; he began masturbating at thirteen, found his one effort at intercourse disgusting, and finally found his true sexual self when a monk initiated him into "the practices of inverted love." The connection is not made clear, but all accounts give details of masturbation as if this were a stage in the development of the full-blown perversion.[18]

Surveillance of masturbation in the public schools of late Victorian England may well have contributed to the making of a peculiar upper-class homosexual culture there. Certainly a sensitive boy first entering this world would have made the link. John Addington Symonds, the future historian and author of a book on Greek "inversions," was shocked at the state of Harrow in the 1840s: "Each good looking boy was someone's bitch or a common prostitute ... one could not avoid seeing acts of Onanism, mutual masturbation, the sports of wicked boys."[19] A generalized worry about homoerotic culture — masturbating on the banks of swimming holes, in dormitories, in shared bedrooms, or anywhere else adolescent boys congregated — was standard fare of pedagogical and medical literature on the solitary vice. And the cure for masturbatory disease would include reversing this tendency: possible marriage — "a heroic measure," says one source, because the onanist is so debilitated; a prostitute if necessary to set desire back on track. She should be "acquainted with the purpose intended"; she should be in good health. But all that being in order, "sleeping with a female revives the natural appetite" so that after a time "even the most debilitated recover their vigour." The notion that "real sex," however morally dubious it might be, was better for a man's health than masturbation would be long-lived. Freud sent his friend Fliess an early manuscript of his work on the etiology of neurosis in which he observed that masturbation causes neurasthenia in men; the more masturbation the more neurasthenia, and, conversely, "individuals who have been seduced by women at an early age have escaped neurasthenia." Freud cautions Fliess to keep this manuscript away from his young wife; this is a confidence between the boys.[20]

There is little of this for girls. The opportunities for group pleasures were fewer — far fewer in boarding establishments, far less opportunity to be off on their own. Still, the theme is there. Mary Wollstonecraft complained about the nasty habit in schools, and she was not the first. Mary Wood-Allen, the American doctor and writer of advice literature for girls, played the same card a century later; her warnings against masturbation and against excessively sentimental friendships with other girls come almost in the same breath.

For a number of reasons — old-fashioned religious connections between sodomy and masturbation, new standards of heterosexuality, worry about secrecy or the wrong kinds of sociability — we have our warrant for linking the two problems, the maintenance of heterosexuality and the danger of onanism. Even the question of the imagination makes its appearance. Baudelaire celebrates lesbians precisely because they are against nature — "great in their contempt of reality" — not in the Thomist sense that theirs is a sexual love that does not have reproduction as its end but because it is so much an act of the imagination. He takes on board the eighteenth century's analysis of what "contra naturum" means but reverses its moral signs. Masturbation might thus piggyback on a more general history, that of how homosexuality came to be regarded as newly threatening.[21]

There are, however, problems with this sort of joint history. First, sodomy and masturbation have been linked, as we have seen, through the ages. Fierce attacks on the one vice did not draw attention to the other except occasionally in a sort of marijuana-in-relation-to-the-hard-stuff way. In the Florentine and Venetian anti-sodomy campaigns, masturbation was not mentioned.[22] Thus we still have to account for why this particular new assault on sodomy should bring with it an unprecedented interest in another secret vice.

Second, there is the problem of gender. Sodomy — homosexuality in the language of some scholars — and a new standard of heterosexuality were regarded as almost entirely issues for men. The anxiety about masculinity and homosexuality finds no parallel in a public anxiety about lesbianism and little about femininity until the late nineteenth century; the dangers of masturbation, on the other hand, seemed acute for both sexes from the beginning. Any explanation will have to account for the novel, and sometimes paradigmatic, focus on girls and women masturbating and on knowledgeable female servants teaching them.

Finally, there is the problem of specificity. Yes, masturbation was seen in the company of homosexuality, but it was at least as often observed with hyper-heterosexuality — for both men and women, boys and girls — as well as with no sexuality at all, a sort of epicene sloth. It was the first step toward sexual excess and sexual degeneracy of all sorts; its role had expanded from being the seemingly innocent beginning of a life of sodomy among monks to being the worm in the bud for almost every evil. Perhaps this story became more floridly skewed toward women by the nineteenth century. Men who masturbated were often thought to be victims of a deep exhaustion that rendered them asexual or, worse, homosexual; women who succumbed to self-abuse were as likely to be diagnosed as hypersexual, because in the whole structure of thinking about female sexuality even the slightest hint of more than usual sexual interest could be interpreted as a sign of excessive desire. Generally speaking, however, in both sexes masturbation seemed as likely to cause, or be a sign of, too much, or too much inappropriate, desire for the opposite sex as too little.

John Marten, in his notorious *Gonosologium novum* — the proto-*Onania* — suggested that in the young of both sexes "the pleasures of love are quick and excessive" but that especially for pubescent girls who frequent men's company and are generally high-living masturbation may be not only benign but necessary for good health. He does not encourage early marriage because "other methods to allay the fury of their desires are better." Earlier, readers had been treated to details of clitoral stimulation. Whatever else might be said about this — there is clearly a fantasy of sex-starved girls living temporarily in a world of erotic autarky — it is solidly "heterosexist" in its general outlook.[23]

Onania is also full of reports of masturbation coexisting with aggressive interest in the opposite sex and worries about its dangers. One man writes in to say that he has been guilty of masturbation but wants medicine for the gleets caused by having intercourse with a woman during her menses. Another says that his father-in-law is making him wait two more years to cohabit with his thirteen-year-old bride and wonders whether "nature's handmaiden" might not see him through; he asks too for his friend, whose wife has recently eloped with someone. (Even our author expresses some doubts whether these stories are true, but that does not affect the point.) Much of this is straightforward adolescent stuff that we would recognize easily in our era: a few hours after being with the ladies, writes one boy, "it's hard to keep one's mind free from sinful, or at least, vain and foolish imagination." The constant refrain of *Onania Examined* is that masturbation is simply another form of fornication and ought not to be singled out, either morally or medically, and that *Onania* is indefensibly wrong in focusing so much attention on it. But *Onania* in its defense does make clear that self-pollution, among its many other evils, is the first step down another slippery slope: "Thousands have been guilty of *Adultry*, as well as *Fornication*, who would never have yielded to those temptations, which over-came them, if they had never been initiated in lasciviousness, and acquired to themselves a habit of Impurity by Self-Pollution." Nothing about masturbation as the bait for worse crimes like sodomy or "homosexuality."

Tissot cites case after case that links masturbation with hetero-sexual excess: the man who dies from his peculiar taste for having sex with prostitutes while standing up — much more demanding than doing it prone — is offered as evidence for how some factor, other than emission, can be harmful to health. He regards hetero-sexual venery and masturbation as on a continuum, the latter more debilitating than the former because it is, as we saw, by nature excessive. One reader wrote to Tissot thanking him for advice on how parents and young people "might preserve themselves from the violence of desires, which hurries them to excesses." (Not masturbating, of course, but eating right and getting plenty of exercise in the fresh air.) Among the surviving letters in the Tissot archives are confessions of patients who thought that excesses with women had compounded the damage of the solitary vice and others who saw it as the first step in their lives of debauchery.[24]

There was a "lesbian" inflection to the story of how, for women, masturbation was particularly dangerous — they forswore the marriage bed and found pleasure alone or in pairs — but more commonly solitary sex was thought to lead in the direction of sexual excess *tout court*. Of course, overt, seemingly uncontrol-lable desire was culturally much more fraught in women than in men, and it is not surprising that it was regarded as a pathology and given a name by the doctors: nymphomania. Before Bienville coined the word in 1768, Tissot had distinguished what he called "masturbation or manual pollution" from "that which may be called *clitorical*." This, he thought, was "sapphic" and seemed to refer to the famous contemporary cases of *tribades*, to whom "nature" had given a "semi-resemblance to men," which they abuse, "seizing the function of virility," "esteeming the gifts of nature, as to think they ought to abolish the arbitrary distinction of birth." The section ends with the claim that women who love women are every bit as passionate and jealous as those who love men but that he will now "conclude these shocking details." Little wonder that Rousseau found Tissot's warning against feminine autarky so appealing.[25]

Tissot's main illustration of these points comes from Juvenal's Satire 6, which recounts the orgies of the priapic maenads.[26] To be sure, these women reveled with one another, but that was only before the young men arrived on the scene. Masturbation as the prelude to a lesbian kingdom is, at best, only one strand in the original. There may be a continuous history of such images, one that still has resonance today. A recent study, for example, documents beautifully the centrality of clitoral stimulation in Renaissance images of sexually deviant and socially marginal women, specifically witches and prostitutes. These women are not engaged in the "solitary" vice, but they are finding pleasure in and among themselves. The threat they represent is, however, not lesbianism but the flagrant rejection of social norms, whether through prostitution or other kinds of deviance.[27]

Bienville's *Nymphomania*, a self-proclaimed almost sycophantic effort to extend Tissot's observations to women's sexual lives more generally, is resoundingly heterosexist. The fury that is nymphomania is, according to its "discoverer," a near relative of masturbation — a disease of the "disturbed motion of the fibres." It attacks those who are, or make themselves, vulnerable to wants that they cannot attain: "the younger part of the sex" whose "desperate passion" for a lover has been thwarted; "debauched girls" who have led voluptuous lives but are now bereft; widows sadly deprived of the sexual relations to which they had become accustomed; women who read "luxurious novels." In short, any female frustrated in her natural desires or those who have fanned the flames of passion into a fury that cannot be quenched will turn to masturbation. It then comes to be understood as both a symptom and a cause of nervous exhaustion: a major way to irritate the fibers without giving them what they really need. To be sure, some nymphomaniacs were thought by nineteenth-century doctors to be on the road to tribadism, i.e., genital rubbing with

other women. But most seemed to have been regarded as inveterate masturbators who lusted insatiably for men; two weeks in a
whorehouse might cure one unfortunate patient, suggested a doctor, half in jest, at a grand rounds.[28]

The story for men is similar. Although masturbation was not
usually thought of as the first step to satyriasis, it was generally
interpreted as both a sign and a cause of excessive and inappropriate heterosexual desire, not of homosexuality or reticence. Do
not be mistaken, pronounced the much-translated early twentieth-century sexologist Auguste Forel: masturbators are "not the
pale and terrified creatures" that tradition holds up to us but
"rather lewd individuals who are early transformed into im-
pudent Don Juans." The whole late-nineteenth-century purity
movement was based on the same assumption that had led John
Marten to regard masturbation as the first step to adultery and
fornication: solitary sex was practice for other kinds. Social purity
can triumph only when men pledge to treat all women with
respect and to keep themselves pure. This meant that, right from
the start, they had to renounce the most egregious of vices: self-
pollution. Here is Catharine MacKinnon's argument *avant la lettre*: impure thoughts and fantasies lead to impure acts. Obscene
companions, inappropriate and exciting books roused sensations
that were "too readily relieved in early life by secret vice" and
later in life by "illegitimate gratification of the passions." The great
amount of prostitution and incontinence in the world, wrote this
well-placed author, was "largely owing [to] the vice of masturbation in the young" — "the *first fall*" — and to the evil influences
that fed desire. Another writer, also connected with the most
prestigious of public schools, thought that masturbation was both
the "principal cause of immorality at schools" — that is, homosexuality — and the basis of all forms of sexual incontinence in adults.
Elizabeth Blackwell, the pioneer woman physician and "Christian
physiologist," thought that all unnatural vices sprang from two
"radical vices" — masturbation and fornication — and that one led
to the other.[29]

If not already in the eighteenth century then certainly by the
nineteenth, masturbation was linked with every conceivable sex-

ual deviance or purported deviance: Mary Cove thought it *both* caused "apathy of the sexual appetites, or its undue violence," and sent hundreds of thousands to their graves prematurely. Krafft-Ebing thought that masturbation led to certain sorts of homosexuality, but he also believed that the critical element that distinguished masturbation from coitus — the essential part played by the imagination — led to all sorts of other perversions and diseases as well. "Psychical Onanism" was, for him, synonymous with sexual fantasy in any circumstance that extended the empire of masturbation still further. Excessive masturbation, but also heterosexual precocity and debauchery at any age, was linked with hereditary as well as acquired madness, with degeneration, erotic paranoia — this more so in women — systemic immorality, and much more besides. Lesbianism, nymphomania, and masturbation merged easily into one another just as they had in earlier nineteenth-century discussions of prostitution. Did a woman become a prostitute because she was sexually insatiable, as evidenced by an enlarged clitoris? Was this congenital or caused by masturbation or by lesbianism? Did lesbianism and masturbation ensue when heterosexual intercourse was no longer satisfying or when it was not available? Or did prostitution arise from poverty with no links to any of this? No clarity here, but masturbation is at the heart of the problem. Every sort of worry about sexuality and society merged into every other: "Civilized man's" degradation of the sexual act — evident in masturbation, prostitution, and marital intercourse using contraception, that is, *all* sex for pleasure — was what produced all the horrible diseases of depravity, thought an influential group of Russian doctors before the Revolution. No end was in sight.

Causation worked in all directions. Onanism might result in homosexuality, but forced abstinence from same-sex partners could also push homosexuals into onanism, which, Krafft-Ebing thought, was itself unhealthy and a bad solution to problems faced by his patients. Some believed that their homosexuality kept them from the far more dangerous practice of masturbation, others that masturbation and excessive homosexual desire *together* led to neurasthenia. (One was so convinced of this, and so convinced that the only solution was castration, that when Krafft-Ebing demurred, he had the operation done elsewhere.) The most elaborate and the most paranoid fantasies grew out of this sort of hodgepodge. One commentator urged especial vigilance of girls and women just after they went to bed, not because of what one might see them do but because they seemed to be doing nothing. Only the most knowledgeable observer could detect the smallest hint of vice. "She has scarcely gone to bed ere she appears plunged in deep sleep," he warns, but do not be fooled. To most people this might be innocent enough, but "to a practiced observer" it is "always suspicious," luring parents into a false sense of security. The "marked exaggeration" with which she pretends to sleep can be exposed by "waking her" and noticing the perspiration not accounted for by the warmth of her cover and the hard, developed pulse. Never mind that no masturbation was noted in this wanton exercise of dissimulation.[30] Very little that might be regarded as deviant sexuality was *not* associated with masturbation, implicitly in the eighteenth century, explicitly by the late nineteenth century.

In fact, all deviancy and degeneration in the eyes of doctors and the general public seemed to have focused on masturbation. We could pile up example after hyperbolic example of individual and social implosion: "The masturbator loses eventually his moral faculties," writes a late-eighteenth-century German doctor, and after still further decline is "sunk to the level of the brutes," a mere shadow of a man. Johann Peter Frank, the father of the idea of a health police — an early version of public health officialdom — thought masturbation dangerous not only to the self but also to society and that the state should therefore figure out a way to put it under surveillance. Writing in the early nineteenth century, Pierre Jean Corneille Debreyne, the international authority on theology and medicine, compiled pages of the most horrendous moral consequences of solitary sex: loss of all the moral faculties, of intelligence, memory, vivacity, health, sociability — everything that makes us human. The great late-nineteenth-century theorists of degeneration could add little to this view. So, when Wagner wrote Nietzsche's doctor to offer his own interpretation of his former friend's physical collapse — in case the doctor had missed the clues — he suggested that the mad philosopher be treated on the assumption that his problems were the result of masturbation. A gifted young poet he had known had gone blind from the practice, and another had suffered complete nervous collapse as well as serious eye disease, Wagner informs Dr. Eiser, and so too the philosopher. Need he say more? Both young men, like Nietzsche, had broken with Wagner. One, he knew, had had a riding accident; the other was a homosexual.[31]

We have come a long way from the original hypothesis which suggested that the rise of concern about masturbation was an aspect of the rise of concern about homosexuality: masturbation became a problem because new boundaries for heterosexuality had to be secured, and any orgasmic act other than with a woman was reprehensible because it breached these fragile limits. It turned out, however, that the solitary vice was associated in the minds of physicians, educators, moralists, and ordinary people not only with sodomy but with every other sort of sexual and moral deviance as well. This does not mean that the histories of homosexuality and onanism are not linked. Both seemed to lie in the shadows of secrecy, excess, and the imagination. And both became newly exigent as the old constraints on sexuality crumbled. As the state and the Church lost their authority over sexual behavior, as sex literally became a private matter, other ways of regulating of all sorts of moral behavior took their place. Political history thus offers a potentially fruitful place to look for an explanation.

We might begin with the observation that *self*-government, which was so central to how masturbation came to be understood in the early eighteenth century, has to be understood as the opposite of the *external* government of mind and morals. In other words, as the purchase of natural restraints and a seemingly natural hierarchical political order underwritten by God and the heavens seemed to wane, the importance of individual reason, restraint, transparency, sensibility, imagination, and education waxed. How the individual was to become part of the new social order is the great problem of eighteenth- and nineteenth-century moral philosophy and political theory. But it could not be avoided, however it was answered. If, as Kant famously said, "enlightenment is man's emergence from his self-imposed immaturity," whose motto was "dare to know," then onanism was its negation: the solipsistic rejection of public life, control, and the imagination in the service of humanity and art in favor of a species of self-generated moral servitude if not actual madness. Neither "the freedom to use reason *publicly*" nor becoming a morally self-governing individual was an easy thing. At the best of times it was difficult, Kant knew, to distinguish between actions grounded in self-interest and those grounded in the categorical imperative. But solitary pleasure represented the worst of times, not only for Kant but also for everyone else who discussed such matters.[32]

The explosion of worry about masturbation is, however, only one — crucially important — aspect of the pedagogical project for creating morally self-governing human beings who are capable of living in the new public sphere of civil society. Contrast *die heimliche Sünde* with *die Öffentlichkeit*, "the secret sin" with "the public sphere," literally the state of being open. In specific political contexts, the question of the solitary vice comes to represent the dangers of the whole political project. It becomes a heated, emotionally fraught microcosm of the anxieties created by the advent of a post-absolutist order, of the *Rechtsstaat*. In Germany, *Selbstbefleckung*, "self-pollution," functioned, as one historian puts it, "as an inventory list where the advantages and disadvantages of the social principles of the Enlightenment were weighed against the advantages and disadvantages of the social principle of absolutism." It was the dark underbelly of civil society, its original sin. All those capacities and possibilities on which masturbation thrived — imagination, the desire for luxuries, reading, privacy — were those most necessary to the new political and social order. And they were at the same time capable of bringing it to moral ruin. The struggle against masturbation through education and through medical bullying was thus a struggle to keep the freedom and the desire on which the new order was predicated within ethically livable bounds. It is a battle that will be fought again and again wherever individual freedom threatens to devolve into social anarchy. What I say about eighteenth-century Germany could be translated to the nineteenth-century United States, where the

Frenchman Alexis de Tocqueville marveled at how civil society seemed to curb the potential excesses of liberty.[33]

It was a moral balancing act, and one can see its tensions in the person of someone who both helped create the new moral and political order and looked with horror on his creation: Joachim Heinrich Campe. Campe was a supporter of the French Revolution but feared the disquiet, or worse, that overthrowing absolutism unleashed. For himself, he preferred a modified old order. One can "live much more peacefully and happily" in a "well-ordered monarchical state under a just and wise prince" who governs not arbitrarily but according to the law than one can in the "tumultuous republic" that was France. He was happy he lived in Brunswick in just such a state under just such a prince. But Campe probably did more than any other eighteenth-century literary figure to fire the fantasy of the young and thus to create the sort of solitary reader who, lost in fictions, stood in mortal danger of self-abuse. If, as so many eighteenth- and nineteenth-century moralists thought, the novel paved the way to the solitary vice, then Campe's translation of Daniel Defoe's *Robinson Crusoe* led millions astray in every corner of the world print culture. Several hundred editions survive in all European languages and many Asian ones as well. But solitude given to fantasy was not the only problem this wildly popular novel unleashed. The lessons young readers might draw from the story are terribly intricate and ambiguous: Crusoe has often been regarded as the prototypical modern *homo economicus*, the man standing alone, free from social and indeed any outside moral constraint. The moral dangers of this character's world were the moral dangers of the masturbator. Into this world of danger that he helped to create Campe launched his collectively written multivolume guide to raising children and, more on point, a half dozen works on controlling the explosion of self-abuse that the new social order had unleashed. Moral self-government — powerfully represented in the capacity to renounce the pleasures one could give oneself alone — loomed large for a man whose work did so much to bring about the new cultural order that produced modern masturbation. His might be understood as a relatively conservative anti-masturbatory commitment, a fear of what masturbation revealed about people who are given moral autonomy rather than the progressive worry about what masturbation said about the effects of this freedom.[34]

There is much to be said for the view that modern masturbation is born from political transformation. Almost all the eighteenth-century literature we have been reviewing was written or published in Protestant or anticlerical circles in places where absolutism and the divine right of kings had lapsed or were under threat and specifically in places where public control of sexuality had collapsed. *Onania* was almost contemporaneous with the Society for the Reformation of Manners — the vice society — which tried desperately and unsuccessfully to fill the place of the Church courts, which until the late seventeenth century had exercised jurisdiction over matters that then became private morals. Thus efforts to control sexuality from within — and masturbation was considered the paradigmatic form of interior sexual desire — might be regarded as the modern alternative to older forms of communal, religious, judicial, and political control.

This political explanation for the rise of masturbation also articulates with the much more general argument made by Michel Foucault about changes during the late eighteenth and the early nineteenth century in how power came to be exercised in the Western world and how this shift played itself out in the making of modern subjectivity. The argument goes roughly as follows: the West witnessed a major shift away from the play of the sovereign's power over the body of the subject to what Foucault called "bio-power," the control by professionals of aspects of the inner being of men and women, boys and girls that these professionals had themselves helped to create as arenas for the exercise of power. This happened over a wide swath of modern society and was by no means restricted to matters of sexuality. Burial, for example, which had been the domain of the Church, became death, recorded and analyzed by doctors and other secular authorities; baptism became birth. And together these became "vital statistics," the raw materials of the census and of all that was built on this newly elaborated instrument. Homosexuality became a medical condition, as did prostitution.[35]

And, finally, doctors created masturbation and the masturbator. Through this new moral and medical scourge, they, and those
riding on their coattails — pedagogues, moralists, experts of all
sorts — came to inhabit the psyches of innumerable boys and girls,
men and women. The state, which licensed and supported this
host of professionals, no longer burned or whipped the sexual
offender but enmeshed him or her, and many others, in the webs
of "bio-power." Put differently, the story of modernity and the
individual is not one of liberation — repression to freedom — but
one in which a new and perhaps more insidious form of power
is exercised. Desire is discursively created in order to be the locus
of control. Masturbation, long slumbering in a moral backwater,
is made over into a major horror, a threat to self and society,
the object of the full power of all right-thinking guardians of
good order.

In some ways, the eighteenth- and nineteenth-century medical campaign against the secret vice is almost too perfect an
example of all this. The evidence is everywhere. One has only to
look to *Onania* — which did more than any other text to create the
onanist — to see that we are witnessing the birth of a society that,
as Foucault noted, dedicated itself "to speaking, ad infinitum
[about sex]" to a "regulated and polymorphous incitement to
discourse," to the "production of sexuality," to the elaboration of
desire in order to insert it in a disciplinary regime. As writers of
confessional and moral-advice literature had long realized, the
more one asks, the more real and attractive sin may become. Temptations might be put before those who would never have encountered them otherwise and therefore they were relatively coy about
their queries. Jeremy Taylor, for example, the best-selling writer of
religious advice books in the seventeenth century, offers but one
instance. (Examples from Catholic confessional literature are, of
course, much more abundant, but this one stands directly in the
lineage that will produce *Onania* a half century or so later.)
"Reader stay," he cautions, "read not the advices of the following
section, unlesse thou hast a chaste spirit, or desireth to be chaste,
or at least are apt to consider whether you ought to be." This is
indeed tempting, but what readers who could not resist actually

encountered if they persisted was pretty tame. Maybe they would get new ideas for sinning, but they would have to work at it.[36]

Not so for *Onania*, which issues exactly the same warning as it invites its readers in and then does not stop. We need to ask why an old convention cautioning silence was honored now only in the breach. Worried that the book might "furnish the Fancies of silly people with Matter for Impurity...I beg the reader to stop here, and not proceed any further, unless he has the desire to be chaste, or at least apt to consider whether he ought to have it or no." But John Marten can only pretend innocence of the fact that the table of contents in all but the earliest editions announces the presence further on of that classic tale of seventeenth-century pornography, the story of the two nuns of Rome whose vastly enlarged clitorises, the product of mutual masturbation, had been mistaken for real male organs. Never mind that *Onania* grew from edition to edition through the letters, real or fictional, that it solicited from boys and girls, men and women who told just how they had learned the vicious practice of masturbation and in what circumstances they subsequently did it. Missives were to be left at a coffeehouse, and the doctor especially welcomed accounts from women, since early editions gave the mistaken impression that they did not indulge in the vice or that it was less dangerous to them than to men.

The first hundred years of anti-masturbatory literature was, in Foucault's terms, one gigantic, international invitation to discourse. Never was a secret vice more public. Tissot justified his 1766 edition's being one-third longer than the previous one by saying, "Since there is less hope of convincing by reasons than of terrifying by examples, one can hardly accumulate too many." James Hodson, who claimed to have the largest sexual-problems practice in eighteenth-century Britain, invited personal calls and letters, which, for a fee, he would answer — and publish. In a phrase made for Foucault, an early-nineteenth-century writer asks that his correspondents "be as MINUTE in details of their cases as possible."[37]

This rhetoric of discovering, describing, and collecting together details of masturbation in young and old continued for centuries; somewhere a crime was being constituted; somewhere the crime — onanism, of course — both revealed a nasty hidden self and fostered further nastiness. Somewhere another innocent criminal was being taught the wickedness of his ways. And always there is the paranoid anxiety that secret sin may not be as easily detected as its enemies boasted. Boys are wholly unaware, writes an English schoolmaster, of the extent to which "their inner life lies open to the practiced eye"; he solicits "the history of their inner life," once he has their confidence; sometimes, when work is pressing, he interrogates only boys "obviously suffering the effects of impurity" and at other times everyone. But despite the falseness of the boys' belief that nothing can betray their secret, some cases escape; seemingly healthy boys turn out to be mastur-bators. Doubly secret, they call for even more vigilance. All of this the well-educated schoolmaster offered as an instance of George Eliot's observation that "our daily familiar life is but a hiding of ourselves from each other behind a screen of fervid works and deeds." The true self — revealed with such purity in its sexual nature — thus awaited discovery and, in Foucault's account, insertion into the grids of power.[38]

The production of "the truth of sex" and of the "masturbator" as a category of pathological sexuality by a medical and more broadly pedagogical "scientia sexualis," to use Foucault's term, was not subtle. "However secret the practice," intones an early-nineteenth-century medical dictionary, "it leaves an indelible mark," so that its votives "can not escape detection from that tact which has been peculiarly distinguished by the term *sensus medicus*."[39]

In a general sense, the profound anxiety about masturbation is clearly part of the transformation of politics and culture that includes the decline of absolutism, the rise of civil society, the creation of a private sphere beyond the reach of the law, and the secularization of morality and its enforcement. It came at the same time as barriers against luxury — long understood as a sign for the abandonment of nature and the corruption of morals — collapsed. Neither a divinely ordained, hierarchical world order nor the sumptuary laws of states any longer defended society against the corrosion of the most readily available luxury of them all. Whether sexuality was a road to modernity or vice versa, they shared a common trajectory. Moral self-government was a cornerstone to governance more generally.

But, that said, changes in politics — or changes in how power made itself felt — as the explanation for why the imagination, secrecy, and addictive excess, the triple threat of masturbation, became so central to moral self-governance takes us only partway. In some measure, this is because of a chronological problem. But there are two further reasons why I turn elsewhere. I do not think that the general view, explicit in Foucault's account in the first volume of his history of sexuality, of how modern subjectivities were created through the incitement of desire and then its domination by new technologies of power is quite right. And this is because the political story — or at least the part that focuses on "the modern self" and not on how power is exercised – is an aspect of another, more compelling one: the story of the joint march of commercial culture and civil society.

I begin with the chronological problem. Yes, self-pollution seemed the evil doppelgänger of Enlightenment in the German states, where a new rule of law was transforming the relationship between political authorities and the sexual body. But it played that part in Switzerland, Holland, England, the American colonies, Italy, and Spain as well, where the political situations were, in each case, very different. Furthermore, the fervor about masturbation did not die down when, to take the German case, the question of the Rechtsstaat was nicely settled. Something more sustained the power of solitary sex to disturb so many people, masturbators themselves and those who sought to limit their indulgence through the thick and thin of political change for two centuries.

And, yes, truths about the body were invented; yes, we can locate the discursive production of one sort of pervert — the masturbator — within "the strategic field of power relations." But the field is far from smooth. The anxiety about masturbation is of a whole different order from its confreres in the disciplining of the sexual body: the "hystericization" of women's bodies; the socialization of procreative behavior (the efforts to direct the activities of the Malthusian couple); the "psychiatrization" of perverse plea-sure (the making of homosexual pathology). Prostitution might be added to this constellation as a separate entity. All came to constitute a subject of knowledge for a variety of professionals but at very different times and in different ways. Masturbation arose as a problem a century earlier; it was the primal vice well before, almost two centuries before, other aspects of sexual life came under the scrutiny of doctors and pedagogues. Unlike the others, it was not regulated by the state: we cannot cite dates when masturbation became legal or illegal, regulated or not regu-lated, as we can for "homosexuality," birth control, abortion, and prostitution. The secret sin worked at levels both more intimate and more universal than all other objects of the new sciences of sex, and it did so over centuries in very different political con-texts. It threatened not just this or that group in society but everyone. It threatened not just the social order or the sexual order but the whole economy of desire in all boys and girls, men and women.[40]

If political change is the main area where we look for the cause of modern masturbation and if masturbation is regarded as part of a larger transformation of how sexuality was mobilized in the interest of power, then chronology matters. Foucault, who thought through the place of solitary sex in relation to the mak-ing of the modern self more deeply than anyone else, focuses on the end of the eighteenth century, when there emerged, in his account, "a completely new technology of sex," of which the attack on onanism was a part. This technology in turn was part of — one might say was caused by — a great shift in the nature of power: "The old power of death that symbolized sovereign power ... [was] supplanted by the administration of bodies and the cal-culated management of life." Sexuality as "a very real historical formation" is thus, in Foucault's story, coterminous with a new sort of power: the replacement of "the privilege of sovereignty with the analysis of a multiple and mobile field of force relations." But this is not the order in which things happened. The masturba-tion problem was making its way through European culture, high and low, in the eighteenth century before "sexuality" existed.[41]

But more important than chronology is the point that the political explanation does not account for *how* things happened and therefore not for *why*. It is true that in a world where there was a genuine growth of autonomy and freedom, there was consequently a genuine need to create the internal mechanisms of self-government that would allow individuals to negotiate the vast array of new choices available to them. It is also true that educators, doctors, and moralists discursively produced desires and then exercised authority by suppressing them. Whether or not this was in every case their explicit or ultimate motif is a separate question. John Marten had to know that his florid accounts of how scores of people learned to masturbate were arousing and thus likely to produce the very vice whose consequences he would cure for a fee. Authority, yes, but in the interests of personal gain, not bio-power. Clearly, pedagogues increased their authority through their endless incitement of talk about sex and subsequent condemnation. But this does not constitute evidence for the more general view that modern society is a creature of dominated subjectivities. In other words, the discursive creation of desire by professionals who thereby exercised authority over it and over the souls of its subjects certainly took place. But this does not elevate it into a general theory.

Foucault scarcely mentions masturbation in his subsequent two volumes on the history of sexuality, those that deal not with the nineteenth century but with Antiquity, and for good reason. As we saw in Chapter 3, masturbation played almost no part in how doctors or philosophers thought about the care of the self and the creation of a morally autonomous being. In the modern world, however, the relation between the self and solitary sex became exigent. This new sexuality is thus primarily made, to put it in Foucault's terms, in relation not to knowledge or to power but to the self.

My Explanation
I will thus offer an explanation in which masturbation became the primal battleground between civilization and libido — the particular form of sexuality in which the success or failure of moral self-

government was most apparent — not through what the state did, or even what professionals with strong links to the state did, but through the work of civil society on its members. To answer the question "why?" I will push one step back to ask about the wider cultural context of the anxieties for which masturbation became emblematic: the imagination, privacy and solitude, excess and addiction. And that context is the civil society that created the new economic activities of the eighteenth century and beyond.

Masturbation, in other words, came to prominence precisely when the imagination, solitude, and excess became newly important and newly worrisome. Private vice is the sin of an era that created the idea of society as the intermediary between the state and the individual and of an economy that depended on the desire for more and always more. This desire was the product not just of discourse but of the entire commercial system. Civilization made its claims felt on the desiring, now morally self-governing subject of this new world in all sorts of ways, but in the sexual body none was more important. As it took on new meanings, it became emblematic of all that was beyond social surveillance, beyond the discipline of the market, all that threatened a well-ordered world. Conversely, the rehabilitation of masturbation in the twentieth century was part of a political movement for a new sexual and a new moral order. Beginning in the 1970s, solitary sex was regarded as a way of reclaiming the self from the regulatory mechanisms of civil society and of the patriarchal sexual order into which the Enlightenment and its successors had put it. It became a sign of *self*-governance and *self*-control instead of their collapse. The history of masturbation is thus the history of the imagination, solitude and secrecy, private and public, excess, addiction, and control in different stages of our developing an individual sexual ethics once it could no longer be found in religion or an organic social order.

I will begin my explanation with an account of masturbation and the marketplace, and then turn to masturbation and private reading, but not because I think economics provide the real frame in which the anxiety about masturbation was created and culture a mere reflection or second-order manifestation. Instead, I want

277

to suggest that the new solitary vice stood as the exemplar of a problem common to both and to modern bourgeois society more generally. Or, put differently, masturbation became ethically central and construed as dangerous precisely when its component parts came to be valued. Never in world history had the imagination figured more importantly in so wide a variety of realms: the economy, literature, the arts. "The pleasures of the imagination" — the phrase is Joseph Addison's — captivated the educated middling sorts of Europe. These delights became the core, the unifying principle, of literature, theater, music, painting, and the other pursuits of "culture."[42]

Never had excess been so praised and democratically sought after. Never had solitude and privacy come so sharply into focus in contrast to the state and to society. Their opposition infused thinking at all levels: private gain could redound to public good; solitude was a time for moral and spiritual refreshment, an escape from the hubbub of an active social world. Finally, pleasure was in its ascendancy: the pleasures of the imagination; the foundation of utilitarianism (humans seek pleasure and avoid pain on the basis of this calculus). In other words, all the elements of what was so terribly wrong with masturbation were themselves widely valued, praised, and discussed. But this made their abuse all the more threatening; one might almost think that if the solitary vice did not exist, it would have had to be created, a kind of Satan to the glories of bourgeois civilization.

Masturbation, Modernity, and the Marketplace
The rapidly growing commercial economy of the late seventeenth and the early eighteenth century did not cause the new problem of masturbation; neither did the new institutions of finance or their failures. But the commercial economy and the imaginative foundations of credit posed the same moral and psychological question as masturbation on the great public stage of history. If masturbation is, as I have claimed, a pathology of the imagination, a practice that seems to have virtually no supply constraints, a satisfaction of endless desire by endless gratification, it might be regarded as a special case of a larger problem: the morally dis-

turbing qualities of a commercial credit economy that magically promised undreamed-of abundance, shakily linked to the concrete reality of real goods and services. Related to this unease was the question whether sociability, or indeed any form of public virtue, could survive the frenzy of private desire and private gain. These issues were most widely debated at first in England, the first great civil society after the Dutch and the one that became exemplary. But they found voice elsewhere too.

Contemporaries spoke of sex and commerce in similar terms. Montesquieu's fictional informant in the Persian court writes back about "the disease spreading until it affected even the healthiest parts of the organism," about "an insatiable lust" that springs up in every heart; even "the most virtuous men" commit "shameful deeds." He is referring not to masturbation but, with transparent disguise, to John Law's "Mississippi Bubble," in which dreams of something for nothing had driven stocks to fantastic heights. The lust was not for sexual gratification but for money. In the next letter, the whole sexual system collapses. The public/private barrier is broken as Zelis drops her veil on the way to the mosque, allowing everyone to see her; Zashi goes to bed with one of her slaves; a youth is caught in the seraglio.[43] Untrammeled desire in one realm seemed to make itself felt in another.

Like masturbation, credit created "constant agonies of mind and fears"; like masturbation, it "impose[d] without appearing to do so" and left its victims "reduced to skin and bone" with their lust not "one bit abated." "Committees of Secrecy" investigated "fictious stock" that lured investors, just as the "power of fantasy" seduced the victims of the secret sin. "Art-magick" raised the value of stocks, just as the masturbator's titillations were "raised by Art." Both inhabited the imaginative world of spurious, fragile realities that fed desires and punished them at the same time. "Bubble," like masturbation, was something unsubstantial, empty, "a deceptive show": "Why should a woman dote on such a bubble?"[44] The problem in both realms was self-generated desire that had no natural bounds. It was born not from some adamantine, foundational need or from original sin but from the imagination and fiction. Desire of this sort was Janus-faced: the driving force both of commerce and credit — the engine of progress — *and* of the solitary sin self-pollution, their doppelgänger in the wilderness beyond culture and society. At stake was a new morality of the marketplace.

In other words, the dramatic, sudden, and radically innovative formulation of masturbation as the pressing problem of solitary and secret, always excessive, and artfully created desire maps precisely onto the problem of the new economy. The expansiveness of this economy — most especially its embrace of credit — called into question the existence of a solid foundation for money, exchange, and value. Chimerical and phantasmal, the unfounded and unlimited dreams of something for nothing seemed as threatening in the economic realm as they did when working their charms on the body. The speculator and the masturbator were playing on the same pitch, but so was everyone who dreamed of contentment through buying just one more thing. There was no escaping it; once the old religious strictures were weakened, a viable moral order depended on making peace with this broad cultural embrace of desire, of private gain and happiness, of fiction and fancy.

Anxiety about masturbation was an expression of anxiety about a new political economic order writ on the body. It was "das Adam Smith Problem," the name philosophers have given to the dilemma of reconciling private gain and public good, in another register. (Smith famously argued in *The Wealth of Nations* that this happened more or less automatically through the workings of the invisible hand, whereas in *The Theory of Moral Sentiments* he emphasized the importance of human interaction, and especially the capacity to feel oneself in the place of another, in moderating greed.) Onanism clearly stood outside the social realm, and the invisible hand could not do its work because it assumed exchange, a system of truck and barter. The solitary vice constituted the abyss beyond permissible selfishness and luxury in a culture whose avant-garde was fanning the flames of desire while at the same time dismantling traditional safeguards against it.[45]

For Tissot and the other creators of the new masturbation, all very much believers in Enlightenment natural ethics, individual

WHY MASTURBATION BECAME A PROBLEM

desires could be limited and reconciled with social welfare by submitting to the wisdom of "nature." "Real need" set natural limits. It provided a guide to appropriate behavior, a brake on excess, and the assurance of harmony in a world in which theological answers had lost their force. "Real need" was what distinguished healthy coition from unhealthy and, more important, masturbatory from other sorts of sexual desire. Nature was the bedrock that anchored social sex; fiction, fantasy, the imagination — false wants — on the other hand, drove the onanist to lunatic excess. Transgression of "reality" — in the sense of going beyond nature — not the violation of the supposed telos of sex (reproduction), made his or her sin "unnatural." "Diseases of civilization" — a common eighteenth-century category — were the result of ignoring these guidelines through excessive consumption of luxuries; conversely, those who adhered to them were living both healthily and morally. There was a parallel realm to all of this with respect to sex. Intercourse based on "natural needs" was thought to be far healthier than intercourse to which a man had aroused himself; even masturbation "spurred only by one's need," as the *Encyclopédie* put it, was not so bad. But self-pollution, as we saw, went beyond this. At the heart of the new medical constellation of masturbatory disease, as a well-respected French encyclopedia put it in 1819, is bottomless demand linked increasingly to "the higher degree of civilization achieved by modern [commercial] societies." Masturbation, thought another doctor of the period, was a "growing evil" as a result of "the diffusion of luxury, of precocious knowledge, and of the vices of civilization."[46]

In this sense, solitary sex might seem just one more evil of luxury, the softness that moral critics had been complaining about since Greeks mocked Persians and Cato mourned the passing of old republican virtues. But it was more threatening now because the strictures against luxury were being relaxed. There were no more sumptuary laws that limited fine things to a narrow stratum of society. Indeed, luxuries were, to a great extent, morally rehabilitated because of the good they were now said to produce. Luxuries made the wheels of commerce and industry turn, and everyone benefited from this; the more people bought them, the better all around. But masturbation was a luxury that had no such compensatory virtues because it was actually *nothing*; it was the fraudulent pleasure.[47]

Tissot's complaint that "we subject ourselves to want without being in want" fits into the old tradition of moral lament but without the new redemptive coda. Masturbation, like the feather pillows and the soft living of idle young men, was self-evidently a luxury: unnecessary and corrupting. The tendency of "men [and the author means here women as well] to subject themselves to false wants" was its root perversion; the real sexual ecstasy of presence was routinely poised against the *jouissance* of culture and fantasy.[48]

Whether there was such a thing as natural desire unmediated by fantasy had long been an open question. Humans, unlike animals, lived beyond their instincts. Even radical materialist accounts of sexual passion like those of the first-century BCE poet and atomist Lucretius, re-discovered in the Renaissance, took notice of the mind and its inflammatory powers. But leaving aside this more general question, everyone writing about masturbation thought that there were natural incitements to sexual intercourse that were rooted in the attraction of bodies and that these could be distinguished from the gratuitous, self-inflicted provocations of the masturbator.

This critical difference could not be sustained in the new economy; fantasy was everywhere, essential and dangerous. Consumption flourished because false wants — the need for something that one did not naturally need — flourished. At every level of society, yesterday's luxuries had become today's necessities as the circle of desire became much more inclusive. Theorists of what was thought of as the "high wage" argued that people worked not because they feared starvation but because they wanted what had earlier been considered luxuries. Broadly understood as "great refinement[s] in the gratification of the senses," so-called luxuries, argued David Hume and others, were the basis not only of a prosperous economy but also of a healthy commonwealth. They — the innocent ones — made us more "human" and more "sociable." They also had a pleasant side effect: in the refined societies where luxuries were widely diffused, "the sexes meet in an easy and sociable manner." "Blamable" luxuries, "vicious" luxuries, on the other hand, were those that did not contribute to sociability. The line between them is not clear. The distinction between the "blamable" and the "innocent" could not "be exactly fixed," Hume recognized, any more than for other moral subjects. But refinement was always the criterion for drawing a border. On this ground alone, the solitary vice would qualify as a "vicious" luxury. But Hume's reevaluation of luxury was part of a much more general reevaluation of the role of the passions in human life. Their role had long been discussed, but they assumed a new centrality in eighteenth-century thought and particularly in economic thought: "Everything in the world is purchased by labour," said Hume, "and our passions are the only causes of our labour."[49]

Over ever-greater swaths of society, the role of the passions, and especially of the desire for material things, was validated. Economic historians have paid a great deal more attention of late to the importance of demand in creating that transformation of the West known as the Industrial Revolution. An "industrious revolution," it seems, pushed more and more people to work and to sell in order to buy things in the marketplace that before they had made domestically or had done without.[50] Everywhere the idea and the reality of a naturally bounded need were in a precarious state, and at precisely this moment masturbation came to be seen as so urgent and so universal a problem. Any theory of the secret vice — as of credit and consumption — would have to be a theory of fantasy and desire. And it would be part of a more general moral theory of the marketplace.

Less than a decade before the publication of *Onania*, a Dutch émigré physician writing in England named Bernard Mandeville boldly proclaimed old views of luxury dead in the process of offering just such a general theory. Today he is known mostly to specialists, but in the eighteenth century he set the cat among some very prominent pigeons. Kant read him seriously and responded directly to his views; Voltaire took up his views and popularized them.[51] No one articulated more clearly the moral chasm in a commercial society between what might once have seemed a divinely ordained social order, on the one hand, and the desires of every man, woman, and child, on the other. But as important for our history is the fact that one of the most influential and widely debated thinkers on economic matters manifestly linked sexual lust with lust for luxuries, that is, the lust for the baubles of the marketplace.

The literary frame for Mandeville's views in his best known work — *The Fable of the Bees*, published in 1714 — was a poem he published in 1705, the same year as John Marten's *Gonosologium novum*, *Onania*'s direct ancestor: "The Grumbling Hive; or, Knaves turned honest." Popular enough to be pirated, it tells the story of sociable bees who live like men "in luxury and ease." The remarkable thing about these lucky bees is that every part of their hive is "full of vice / Yet the whole mass a paradise." Everywhere there is deceit and chicanery, but instead of producing individual misery and public collapse, the opposite happens. The whole colony has

> made friends with vice: and ever since,
> The worst of all the multitude
> Did something for the common good.

This paradox was the subject of the much longer and more famous 1714 tract, in which Mandeville offered extended commentary on the poem, expanding on it line by line in muscular, ironic prose that hammered in the argument he had first made in verse. The most notorious redemption of "private vices," as he called all this selfish seeking after one's own advantage, was thus published more or less at the same time as the most famous, and also the first, commercial attack on "*the* private vice." There is a delicious back-and-forth play in this conjunction.[52]

Pleasure, Mandeville argued, was not an abstract notion of the philosophers but something far simpler: "An Englishman may justly call everything a pleasure that pleases him." Real pleasures are not what men say are best "but such as they seem to be most pleased with." Almost all pleasures, even supposedly sinful pleasures, satisfied imagined needs, ones born of civilization and ingenuity. In fact, he thought that natural needs were so primitive as to be irrelevant to the discussion; the poor today lived better than the rich in earlier days. Thus not basic necessity but the unending human capacity for enjoyment made the hive prosperous and stimulated the new economy. Perhaps, Mandeville admitted, his definition of a luxury as "everything... that is not immediately necessary to make man subsist as he is a living creature" was too rigorous. But once it was broadened, once anything beyond this absolute minimum was admitted and counted as a necessity — a real need — the game was up.[53]

And, of course, his point was that even the most impoverished of cultures were evidence for the impossibility of maintaining a luxury/necessity distinction: "not even among the naked savages" are luxuries absent. Plentiful beer, meat, and feather pillows, not to speak of decent burials and much, much else that was once an unexpected luxury for the poor, were now necessities. History seemed continually to move the threshold: the richest men of the distant past "were destitute of a great many comforts of life that are now enjoyed by the meanest and most humble wretches." It was, Mandeville seemed to be arguing, the work of culture to inflate desire, and a good thing too.[54]

Mandeville did not deny that natural passions existed; to the contrary, he argued that humans were driven by them and that they governed us "whether [we] will or not." His infamous defense of public stews (brothels) — a commercial sexual marketplace — began with a long historical summary of evidence — page after hilarious page — that even philosophers were driven by the "irresistible force of love" and that it would be foolish to try to suppress it. Socrates confessed that even in old age he was affected by a girl's touch on the shoulder; Aristotle had a son by his concubine; Zeno was famous for his modesty because he rarely made use of boys, but he took his maidservant to bed and argued for a commonwealth of women. There are many more examples. Public policy, Mandeville concludes, should acknowledge that if the demand for sexual intercourse could not be repressed in the most virtuous and reasonable of men, it would be foolish to try to do so among more ordinary mortals.[55]

He specifically denied that the old moral constraints, the old strictures on vice and the old guardians of virtue, could control passions that even philosophers could not manage. Nor should they. "The nearer we search into human nature," Mandeville said in innocent anticipation of the far more biting attack that would be launched by Nietzsche, "the more we shall be convinced that moral virtues are the political offspring which flattery begot upon pride." And conversely — deeply connected to the psychological role our subject would play in the modern world — was the other side of this maxim: "It is incredible how necessary an ingredient shame is to make us sociable." Pity will not make us virtuous; nor will reason; nor will religion. For ages it was believed that "it would be more beneficial for everyone to conquer than indulge his appetites, and much better to mind the public than what seemed like the private interest." This simply is not true, he argues. The pleasures we seek for ourselves, not the supposedly good things we do for others, make us social beings and provide the glue of society. They keep the hive buzzing happily and their re-pression would render it lifeless and dispirited. Our desire to be flattered and praised — even when we know through reason that neither is deserved — is more conducive to virtue than all the maxims and exhortations of preachers and moralists. Actions based on how we would imagine their redounding to our own benefit are far more likely to produce good than those based on the precepts of public moral. Everywhere, in short, private satis-faction, prodigality, and selfishness seemed — contrary to every-thing that had been believed for millennia — a very good thing indeed.[56] Thus the moral status of precisely those features of mas-turbation that seemed so troubling after 1712 — selfishly seeking pleasure for its own sake, imaginatively finding ever more things in which to take delight, endlessly, even excessively desiring — was high on the agenda of the first great theorist of the morality of the free market. His conclusion was — famously — that private vices produce public virtue. He did not say *the private* vice, but his plural private vices must have resonated with the newly an-nounced singular one of the same decade.

Even the lowest and shabbiest of vices, like gin drinking, prostitution, and thievery, added to the common welfare, Mandeville argued. And the luxuries that had so long and so irrationally been condemned by moralists — all the things one might imagine, dream about, or wish for — were precisely what made a community prosperous. Conversely, when private vices are suppressed, public virtue collapses; the happy beehive falls into disarray when the supposed virtue of self-denial becomes temporarily triumphant. Exchange stops, the economy collapses, the prosperity of all who live by buying and selling ends. But then what some might condemn as wasteful and excessive but what Mandeville regarded as the life-blood of the community returns, and affairs take a turn for the better. "Prodigality I call a noble sin that agreeable and good natured vice that makes the chimney smoke and the tradesman smile."[57]

Mandeville had nothing particular to say in *The Fable of the Bees* about masturbation, but his *Defense of Public Stews* puts sex and sexual pleasure solidly in the same category as all the other things we might want and enjoy, including sex with ourselves. Diogenes is offered as one example of a philosopher who could not suppress his sexual desires. In the voice of a character named Phil-Porney (literally, "lover of harlots"), he suggests that we give up trying. Mandeville proposed that the world would be far better off if, instead of trying to stop prostitution — to take the case in point — public stews were allowed their niche in the marketplace. (Pornography, "writing of harlots," as we shall see, was also a creature of the revolution of desire that drove both the new consumer culture and the new vice of masturbation.) The specific point is that the alternative — trying to stop the unstoppable — had a very long history of failure. But more generally, Mandeville's argument in the *Defense of Public Stews* is the same as in *The Fable of the Bees*: private vices redound to the common good. Avarice and prodigality, for example, he thought of as "two contrary poisons in physic," the noxious qualities of the one offset by the other so that "they make good medicine between them." Men of an amorous sort, for example, would be far better off gratifying their sexual desires before those desires take over their brains — from "the glans penis to the glandula penealis" — and before abstinence makes their lust still more insistent. And it would be better for society that such men go to brothels than that they corrupt modest girls or spread diseases that are endemic to ill-regulated stews. And of course more commercial sex is good, just as all commerce is good; prostitutes, after all, are also consumers.[58]

Arguments for the free circulation of sexual pleasure apply to all other objects of desire. Far from it being a virtue to dress appropriately to one's station, the irrational efforts by rich and poor alike to be something other than what they are work to the public good. The poor woman will starve herself and her family to buy a secondhand gown; the woman of the middling sort will ape her betters; and so on up the social scale in an epidemic of emulation and continual striving. "Envy and vanity itself were ministers of industry." So, precisely the danger of masturbation — fantasy, the lush imagination, and the unnatural needs that were at the root of its evil — were rehabilitated in the marketplace. There they served both the public and the private good.[59]

Mandeville's system of self-regulating evil — public welfare from the gratification of selfish desire — was, of course, a version of Adam Smith's invisible hand *avant la lettre*. The moral magic of the marketplace transformed private greed, privately pursued, into public good; buying and selling turned the sow's ear of self-ishness into the silk purse of virtue.

Of course, Adam Smith did not think the market could do it alone, which is where sentimentality and sociability come in. His theory of moral sentiments understood virtue as the product of some combination of physiology (a natural propensity to feel the pain and suffering of others), imagination (one could think one-self into the place of others), and community (one wished to live in such a way as to be regarded with approval). In this account, sympathy more than truck and barter made men moral in a com-mercial society in which the private was defined as that sphere in which each of us pursued our individual desires. But the point is that for Smith and many other thinkers of the age of *Onania*, as for Mandeville, the marketplace provided the necessary if not the sufficient tissue of connectedness. How this happened was a central question of social theory during the eighteenth and nine-teenth centuries; some denied that it happened at all and argued that the cash nexus was a poor substitute for community. Still, even if the market did not protect against loneliness and anomie, it did depend on exchange; there are no markets of one. There was some minimal reality "out there" beyond that of a desiring social atom.[60]

Social sex — that is, sex that involved two or more people of whatever gender — however private it might be and however fiercely some resisted the idea that it could be treated as a commodity, was nonetheless moderated, and understood to be moderated, by the forces of supply and demand, by a calculus of pain and pleasure that involved others. Yes, as Mandeville argued, perhaps unrestrained private desire ultimately produced public good. Supply and demand did not, and ought not to, restrain the search for luxury. Even pride, which comes close to pure egocentrism, had its virtues. But in the end all of this depended on a social, institutional, and biological reality. The availability, social cost, health risks, and much else constrained both supply and demand of all those many sources of pleasure, including sexual ones. The term "marriage market" seems to have been first used in a book title in 1846, but the concept had been around since the late seventeenth century. Offering and accepting goods and services out there in the marketplace always had a cost.

Of all forms of sex — perhaps of all forms of pleasure — only masturbation escaped this bottom line, and Mandeville knew it. It was unstoppable. First, the world offered it no resistance: "The privacy, safety, convenience and cheapness of this gratification are very strong motives." ("Putative safety," *Onania* would have said.) Second, because it was not just cheap but free, it could not be "prudently managed." Every day boys commit "rapes upon their own bodies"; they "attack themselves" — masturbate — because they have neither a real inclination nor the ability to attack a woman. They are rendered impotent or worse by the constant and habit-forming friction. Public stews, Mandeville concludes, will keep boys from "laying violent hands upon themselves." Obviously, much of this is tongue-in-cheek, illogical, and comically hyperbolic; self-rape is an oxymoron; if the boys really lack inclination or ability then brothels would not help. But in his

289

worry about the absence of a bottom line in the masturbatory economy, Mandeville is totally conventional.[61]

The authors of anti-masturbatory works decried with one voice the absence of any such constraints as the reason why this particular private vice was so dangerous; not shame, not guilt, not fear of rejection, nothing restrained the onanist unless he or she would listen to all those doctors, teachers, and philosophers who taught that there was, contrary to what seemed to be the case, an enormous price to pay. If solitary sex was not moderated by the forces of supply and demand, then death was — had to be — the only bottom line; physical and moral collapse lay hidden like shoals before the final, fatal rocks.

With respect to heterosexual intercourse, this was precisely. Thomas Malthus's point. Nothing was more attractive, he understood, than the pleasures of "virtuous love." He meant by this the sexual pleasures of the marriage bed, but the point goes for illicit relations as well although he would never have said so. Even for the scholar, that most intellectual and high-minded of creatures, his fondest deathbed recollections would not be of his many hours of quiet study, but of far more fleshly delights. No question, he thought, what one remembered most warmly in the cold of one's last moments.

With something so terribly seductive as sex, only the scourges of famine and disease would bring men and women back to the hard truths of the reality principle: one could not have sex for free. Malthus believed, of course, that intercourse without the possibility of conception, that is, using birth control, was a moral impossibility, and so the only alternative he envisaged — not at first, but in later editions of his most famous book — to the positive checks of famine and disease was the moral check of abstinence.[62]

Tissot and those who followed him tried to create the Malthusian scourge before Malthus; their constant refrain was that masturbation killed even if it seemed safe. (One of the ideas that seems most ludicrous today is that the risks of pregnancy were minor in comparison to those of self-abuse.) Hidden costs had to be made manifest; something had to check newly liberated desires. There had to be supply- or demand-side constraints or mechanisms that would moderate infinite wants: the invisible regulator of the marketplace, dearth, death, sensibility; an interest in how one might look in the eyes of others whose respect and admiration one craved; the principle of utility or some other con- sequentialist ethic; some overarching principle of reason — the Kantian categorical imperative — which showed that selfish indul- gences were simply ridiculous. Only this last idea existed inde- pendently of society, and even it was embedded, for Kant, in a complex account of marriage.

Masturbation presented the ultimate challenge to all such views of how selfish desire might be socialized, the limit case, the exemplary case for the challenge it posed. In courtship, there was at least a universe of two, if not hostile parents and a hostile envi- ronment, to create resistance and ensure that only the virtuous ultimately triumphed. This was what novels taught and reality to some extent reinforced. If virtue did not always win, there were certainly lots of problems to overcome. At the very least, one's partner could refuse and thereby limit venereal excess. Not so with masturbation. As Rousseau most famously reported — and his words found many echoes and antecedents — the solitary vice allowed its practitioners

> to dispose, so to speak, of the female sex at their will, and to make any beauty who tempts them serve their pleasure without the need of first obtaining her consent.[63]

"The dangerous supplement" escaped an economy of scarcity; for the masturbator, demand was endless but so was supply, limited only — if at all — by the seemingly irrepressible powers of the imagination and perhaps ultimately, so doctors tried to convince their patients, by the rebellion of the body. The point of so much moralizing and pedagogy was that guilt and fear would stop the evil practice before death intervened. One might argue that, in the absence of divine authority, the need for a new guilt about solitary sex arose because there was nothing else, nothing external, to restrain solipsistic pleasure. Here was one arena in which even Mandeville could find nothing redeeming. In the masturbatory economy of excess, the unnerving truth was that *nothing* turned private vice into public virtue. It went against the founding axiom of all economic life: there really might be a free lunch.

Not until the twentieth century did someone — Freud's colleague Wilhelm Stekel — finally make a case for how the Mandevillian magic might work. Stekel argued that "if masturbation were entirely suppressed the number of sexual misdeeds would increase to an immeasurable extent."[64] All sorts of forbidden yearnings that might have led to rape or pederasty found a healthy outlet in onanism. And even this might not be true if we believe Catharine MacKinnon. Quite to the contrary! But more on this later; in the eighteenth and the nineteenth century, no one proposed redemption.

When viewed through the prism of the debate about the morality of the marketplace, the logic of masturbation was remarkably close to the logic of new economic realities with respect to the imagination, private desires, luxuries, and excess. But the paradox of dire warnings in one realm and high praise in another has wider resonance. The talk of false needs and of succumbing to fictions of desire that permeated discussions of solitary vice also permeated, for example, talk about credit. The diseases of the masturbator were very much like those of the commonwealth addicted to the new fictions of paper. Both self-pollution and credit were, and were understood to be, predicated on the imagination. Both threatened the real social order; both were haunted by phantasms; both ran counter to the epistemological order of things. Whether, as conservative critics — the "country party," in the English context — claimed, credit destroyed real value or whether, as its champions argued, it was bad only when we gave in to it excessively and otherwise was compatible with virtue, no one doubted that it depended on believing in something that was not actually there. And in the case of stock speculation, it depended on being swept up in the excitement of a double fiction: that paper could be money and that one could get something for nothing.[65]

The parallels between sex and finance are uncanny. Addison and Steele's *Spectator*, a journal many educated eighteenth-century English men and women would have seen as the key to understanding modern city life, goes on a long riff, for example, in which it might as well be the onanist as the state that is addicted to false needs. Public Credit is sitting on her throne, plump and healthy as long as the bags of money that surround her are filled with real gold. (How gold became money is another leap of the imagination, another bit of cultural alchemy, but that one happened far enough back that it no longer seemed peculiar. To the Greeks it had seemed odd, but by the eighteenth century it had become part of the way things were.)[66] But Public Credit's florid complexion vanishes when air fills the once-weighty bags. Now she becomes like a skeleton, devastated, suffering, like the masturbator, from a "wasting Distemper"; the most "hideous phantoms" march into her reveries "in the most dissociable way." Temptations to create the windy, inflated fiction of paper are all around her: "The Lady often smiled with a secret pleasure" as she looked upon the acts of Parliament — pieces of paper tacked to the walls — that had created the public funds, that is, long-term borrowings. But then reality reasserts itself, and all is well again: the inflated money bags, "full of wind" and "notched sticks" (the promises of future revenues for which the treasury obtained present funds), turn back into something real — into gold — and "the Lady was well again."[67]

Credit and masturbation traveled in the same linguistic circles. Archibald Hutcheson, a leading commentator on early-eighteenth-century finance, wrote about the "imaginary value" of South Sea stock, the "amusement of a pleasing dream"; Anthony Hammond, a prolific writer and editor, pointed to the slow emergence from "infatuation, lunacy, or phrenzy" that followed the bursting of the bubble in 1719, the reeling from "fictitious losses," the dangers of "evanescence" versus "the weightiness of the real." Credit was born of the imagination and died by it, as the novelist Daniel Defoe made abundantly clear in a raft of pamphlets, and he was a man who knew something about fiction making. It worked insidiously, destroying its votives without their knowledge; credit, like masturbation, was "an invisible phantom." It substituted whimsy for reason, "bewitched thousands to fall in love with her tho she reduced them to skin and bones." The dangers that came to be

293

attached to masturbation for the first time around 1712 were deeply and newly attached to specific, epochal changes in economic life. Perhaps public credit was not secret, but it certainly captured the souls of those devoted to her.[68]

Adam Smith was Tissot's exact contemporary, and what he writes about credit could easily be transformed, with a word change here and there, into one of the Swiss doctor's attacks on the solitary vice. Paper money that was not "abused," the political economist says, would automatically conform to a metallic standard if "reality" were always foremost. The problem is "excess paper" in a way that suggests that "the dangerous supplement" haunts both the masturbatory and the fiscal realm. And the solution is to ground moderation in reality, to eschew fantasy and representation; credit, like masturbation, is not so bad if it is in response to real needs and if something, out there, maintains an equilibrium:

> When a bank discounts to a merchant a *real* bill of exchange drawn by a *real* creditor upon a *real* debtor, and which as soon as it becomes due is *really* paid by that debtor, it only advances to him a part of the value which he would otherwise be obliged to keep by him unemployed. . . . If the paper money which the bank advances never exceeds this value, it can never exceed the value of the gold and silver which would necessarily circulate in the country if there were no paper money; it can never exceed the quantity which the circulation of the country can easily absorb and employ.

The wrong sort of credit, like masturbation — and like the novel, as we will see shortly — has what critics regarded as a false epistemology: a disregard for reality and, worse, willful distortion. Public credit allowed governments to fight wars that were acceptable only because their true costs were hidden behind a veil of debt; citizens were simply spared a sacrifice that future generations, unborn and voiceless, would have to make. Private credit allowed people to spend beyond their means or, rather, not to know what their means were. Credit, as the novelist Maria Edgeworth said, was "that talisman which realizes everything it imagines and which imagines everything."[69] Money, in other words, is the same sort of fetish as the object of masturbatory desire. Paper money, bills of exchange, and the like, on the one hand, and free sexual pleasure born in the most fertile reaches of the self, on the other, share a weird and disturbing magic.

Real exchange, like real sex, stimulates manufacturing and sociability; false commercial paper, like masturbation — sex *with* no one — does the opposite. But it was not so easy to sort out the good from the bad ways of being alone or with people. Conversation and sympathy, the Scottish Enlightenment philosophers tell us, bridge the atomizing tendencies of market self-interest. Sociability seemed to keep the bad kind of imagination at bay, whereas solitude allowed it to flourish. But solitude also offered relief from the ceaseless demands of sociability. So the problem, taken up by some of the same people who created the modern problem of masturbation, was to find a balance. Solitude is "the state in which the mind voluntarily surrenders itself to its own reflections," writes Johann Georg Zimmermann, the German doctor, physician to kings. This sounds dangerous and in another context — Zimmermann's writing on masturbation — could well be the beginning of a jeremiad against the solitary vice. But in his international best-seller on solitude, it was the opening shot of a long reflection on how the mind's surrender to itself opens the heart, prepares one for labor, and offers solace from "the spiritless and crowded societies of the world."[70] One needed to stand outside the world of exchange — social or economic — but one had to do it in the right way. And here, too, masturbation was the limit case. Nothing good came of the masturbator's solitary surrender to what was on his or her mind, whereas in other circumstances solitude might provide peace and a renewed capacity to be social. Some kinds of sociability are virtuous; other kinds — the young away from responsible supervision, for example — produce the secret vice.

The tension between those things that were identified, on the one hand, as the essence of the masturbatory problem *and*, on the other, as the foundations for a new order is everywhere in thinking about economy and society: the pleasures of the imagination versus its perils; the right kind of sociability and solitude versus the dangerous sort; desire as the engine of commerce versus desire as addictively generated by willful self-indulgence. Modern masturbation and the moral reconfiguration market society demanded were of the same generation. The same thinkers engaged in both the sexual and the broader cultural variations of the problem; put differently, they responded to the challenge thrown down by Mandeville in both registers. Thus Rousseau, for example, worried that natural self-sufficiency was being destroyed by the false needs created by commerce and sustained by a currency whose value bore no relationship to anything concrete and substantial. It sounds familiar: an eighteenth-century version of an old conversation about luxury that had taken a dramatic turn in the years around the publication and spread of *Onania*. But self-sufficiency too had its dangers. False desires and imagined pleasures were what enabled the sexual self-sufficiency that Rousseau found so terrifying were it to ensnare his pupil in *Émile*. Luxury in the context of "the dangerous supplement" may have destroyed self-sufficiency in one register, but it also made it dangerously irresistible in another. And self-sufficiency was a mixed blessing. The masturbator was lost to society; artifice and excessive imagination corrupted. But imaginative literature also elevated its readers. No one did more than Rousseau in his novels to create the sorts of fictional longings and sympathies that were meant to make men and women more moral, more social creatures. His *Julie ou La Nouvelle Héloïse* is all about the ebb and flow of desire fanned by absence and adversity and sustained by imagined bliss. Fictions — luxuries of the aesthetic — created social bonds if directed outward; turned inward, they collapsed into the solipsism of private vice.

These themes resonate in earlier and less celebrated literary circles as well. John Armstrong, now forgotten but in his day a famous and much-published doctor-poet, wrote a long, popular (at least thirty-four eighteenth-century editions) blank-verse treatment with a revealing title — *Oeconomy of Love* (1736) — that illustrates the problem of desire in its two registers. Much of the poem consists of soft-core pornographic gushing about the wonders of sexual excitement — "parting breasts, wanton, exuberant and tempt the touch" — and the rightness of giving in to it: "Nor thou, fair Maid, refuse indulgence." But should no "fair Maid" be available, the aroused reader should resist a substitute; Armstrong mounts an aggressive twenty-line attack on "the Vice of Monks recluse." Masturbation represents the limits of gratification in a poem that admits of few others. The circumlocution is itself telling: standard anti-Catholic stuff going back at least to the early seventeenth century but with the emphasis on the monks' withdrawal from an economy of any sort. The problem is not just that monks masturbate instead of having healthy sex. It is that they are antisocial — reclusive — about it. Pleasure, suggests the poet, was not meant to be solitary. Did nature, he asks, "for thy narrow self grant thee the means of Pleasure"? Certainly not.

Nature in fact was displeased except when "the swelling mingling Tumult of Desire" "from active soul to soul rebounds." She valued exchange, whether of sexual favors or anything else. Second-best would be the whore bought for gold, however bad she might be for a young man's health; better a brothel than solitary satisfaction: before you sink to masturbation, "visit thou those haunts of publick Lewdness." Decidedly the worst option was to succumb to the temptation of satisfying all that pumped-up desire alone: "Banish from thy shades / Th' ungenerous, selfish, solitary Joy." Enjoy the fruits of the imagination, but enjoy them socially. (In addition to the many eighteenth-century freestanding editions of Oeconomy of Love, one was published with a long poem titled The Pleasures of Imagination by another doctor-poet, the prolific Mark Akenside.)[71]

Efforts to create a new moral framework for desires, luxuries, and gratification as the root of good and of evil followed different trajectories for men and women. Gender figured prominently because, from Onania forward, it was clear that the sexual economy worked differently for women and for men; "always there is desire that impels and a convention that restrains," as Flaubert wrote. He meant a particular restraint; the quotation is from Madame Bovary. And the impulses were different as well. Women as consumers were construed both as necessary to keep the exuberant consumer culture of the day flourishing and as dangerously absorbed by these desires. I will take this up more concretely in my discussion of women and the marketplace in the section on reading and fiction that follows this one. The general point is that consuming, reading, self-discovery, and eros were deeply intertwined through the centuries. D.T. de Bienville, who created the new disease of women's desire — before there had been only satyriasis — laid the blame for masturbation and nymphomania, as we saw, squarely on the imagination, "the chief minister of self-love." First among his examples of how the imagination works is not sexual passion but excessive desire for food and things: in the glutton, "the imagination augments his passion for high living, and makes him sacrifice everything to indulge it." Masturbation, gluttony, and the compulsion to consume represent the collapse of what in another context was called market discipline, what Freud and his colleagues understood as the reality principle.[72]

Kleptomania, a disease largely of women, takes this on specifically: like masturbation, it is a disease of artificial desire. Display cases, like the phantoms of the imagination, seemed to exist "in order to arouse desire; they are," as a nineteenth-century doctor put it, "the preparation for an illusion." If the overwhelming impulse to find pleasure in one's own body was indeed a product of "the higher degree of civilization achieved by modern [commercial] societies" (see above, p. 281), then so was the overwhelming desire to have what was on display, or simply to have. There are, of course, other interpretations of the link between masturbation and kleptomania. Freud's colleague Otto Fenichel, for example, suggests that stealing may represent "doing a forbidden thing secretly" and offers the case of a woman who reported that she was sexually excited whenever she stole, orgasmic at the moment of theft, and frigid in sexual intercourse.[73] But my point is that autoeroticism has been linked with the dangers of commercial society since the eighteenth century and that it is here linked specifically to consumption by women. Broadened to include consumption as well as production, commerce opened up a vast world of self-exploration and self-expression, of which solitary sex was but a part.

Finally, the problem of masturbation is linked in recent world history to what might loosely be called modernity in both its economic and its political dimensions. The link is loose and so, of course, is the concept of modernity; but, still, the connection is there. The European suspicion of masturbation and the late-nineteenth-century claim by Krafft-Ebing and others that it was a form of perverse sexuality that included homosexuality was introduced to Japan during the Meiji Restoration, the period of Japanese industrialization, through Western medical writings. Only then did solitary sex become a matter for policing and not, as it had been before, a universally practiced substitute for other sorts of sex, an exercise in fantasy, a part of a larger world of eroticism. Before then erotic images were used for masturbatory purposes and fit, with no major moral problems, into the homoerotic and heterosexual regimes of urban centers (see figures 5.1a and 5.1b). More generally, doctors and pedagogues — and by the first decades of the twentieth century a large lay audience as well — came to regard sex education and hygiene as an important aspect of progress. (Opponents argued that the Japanese were by their nature, or in any case by virtue of their bodily habits, different from Western people; less meat and drink, for example, meant less sexual desire and therefore less need to channel it appropriately.) Proponents argued, to the contrary, that there was plenty of desire among the young and that sex education was necessary primarily to avoid the "horrible consequences of masturbation." Taking on board Western medicine and the view that national strength depended on the science of bodies meant taking on the solitary sex problem.[74]

We have other hints too that solitary sex becomes a problem in connection with Westernization. Indian girls who live away from home and have highly educated mothers are more likely to masturbate and to report feeling bad about it. Russian doctors from the 1890s to the early twentieth century, the period of maximum prerevolutionary industrial development, thought that increased masturbation — as well as prostitution and other sexual perversions — was the product of economic and political development. And if onanism was indeed the perversion of bourgeois alienation

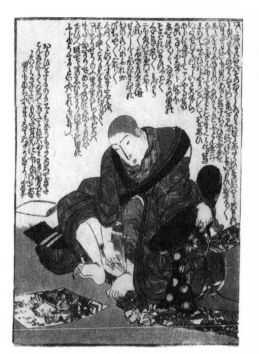 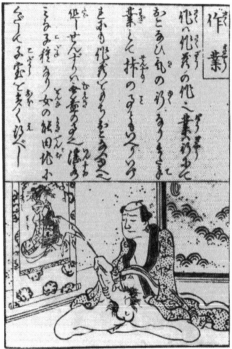

Figures 5.1a and 5.1b. Men and women masturbating. On the left is a nun using a portrait of Matsumoto Kōshirō to masturbate; on the right is a man masturbating while contemplating a picture of a prostitute. Both are in a tradition of erotic pictures in which images of masturbation are but a very small part. (Left: Utagawa Kunimaro, *Nun Using a Portrait of Matsumoto Kōshirō [?]*, multicolored woodblock page from a *shunga* album, Ikurasemu [c. 1830s]; right: Anonymous, *Produce,* monochrome woodblock illustration for *Teikin warai-e shō* [c. 1830]. Private collection.)

and selfish individualism then a proper socialist, proletarian education — so the Communist revolutionaries after 1917 hoped —
would wipe it out. Research seemed to confirm their optimism:
one study found a drop in masturbation from seventy-three to
fifty-three percent among boys and a more encouraging decline
from fifty-two to fifteen percent among girls; another found that
women on a collective farm masturbated only a fifth as much as
the girls at a local polytechnic college. The cure for masturbation,
in short, was socially valuable work and specifically membership
in a communist youth organization. As social science, we can not
judge these findings or views, but we do know that solitary sex is
consistently recognized as a problem in the context of the cultural
challenge brought about by rapid social and economic change.[75]

In early-twentieth-century Shanghai, the city where young
women bobbed their hair, smoked cigarettes, and acted the part
of their supposedly liberated Western counterparts, a young
writer took Flaubert's *Madame Bovary* deeply into her consciousness and prose. No novel of the nineteenth century links the
psychic economy of goods and of the pleasures of the body more
intimately; none is more subtle on the relationship between wanting the latest novels or fashions and wanting sexual gratification.
The young writer was Ding Ling, the most prominent woman
author of the May Fourth generation, the group of intellectuals
and politicians who brokered the cultural transition from the old
regime to the new and who, as writers, took on critical aspects of
the eighteenth-century Western European literary project: self-
exploration, the creation of sensibility, the embrace of fiction as a
map of a new kind of person. For Ding and her contemporaries,
Rousseau's *Confessions* was a crucial text in thinking through what
it meant to be modern; sexuality was a key to feminine liberation.

This avid reader of Rousseau and Flaubert sits in China's most
prosperous, commercial Westernized city, self-consciously struggling to develop a voice in which to ask "What is love?" and to
articulate the paradoxical and contrary answers. One of her protagonists is ill; strange thoughts run through her mind; the wind
blows; she is in her room with nothing to read. She cannot sleep.
She masturbates:

As the sunlight hit the paper window, I was boiling my milk for the third time. I did it four times yesterday. I'm never really sure it suits my taste, no matter how often I do it, but it is the only thing that releases frustration on a windy day.

It is a familiar story of the complex relationship we moderns have to the autarky of solitary pleasure that the eighteenth century found too dangerous to contemplate except by condemning it wholesale:

Actually, though it gets me through an hour or so, I usually end up even more irritable than I was before. So all last week I did not play with it. Then, out of desperation, I did, relying on it, as though I were already old, just to pass time.

And then, after masturbating, she reads the paper: about national and local news, education, propaganda, economics, the stock market.[76]

"Consumption," as the anthropologist Mary Douglas noted, cutting to the chase, "is about power." And its history is thoroughly intertwined with the history of yielding to the imagination, of imitating and procuring, which figure so prominently in the very first articulations of the dangers of masturbation. In the old regime, ordinary people had lesser needs than "kings or great ones," because "they [were] bounded with a more lowly pitch of Desire and Imagination." Masturbation became a problem — the exemplary version of the problem of desire and the imagination in the economic sphere — when this view could no longer be sustained.[77]

Books, Reading, and the Solitary Vice
The point I made at the beginning of the previous section applies here in a new context: just as stock-market crashes, new credit instruments, and new attitudes toward luxury did not cause the advent of modern masturbation, neither did new reading practices — private, silent, absorptive — new kinds of reading matter — novels and pornographic novels in particular — or the dramatic

expansion of the economy of print — the producing, buying, and selling of the printed word or image. But the cultural energy of certain sorts of reading and books — creatures of the marketplace themselves, crucial in the creation of desire and in its ethical management, predicated on solitude, fantasy, the free play of the imagination, and the capacity to dwell within the self — was the cultural energy of solitary sex. Novels were even more threatening than the world of commerce; they were more purely the counterpoint of masturbation. Markets, however wild and speculative, had a bottom line, however hidden: bubbles burst; credit collapsed. No reassuring reality principle governed the world of novels.

Print culture, the essential communication network of civil society and the teacher of its most basic ways of being and feeling, depended on and encouraged precisely those qualities that made masturbation seem so threatening. In the intertwined world of books and images, solitary sex represented the dangerous, dark side of new ways of thinking and being. Or more precisely, the solitary vice was where literature both as a practice — writing and more often private reading — and as content could lead if it were not civilized. Pornography was the sign of uncontrolled content, masturbation of excessive self-absorption, imagination, and solitude. In other words, masturbation becomes a problem, because aspects of print culture become a problem, and this happens because the dangerous dark side of the much-extolled imagination and fantasy, of the capacity of always wanting more, and of the newly created realm of the private is solipsism, selfishness, and complete moral collapse. Civilization depended, in short, on what it also feared.

That masturbation might represent broader cultural developments in media cannot be surprising to us moderns of the twenty-first century. The day I first wrote these sentences a letter appeared in the *New York Times* from a Yale Law School professor who bewailed his own addiction to the Web — so powerful, he says, that he had put in filters to do what his willpower could not do. He also complained bitterly of his students who check their e-mail and engage in other solitary electronic pursuits while in class, which made me think of Tissot's account of the bored seminary students who masturbated during lecture and of similar contemporary stories of self-absorption.

More specifically, the connection between literary practice and the content of literature, on the one hand, and masturbation, on the other, is one that modern scholars have shared with us now that solitary sex has been at least partially rehabilitated. "In graduate school," writes one of the more self-revelatory of their number, "I read Rousseau's *Julie*, noting in the margin each time I cried." In this, she was not very different from eighteenth-century women readers who worried that they had perhaps not cried enough; unlike them, however, she planned to write a paper on when she cried and why. It was a fantasy project, she goes on to say, that was akin to writing on Sade, "a text which moved me to masturbate." Once again, Rousseau and "the dangerous supplement" come together. Like so many eighteenth-century readers, this critic was fascinated by the sheer physical pleasures of reading, by what it did to the body. To get right to the point, she focused on "the connection between these two productions of bodily fluids — tears and arousal" — which, in turn, maps onto the connection between "the sentimental (coded as feminine) and the pornographic (coded as masculine)."[78]

Eighteenth-century commentators would perhaps not have been as sure about which gender to associate with pornography as modern researchers, but the link between masturbation and the modern literary enterprise was there from the beginning. (A noted authority says that pornography today exists to produce sexual fantasies "that initiate or accompany male masturbation" and that if a similar need existed among women there would be more pornography written for them.[79]) But reading as a physically powerful act, one that engaged the imagination, one that invited the sort of pleasurable, secret, potentially addictive self-absorption that contemporaries identified as the core of the private vice, was certainly something women did. The rise of silent reading and the novel did not, as I said, cause the dramatic new exigency of solitary sex. But solitary sex was the exemplary case of the moral challenges they represented.

Neither I nor Jane Gallop, the distinguished professor at the

University of Milwaukee who masturbated while reading Sade and wept while reading *Julie*, invented this conjuncture. Dr. Johnson was on the same track in the eighteenth century. He noted that the most reclusive people are not necessarily the most studious nor the most capable of keeping their inner lives in good moral order. Many "give themselves up to the luxury of fancy." They manipulate in their minds the past and the future; "they place themselves" like the Rousseau of the *Confessions* "in varied situations of happiness." "Invisible riot[s] of the mind," Johnson called these reveries; they were, he said, "secret prodigalit[ies] of being," which were "secure from detection, and fear of reproach." The roaming, unsecured, and undisciplined mind free to imagine as it wished, free to create worlds of its own, seems very close to the secret life of the sexual, desiring body. Johnson's "secret prodigality of being" is the threat of solitary sex.[80]

I claim no originality in making this observation. Tissot beat me to it by more than two centuries. "The self-polluter perpetually abandoned to his obscene meditations," he wrote less than twenty years after Samuel Johnson, "is in this regard, something in the case of the man of letters, who fixes all his attention on one point." And, he adds, it is "rare that such excess is not pernicious." In fact, the "diseases incidental to literary and sedentary persons" are perhaps the prototypical, the purest form of masturbatory disease, and the intensive, self-absorbed work of the literary man, the prototypical form of solitary vice. In "studious men," Tissot explains, there is a "perpetual dissipation of the nervous fluids which springs from the incessant action of the nerves," without hand being put to genitals. Semen, that is, "the most important liquor, the Essential oil" — by which he and his contemporaries meant something like nervous energy, life force — is lost most straightforwardly not through ejaculation but by thinking too hard. It is not the hand but the brain that is "either unstoppable or incapable of action" both in the man of letters and in the masturbator. Both physiologically and morally, the solitary vice is a special case of solitary mental work, and specifically of literary engagement. Tissot might not always have understood the question quite as broadly as I will construe it here, but the men who created modern masturbation understood that they confronted a far larger issue than self-induced orgasm, one that went to the heart of what it was to be a modern person as they understood this creature.[81]

The connections between literary practices and masturbation are deep and extensive. Masturbation's evils — suspicious solitude, dependence on the perfervid and unbounded imagination, the seeming inevitability of addictive excess — find parallels in the silent but far-reaching revolution of consciousness that private reading both reflects and helped create. There is, however, a difference between private reading and private vice. As far as we know, people have always masturbated. They have not always read silently in private, and they have not always read a form of literature whose pleasures were the result of its fictionality, its absorptive power, its capacity to inscribe new sorts of pleasures onto the soul. Private vice becomes morally exigent as one aspect of the far larger and specifically modern problem of privacy in general and private reading in particular.

The trajectories of these questions are somewhat different: private reading has a longer and more continuous history than masturbation; it had no clear 1712. But it did come into its own in the generation before *Onania*. Whereas solitary sex was only rehabilitated in the late twentieth century, private reading was more quickly tamed. By the middle of the eighteenth century, everything removed from the public eye had ceased to be regarded, as it once had been, as uncivil. And private reading in particular, though always suspect in some circumstances and never wholly policed to the satisfaction of some, became acceptable if not always praiseworthy. Even the novel, the most threatening form of literature routinely read in private, had been morally domesticated by the late eighteenth century except in the most suspect of circles. (The American purity reformer Anthony Comstock, for example, was never quite reconciled to any fiction; his usual line was that the trash most people read never induced them to read anything better and, in any case, many books of the classical canon like Boccaccio were as bad as half-dime novels.)[82] Masturbation, however, continued to represent the evils of both private reading and imaginative fiction, and even when they stopped being acutely threatening, the horrors of the private vice remained as their legacy: the dangerous, resistant "first darling sin" of selfish desire.

The reading part of the story stretches back thousands of years. We know that in Antiquity — when masturbation was of minor interest — reading was usually public and aloud; or, if individual, the reader generally spoke in a quiet voice. Reading without saying the words was thought prodigious; famously, Augustine was amazed at Ambrose's ability to do what every elementary-school student can do today — read silently — and the learned bishop must have done it haltingly at that. In fact, the very transcription of language without spaces between the words — as it was done before the High Middle Ages — made silent reading at anything approaching modern speeds extremely difficult. It is all but physiologically impossible to read unseparated writing without saying the words aloud. And conversely the rise of our modern form of transcription — a set of graphic conventions for the separation of words — along with new syntactic forms of Latin made it possible for silent reading to become routine. It had happened in literate — primarily clerical — circles by the thirteenth century, and then spread into aristocratic lay society.[83] Reading became a far more intimate matter than it could have been before, a way of communing within oneself with the ideas, passions, fantasies of others and making them one's own.

Silent reading was, of course, not necessarily private reading. When the fourteenth-century historian and poet Jean Froissart gave Richard II a manuscript copy of a book of his verse, the king took it into his chambers only after skimming through it and then reading parts aloud to courtiers. And even in his private quarters, he would most likely have been in the company of retainers and close advisers. The luxury — and the political possibility — of reading silently, in seclusion, in the quiet of one's bedroom, even in bed, was possible at first only for a very few. By the fifteenth century, however, it had become more widespread in wealthy lay as well as clerical circles; intimate solitary reading had become a real possibility and pleasure.

The moral implications of this revolution were clear from the beginning. On the one hand, it made possible a more direct and personal relationship with God, a closeness through the contemplation of religious texts; books meant to be read in one's closet for the benefit of one's soul proliferated. Not only Protestantism was nourished by private access to sacred and devotional literature, even if reading has always been associated with reform. (In fact, the geography of literacy follows closely the geography of Protestantism, but that is a larger question we need not take on here.) On the other hand, private silent reading was manifestly dangerous. It made it much easier to encounter sexually exciting material free from observation and restraint; it sustained private fantasy and incited private desires. Images of potentially salacious biblical scenes began to make their way into illuminated manuscripts — David and Bathsheba, Susanna and the Elders — but movable type enriched the erotic, as well as religious, inner life on quite another scale. Here was a technical innovation that could really penetrate to the quick.[84]

Printed books, hundreds of times cheaper than manuscript, were filled with all sorts of stuff — heresy, politically and religiously dangerous thoughts, romances, erotica — all of which responded to the public demand for the previously unthinkable luxury that we in the modern age take for granted: reading alone. It was a blow for freedom of thought with all its attendant thrills, dangers, and contradictions. Among the first really big press runs — four thousand or more — were Luther's Bible and Aldus Manutius's introduction to the erotic Latin poetry of Catullus.[85] Giulio Romano's images of the sixteen positions for making love, the so-called *modi*, first circulated only among connoisseurs, but then they went into print, making the private contemplation of erotica far more widely available than ever before to an eager and ever-growing audience. Cheap versions were still circulating in late-eighteenth-century London among the popular classes. Ultimately, these lewd poses were married to Pietro Aretino's lewd sonnets in praise of copulation and sexual organs to produce the first — and most long-lived — book in the Western erotic tradition. Maybe the prints were studied by couples, perhaps they were contemplated alone. But it was a book for one's time alone, for those moments of quiet and solitude that allowed readers and viewers to turn inward. Erotic printed material gave readers and viewers the opportunity to meditate, as one historian has put it recently, "on the way in which all forms of sexual experience were self-referential."[86] *I modi* was also a direct challenge to papal authority, censorship, and the politics of the Church generally, a model for how the private world of sexual stimulation came to be regarded as so powerful a threat to society. Of course, this sort of contemplation need not be of images in print. The men who commissioned the now-canonical paintings by Titian and Giorgione, for example, of Venus with her hand on her pudenda — masturbating perhaps — for their private spaces did not threaten anything, but they were engaged in a complex new relationship to art and representation that mechanical methods of reproduction made enormously more widespread than before.[87] (See figures 5.2a and 5.2b.)

This is all still the prehistory to the "reading revolution" of the late seventeenth and the eighteenth century. By then its impact on politics as well as on the inner life of a broad swath of the literate population would be profound. Policing the act itself — private, silent, intimate secret reading — as well as the content of what was read — sorting out the innocent from the pernicious — became a major cultural project. (The whole discipline of literary criticism grew up to help with the task.) For the generations that followed the publication of *Onania*, autoerotic sexual pleasure continued to be construed as the evil twin of the secret pleasures of reading works of the imagination: the unassimilable double of one of the great cultural triumphs of modernity. Private reading, even private reading of imaginative fiction, had been tamed by the late eighteenth or early nineteenth century. Masturbation, however, and the one form of fiction with which it had always been explicitly linked — pornography — were left as residues that found few defenders until the late twentieth century. I will discuss their joint, and sometimes separate, rehabilitation in the next chapter.

For now I want to consider private reading as a process distinct from its content, in the sense that we worry about the impact of TV or the Internet without specifying the content of programs or Web sites. Of course, this separation is difficult. At one extreme,

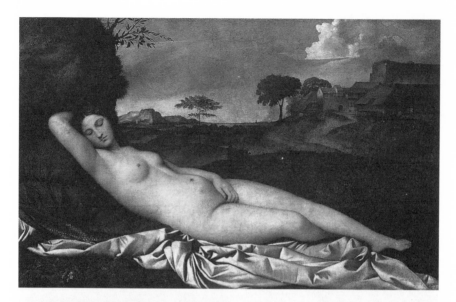

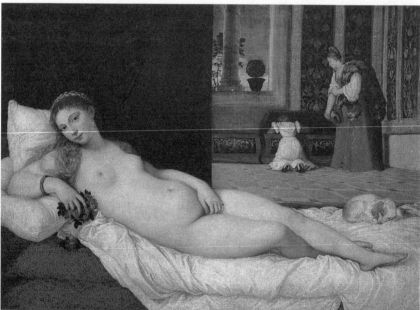

Figures 5.2a and 5.2b. Pictures from the great tradition of high art like these, with their suggestive placement of the model's left hand, were painted for the private rooms of gentlemen. Printing technologies made more explicit erotic pictures far more widely available for private contemplation. (Top: Giorgione, *Sleeping Venus*, 1510 [Alinari/Art Resource, New York]; bottom: Titian, *Venus of Urbino*, 1538 [Alinari/Art Resource, New York].)

certain kinds of reading, like certain kinds of TV watching or Internet surfing, seemed entirely unproblematic. Whether one read manuals on coach making, coppersmithing, or penmanship silently in private or aloud in public was morally neutral because the things that the imagination reassembled from words on paper were essentially public anyway and had little effect on the inner life. Also, the technology itself was never condemned wholesale. People were quick to pick up on the good that could come from the widespread, revolutionary technology of silent private reading and thought that they could turn it to ethical advantage, however dangerous it might be politically, socially, or morally. In some measure, this meant controlling the setting and the sociology of reading, just as other activities were policed. We have already seen, for example, how the constraints of class and proper breeding were thought to mitigate the dangers of closet prayers in the seventeenth century. Certain sorts of reading material and situations were thought dangerous to some but not to others. Reading itself was enlisted to counter its own worst effects; fire could be fought with fire. Proper reading could be an edifying — indeed a vital — way of touching the consciences of individuals deeply and directly; good books inserted good thoughts and good ways of thinking and feeling straight into the consciences of readers. Good books not only taught but stimulated sympathy; the right sorts of books produced feelings of horror and revulsion against evil. They created a new moral sensibility. And this is what the burgeoning literature against masturbation — that which was not purely advertising anti-masturbatory products in any case — was about: private, silent solitary reading was mobilized as prophylactic against its own worst dangers, private, silent vice.

As Chapter 2 showed, print culture was essential to *how* masturbation became the primary sexuality of modernity: commerce in books and pamphlets spread the word about the new vice of commerce. But more specifically, private, silent reading was essential. In fact, it is hard to imagine how a secret vice that could not be spoken about would have made itself known otherwise. Kant "consider[ed] it indecent even to call it by its proper name." *Onania*, Tissot, and all the pedagogues and doctors and moralists had access to the inner reaches of the mind through books without embarrassment or lapses of decorum, in much the same way as modern researchers, too embarrassed to ask about masturbation, inquire about it through written forms. Private reading was the perfect vehicle for propagation of the knowledge that solitary sex was indeed a *secret* vice, because the act itself reinforced the message: anything so bad, so embarrassing and horrible, that word of it could not be breathed aloud had to be a deeply guilty pleasure. Reading secretly about a secret was guaranteed to make it seem all the more dangerous and perhaps all the more delicious. This was the age of secret histories, of behind-the-scenes views of politics and social life. It was also the age of the epistolary novel, which worked by giving the private reader the illusion that she had access to the secret letters, and thereby the inner thoughts, of its characters. The letters that fill the published eighteenth-century record of masturbation — testimonials or inquiries — must have had much the same effect. They described what people did that could be revealed nowhere but in correspondence with a doctor. But more on the connections of masturbation to other literary forms in a moment; the point now is that we know that private reading did, in fact, play an essential part in creating the secret vice.

Almost no one reported what confessors and writers of books on morality had so long feared: that they learned to masturbate from books or warnings. But from the twentieth century back to the eighteenth, the book was crucial to making masturbation morally exigent, to teaching both that it was wrong and dangerous and that the battle to conquer it was a test of real character. Not masturbating was portrayed as the victory of triumphant willpower, whereas continuing to do it as a sign of moral weakness and defeat. The whole gigantic market in the literature on masturbation rested on the notion that something more than preaching or word-of-mouth advice was necessary to propagate an awareness of moral danger; many a guilty conscience seems to have been born from print.

Examples abound. A Russian peasant responding to the queries of a researcher in the 1920s said that now that he had *read* about how bad masturbation was, he would stop; without a book, he might never have known that a lifelong practice was a lifelong vice. Many of the people who wrote for advice to Marie Stopes, the birth-control advocate and author of a best-selling guide to mutually satisfying sex, were similarly beholden to their reading. Miss L. said she was single and had been "the victim of masturbation from an unknown beginning until about three years ago." Her moment of enlightenment came when she read Edward Carpenter's *Love's Coming of Age* and, "*for the very first time* [emphasis in text] understanding, stopped after a very long struggle." (Instead of masturbating, she took up heavy petting with her boyfriend, which she felt was probably not so good either; Stopes advised that she stop that too and marry her beau as soon as possible.) Another correspondent wrote Stopes to confess that he learned to masturbate as an ignorant boy, that the habit had nearly wrecked his life, but that he had found out just in time "the real nature and danger of my course" from reading Stopes's *Married Love*. He had been ashamed of what he was doing but was afraid to ask advice; he wrote that he felt sure Stopes would have sympathy. C.H.G. learned self-abuse as a schoolboy and did it for years but recognized the error of his ways when he accidentally came upon a popular sex-education book, *Knowledge a Young Man Should Have*, bought it, and read about how much harm he had done to himself. (His father, he wrote, would not talk about sex, and grown men told him it was good for him.) As we have already seen, by reading a much-reprinted German anti-masturbatory tract of the early nineteenth century, the playwright August Strindberg learned that what he was doing was a horrible vice about which he ought to feel guilt. Bishop Sixt Karl Kapff's book worked as intended; August was plagued by his conscience for years. Tissot tells us, and his archive supports his claim, that the publication of *Onanism* unleashed a torrent of letters from readers whose lassitude, pimples, sweating, and various cardiovascular complaints were due, so the writers thought, to their "infamous habit" during childhood. Readers were ready to find in books the clues to self-diagnosis: their suffering was the result of their secret vice. *Onania* reprinted letters from readers who told about how they first learned that masturbation was a vice from newspaper advertisements and then tried, sometimes three or four times, to buy the book so they could learn more. This has been, over the centuries, a bookish vice.[88]

But there is another side to all this. Private reading also bore all the marks of masturbatory danger: privacy and secrecy, of course, but also the engagement of the imagination, self-absorption, and freedom from social constraint. The private reader was, at least for the moment, an autonomous if not autarkic being. Modern writers are remarkably clear on this. The novelist Josef Skvorecký described reading in bed when a boy in Communist Czechoslovakia as a forbidden act: hidden under the blankets, "cuddled in my bed . . . [I] indulged in the pleasures of reading, reading, reading. . . . I fell asleep from a very pleasurable exhaustion." Colette veritably gushes about the sensual delights of silently reading novels in bed when a girl. But the connection of private reading to private pleasures goes back much further. It was certainly more fun than a board game, thought Chaucer's insomniac lady in *The Book of the Duchess*; do not imitate "certain persons who busy themselves in reading and other matters" in bed, warned the Catholic educator and saint-to-be Jean-Baptiste de La Salle in 1703.[89]

And, of course, warnings about the dangers of private reading of imaginative literature had a long history. (Perhaps reading in dangerous company, reading away from the full light of public scrutiny, would be a better description.) Recall Canto 5 of Dante's *Divine Comedy*: "We read of Lancelot, by love constrained / Alone, suspecting nothing, at our leisure," answers Francesca to the question of how "Love did first show you those desires / So hemmed by doubt."

Sometimes at what we read our glances joined,
Looking from the book each to the other's eyes,
And then the color in our faces drained.

But one particular moment alone it was
Defeated us: *the longed-for-smile*, it said,
Was kissed by that most noble lover: at this

This one, who now will never leave my side,
Kissed my mouth, trembling. A Galeotto, that book![90]

Clearly, what the two lovers read matters a great deal; but the intimacy of reading alone together is what leads to further intimacy. Private reading, in other words, was a way of being intimate with oneself or with another; in the balance between individual and society, it was very much over on one side. Quite apart from content, the act itself posed a threat, one that was ever more pressing as the practice became widespread.

Its connection to the private vice was manifest to contemporaries. "The patient should never be left alone, never suffered to read, never have time to reflect," advises a mid-eighteenth-century tract on the treatment of masturbatory disease, because this is precisely what got him in trouble. On the authority of a colleague, Tissot offers the same advice: "Patients should never be left entirely alone; . . . they should not be allowed to meditate, to read, or in any way to occupy the mind." The reasons for this are several. To begin with, reading reproduced the situation that got the masturbator in trouble in the first place: "Nothing is more pernicious to people inclinable to a single idea, than idleness and activity"; all books that require application "may recall those ideas to their imagination, the remembrance of which should be entirely obliterated." Moreover, reading makes the symptoms of masturbatory disease worse: already weakened sight is further strained; already weakened nerves are further stressed. The suspicion that solitary reading put one in danger of solitary vice thus had a long history that continued to have influence even when private reading became commonplace and generally accepted.

The act itself never quite shook its legacy of unpoliced pleasure; perhaps not until television replaced it as the new antisocial medium was it fully rehabilitated. And television in turn now seems tame compared with the Web. One read alone — in bed, under the covers, in one's own room, luxuriously and out of sight. A long footnote to the Italian edition of Tissot recounts the story of a young man who ended up "languishing in fantasy" and couldn't let a day go by without self-pollution; he knew full well

315

that to be cured he ought not to stay in bed once he had awakened; instead of exercising his imagination, he ought to get up and
"rejuvenate his machine."[91] Serious Victorian writers on addiction
took reading as their subject and offered advice on how it could
be turned to social good. It was simply useless, "a way of spending
our limited capital in time," wrote Herbert Maxwell in "The
Craving for Fiction," unless one did it seriously and kept notes so
that something was transmitted to the future. That is, if one read
alone not for pleasure but for some utilitarian purpose, it might
not be "addictive." Maxwell was writing in the decades when
"wanker" became the common slang for "masturbator" and took
on the connotation of someone engaged in useless effort. "The
vice of reading," argued another Victorian, Alfred Austin, in the
context of a discussion about addiction, was the result of doing it
for its own sake. Austin thought that reading fiction in such a way
that the imagination was exercised to produce disenchantment
was a good thing, since it led to social change. But in general the
problem was that reading anything was potentially like masturbating: done for no purpose but pleasure.[92]

Some argued not that reading led to masturbation or that, as
Maxwell and Austin suggested, addictive reading was a homo-
logue of masturbation but that "reading disease" and masturbatory disease were more or less the same thing and had the same
cause. Isaac Ray, the nineteenth-century American forensic psy-
chiatrist, for example, seems to say that reading almost anything
fictional literally inflamed the imagination, even if the books
were not filled with explicit sexual themes. The reader becomes
sick in the same way as the masturbator; imagination infected
them both, and then the two, jointly produced pathologies made
each other worse. The mind of youth, Ray wrote, was "enfeebled
by an incessant repletion of juvenile literature," which left it
"unconscious of any manly thoughts." A boy "abandon[s] himself,
body and soul," to the allurement of books, which seduce "the
sense with their fantasy." "Violent mental emotions thrill through
the bodily frame." Body and mind work together, and soon he
may as well be masturbating, which in fact he is led to do. Masturbation seemed a handmaiden to the even worse vice of litera-

ture, whose "debasing effects" were "constantly assisted by the habit of self-indulgence."[93]

Ray was not alone. Important American educators thought that omnivorous reading had a tendency to feminize males and, more specifically, that if this potentially useful activity was not carefully regulated it could easily tip over into onanism. The eugenics movement of the early twentieth century picked up these themes. In boys and girls, cautions a writer on maintaining racial strength, "one would be inclined to regard such a dislike for the ordinary vigorous mode of life which normal adolescence demands and enjoys" in favor of staying indoors, lounging on a sofa reading or daydreaming, "as indicative of self-abuse or psychic masturbation."[94] One of the main expositors of Freud in America noted that some boys and girls begin to masturbate while reading, and not necessarily books of an erotic nature either: brutal scenes in *Uncle Tom's Cabin* might do it for boys; girls apparently resorted to masturbation after reading sadistic or masochistic scenes. Nerds — that is, those who live in their minds — are likely onanists.[95] The reading revolution never quite shook off the vice that it helped to create. It had put privacy, secrecy, and solitary pleasure on the moral agenda of the age, and even when it itself was tamed, its evil twin continued an unruly life of its own.

The imagination, the first great villain of the solitary vice, was also the faculty that first came to prominence in the eighteenth century both in thinking about philosophy, ethics, and art and in the day-to-day lives of all but the poorest. The "pleasures of the imagination" were intended as democratic. There was no moment of origin for this revolution as there was for solitary sex; but we might make something of the fact that Addison's enormously influential essay "The Pleasures of the Imagination or Fancy" — the pleasures that, he said, arose from contemplating actual visual objects or from calling them to mind through any sort of representation, including images, statues, or words — was published in 1712. (Addison uses the terms "imagination" and "fancy" more or less interchangeably, both going back at least to Augustine, who used *imaginatio* and *phantasia* as two versions of the same thing: the former a faculty of reproducing in the mind something that was no longer present, the

317

latter what one historian of these concepts calls "the light, airy play-ful activity of mind in its freedom.")[96] Whether the objects were present or not, the imagination — the evil genius of masturbation — made them available for self-arousal. It was poised to become the most praised and the most fraught faculty of the century.

The imagination is everywhere in eighteenth-century think-ing: in discussions that range from the economy and credit to sen-sibility and morality to epistemology and aesthetics. It was, quite simply, at the core of modern humanity, an absolutely fundamen-tal and irresistibly attractive faculty linked to novelty, change, and freedom:

> Our imagination loves to be filled up with an object.... [T]he mind
> of man naturally hates every thing that looks like a restraint upon it
> and is apt to fancy itself under a sort of confinement when the sight
> is pent up in a narrow compass.... [E]verything that is new or
> uncommon raises a pleasure in the imagination.[97]

Addison, of course, was not thinking of the pleasures of "yielding to filthy imagination" that *Onania* warned against when he wrote his essay more or less simultaneously with John Marten's alto-gether less edifying tract. It would probably never have occurred to him in so elevated a context. But the enormous expansion in what was expected of the imagination made solitary sex morally exigent; here, as in the economic context, the new secret vice came to define the limits of a vital but dangerous new exercise of individuality and freedom.

How the imagination went from being a decidedly second-rate faculty — useful at best in mediating between sensation and rea-son, dangerous at worst in allowing humans to mistake repre-sentation for reality — to its place of honor in the eighteenth and nineteenth centuries is a long story told in other books. But from whichever angle the story is told, the end is the same. By the time of the Romantics, the old rankings had been turned upside down: "Reason is to the imagination as the body to the spirit, as the shadow to the substance," wrote the poet Shelley in *A Defence of Poetry* in 1821. It was now what most defined the particular human genius. Fifty years later, Darwin is rapturous about it: "one of the highest prerogatives of man . . . [the faculty that] creates brilliant and novel results."[98]

The story from minor role to star player might begin with the problem of explaining conscience, amiability, or the very possibility of an aesthetic response in the epistemological revolution started by John Locke, a set of questions that were answered when his successors elevated the imagination to a place coeval with reason and understanding. It might have a big chapter on its role in Hume's epistemology, in his insistence that to reject the imagination's trivial suggestions while embracing its supposedly well-founded suggestions "wou'd be most dangerous, and attended with the most fatal consequences." It was not so easy to hive off fancies in a philosophy that insisted that so much of what we hold dear is, in fact, based on them. Likewise, we might pause and consider the importance of the imagination in the moral philosophy of Hume, Smith, and others of similar persuasion, for whom it was the ability to imagine the consequences of an act well into the future and through an elaborate set of situations that made moral behavior possible. It, along with nervous physiology, was the basis for sympathy, which the great opponent of masturbation Jean-Jacques Rousseau, among others, thought was the foundation of morality. There would need to be a big section in such a history on Kant, for whom imagination was not, as it had been, opposed to reason but reason in its sensuous form. And this outline leaves out a great number of possible topics.[99]

Alternatively, we could approach the question by rehearsing all the things the imagination was said to be by various eighteenth- and early-nineteenth-century thinkers: the central guiding principle of the continuity of the person which allowed us to connect our pasts, presents, and futures; the link between reason and the senses or between the body and the mind; the foundation of art and of economic desire; the core concern of a new branch of philosophy–aesthetics; the key to how ideas were understood to be connected in associationist or perhaps any empiricist psychology, among much else. If reason was not entirely dethroned from its place in the hierarchy of the faculties, it now had stiff competition.[100] And though it may be difficult to sort out the many diverse and complex meanings of the faculty that also constituted the core danger of solitary sexual pleasure, its centrality to a broad range of cultural concerns is clear enough. What doctors and moralists identified as the biggest problem with masturbation became at the same time an essential quality of a cultivated human being.

We need not confine ourselves to high intellectual history in following through this curious juxtaposition. The pleasures of the imagination were everywhere and were closely tied up with reading. Through certain works of the imagination — through the fictions called novels — men and women were supposed to learn how to harness their capacities for fellow feeling, how to suffer empathically what others suffered, how to feel a common humanity, and more generally how to navigate the new world of love and commerce. Novels, the imagination, and modern solitary sex took a major turn together. The attractions of the great literary genre of the age were precisely those that entrapped the masturbator: the pleasures of tricks and deceits. Or, more precisely, the pleasures of the novel — "nobody's story" — were the pleasures of fictionality itself: the frisson of absorption in a reality that was known to be artifice. The elaborate novelistic confections were perhaps more complex and elaborate than the average masturbatory fantasy, but the seductiveness of "nobody's story" was not so very far from the seductiveness of sex with nobody.[101]

We are now ready to think more about the problem of content and genre that added to the intrinsic dangers of reading alone. In the wide-ranging discussion that swirled around the question of how to civilize the imagination, no topic was more prominent than the novel and solitary novel reading, and most especially women reading novels alone. (Reading novels aloud or in libraries, though not entirely regarded as safe, was never seen as quite so threatening; in these public situations, reality had at least a toehold.) If "fictionalizing" in general is a way of being present to ourselves, a way of self-grasping and a way of escaping, of overstepping and of creating boundaries, then the stakes in reading a particular form of fictionalizing — the novel — are great: reading novels could create new ways of being morally present to oneself for good or ill.

On the one hand, they were said to be not only pleasurable but also edifying. In them, virtue triumphs and wickedness gets its just reward: by resisting temptation, Pamela triumphs and makes a better match than the one she rightly rejects. Sensitive, virtuous heroines, like their real-life counterparts, make manifest their goodness by the right kind of reading. Moreover, the moral wheat could be separated from the chaff. Critics and journals began to sort out the good novels from the bad, sound thinking from skeptical philosophy. As a technology of practical morality, a school for affection, love, and sympathy, the genre always had its defenders, including that scourge and victim of the masturbatory imagination, Rousseau. The novel, in short, was absolutely critical to the making of civil society, and contemporaries knew it. *Lesewut*, *Lesesucht*, and *Leseseuche* (the craze, the passion or addiction, the plague of reading) were everywhere; not a woman's room and scarcely a worker's quarters were without print. So, whatever ill wind might blow, this was how the modern world was, and fictional literature could help one live morally in it.[102]

But there was also always a cloud over fiction, the same cloud as over solitary sex. The danger of forsaking the real for the wasteful and illusory, which Tissot put at the heart of onanism, is there too in critiques of "novelism." "When a farmer's daughter sits down to read a novel, she misspends her time," writes the *Critical Review*, a journal whose purpose was to sort out good from bad reading; it is time that she ought to employ in "real service." (We might be reminded again of the historian Alain Corbin's characterization of masturbation as "the supreme symbol of individual time.") Novels, like masturbation, created for women alternative "companions of their pillows"; novels, like masturbation, inflamed the passions of youth and probably contributed to the increase in prostitutes. As the prolific eighteenth-century literary man-about-town George Colman put it: "'Tis NOVEL most beguiles the female heart. Miss reads — she melts — she sighs." In short, novels, like seductive whispers and dirty talk, turned women on, made them forget their honor, and led to

every sort of deviant sexual practice. And novel writing, especially for women, had about it a sort of harlotry: a public woman
of letters was all too close to a public woman.[103]

The moral pathophysiology of novel reading and masturbation
was also similar, an example of the general and large category of
diseases caused by the inappropriate exercise of a faculty, the
imagination, whose vividness, immediacy, and unalloyed attraction could wreak havoc on the nerves and all that they touched. In
the eighteenth century, the imagination did immense amounts
of epistemological, ethical, and aesthetic work. Its powers were
great. Imagination "revives the perceptions themselves," as Condillac put it, whereas memory "only recalled the signs." It is perversely creative, able to make "new combinations at pleasure." It
can play all sorts of tricks that amount to disposing our ideas
"contrary to truth"; madness lies at the end of this path. It is thus
a terribly vulnerable faculty of the mind, a weak link. "Little by
little we will take all our chimeras to be realities," says Condillac,
and therein lies the danger of novel reading, especially for poorly
educated girls who have trouble anyway telling the real from the
fictive.[104]

The problem with the novel and with masturbation is not, of
course, that those who engage in fiction reading or in erotic self-
stimulation literally cannot tell, or are mistaken about, the onto-
logical status of fantasy. No one would claim that a character in a
novel or the imagined objects of desire really exist, although one
might for a time act as if they do. What Condillac means, and
what was worrying moralists generally, is that the fictional quality of the characters in a novel or masturbatory fantasy made
them more real, more compelling, more able to arouse sentiments than so-called real characters or real sexual partners. In
any case, it made them infinitely more accessible and free from
control. The danger lay in representational excess, in fiction or
artifice coming to supplant nature with its in-built structure of
constraints.

Now we have masturbation solidly in the realm of reading. If
insanity could be due, as Alexander Crichton, the first great theorist of alcoholism, put it in 1799, to "disproportionate activity of

the representative faculties" arising from "causes that exalt imagination" — that is, the faculty of fiction too frequently exercised" or "strong passions" — we are in a position to understand not only religious manias — Tissot cites the case of an insane Moravian — but also masturbatory madness, the mental illnesses of novel readers, and all the other ills caused by overstimulated nerves.

If reading books had somatic consequences, the far greater mental excitement of masturbation would not go unnoticed by the flesh. In 1802, Thomas Beddoes, the radical physician, chemist, prototypical late Enlightenment character, and father of the Romantic poet, attacked "books which act perniciously upon the constitution ... novels which render the sensibility more diseased." He thought that circulating libraries accounted for many sicknesses because "the power of certain ideas to irritate organs ... requires no illustration." The dramatist Richard Sheridan regarded them as "an evergreen tree of diabolical knowledge." Readers of *La Nouvelle Héloïse* wrote the author about "sighs and torments" they experienced, about their hearts "beating faster than ever," about being driven to bed and nearly mad, about weeping and being convulsed by such sharp pain that they had to put the novel down. Masturbation and novels thus worked in the same way. Coleridge thought that reading novels "occasioned the entire destruction of the powers of the mind." An eighteenth-century commentator thought that they intoxicated the mind with "morbid sensibilities," — that is, they rendered it exquisitely vulnerable to moods, feelings, and stimulus — they were to the mind "what dram drinking is to the body." Novels "affect the organs of the body," "relax the tone of the nerves," and along with music have "done more to produce the sickly countenances and nervous habits of our highly educated females than anything else." We are getting very close to masturbatory disease. And if we add the view that "novelism" — the *Methodist Magazine*'s term — produced vacant countenances, continually fed the imagination, ruined the lives of women by, among other things, becoming alternative "companions of their pillows," — the same phrase again — "tickled the imagination," and set up irresistible discontent, it seems ever closer to its contemporary onanism. Novelism, like onanism, was

323

dangerous because its protagonists were not really there and were all the more stimulating for their absence. Both offered desire all too free a play. The difference is that, much as they had in common, fiction had its virtues and self-abuse did not.[105]

The new "trouble and agony of a wounded conscience" of those who gave themselves over to solitary sex was born at the same time as the imaginary literature that helped produce the urge to do it, the guilt, and a remedy of sorts in safe fantasy. *Onania* began with a moral peroration, but it quickly moved into the epistolary mode; edition after edition of it and its *Supplement* grew from letters. They harked back to the "letters" on questions of love, marriage, and repentance that filled the magazines of the 1680s and 1690s. "It was," for example, "my calamity to be seduced, as to give up the very soul of beauty, my Honour, to a lewd and infamous Rifler, with whom I secretly continued the vile and unhappy conversation, for twelve months together," writes "a very young woman, born of parents of some little quality," to the *Ladies Mercury*. After this affair was over, she says that she married "the most passionate of men," a man of great worth, honor, wealth, and virtue, with whom she would be happy were she not plagued, a hundred times a day, by the "rueful remembrance" of her sins. The problem is not only the "delusion and pollutions" she brings to the marital bed but a further deception: "I practiced even the vilest of Arts in his Bridal Night Joys, being in that dearest scene the highest of counterfeits." That is, she pretended to be a virgin. What to do?[106] Written by men who claim to be dedicated to the service of women, this is itself a most artful literary production: voyeuristic, primly salacious, and yet moralizing, said to be true but pretty clearly fiction. It is almost exactly the tone of *Onania* and of early novels as well. This is meant to be edifying stuff with just a bit of a kicker.

If the *ur* text of the solitary vice looked back to the news sheets out of which the novel grew, it also looked forward to the seduction or would-be seduction scenes of eighteenth-century novels with their morally edifying resolutions. Even the eponymous heroine of John Cleland's *Fanny Hill* finds true love and monogamy at the end of her adventures. Her literary ancestor in

Onania is perhaps not so fully developed, but Marten paints her wickedness in considerable novelistic detail, and she, too, comes to see the error of her ways. In a long letter, a correspondent confesses that she was taught the "folly of self-abuse" when she was eleven. (To be precise, she should have said that she was taught self-abuse; she learned it was a folly only much later.) Like Fanny, she shared a bed with the woman who initiated her into the pleasures of sex, not for a few nights, as Fanny did, but for seven years! Unlike Fanny, she did not move on to men but practiced with her maid "all the means we were capable of to heighten the titillation and gratify the sinful lusts the more." Our heroine, classically educated — she would not be in this fix, she says, if she had read more of the Bible and less Juvenal, Ovid, or Martial — and the chambermaid were encouraged by Aristotle's pronouncement that they could procure for themselves "*cum digits, vel aliis Instrumentis*," a sensation "*non multo mino Coitu Voluptas*." Indeed! (The letter writer is referring not to the real Aristotle, who, as far as I know, never wrote on this subject, but to the author of a book called *Aristotle's Masterpiece*, which was a major source of sexual information or misinformation from the late seventeenth through the early twentieth century.) Now, after all these years, she confesses that her clitoris is the size of a thumb and asks, "What should she do?" Not to worry, says Dr. Marten. Read Dr. Carr's account — duly reprinted — of two nuns who were thought to be hermaphrodites but instead had each enlarged her clitoris by excessive masturbation and lesbian rubbing.[107]

I will return to the manifestly pornographic quality of Marten's story in a moment. The point for now is that this little novelistic snippet was, at least on the face of it, meant to teach virtue and was taken by later writers in this spirit. Growing from edition to edition through letters, *Onania*, like an epistolary novel, was the most literary of productions: a compilation of intimate revelations, full of secret details and extraneous flourishes, that were said to be in the service of virtue. The putative malformation of the letter writer was meant to instill fear of vice and very well might have. All sorts of writers, not as venial as Marten, told stories like this with the intent to terrorize. And his specific gambit had a long history; modern diarists as well as medical texts report the fear that masturbation was evident in the genitals. It could not be hidden from the *sensus medicus*, so the masturbator's supposedly secret guilt was in fact all too manifest on his or her body.

Understanding all this perfectly, Tissot approached *Onania* as if he were a literary critic. The book is "perfect chaos"; he omitted in his extracts, he said, many of those parts that best represented "the vivacity, the pathetic expression of pain and repentance" of onanism's victims but reminded his readers that it is on facts like these that "the impression depends." Critics of Tissot, in turn, picked up on these literary themes. A certain M. de Lignac, the author of a successful book on the physical differences of men and women as they are relevant to marriage, praises him for making his readers "shudder with horror," for being the "great master" who has painted "pictures so doleful" as to "efficaciously approach his readers." The translator's introduction to Tissot's *Essay on the Disorders of People of Fashion* says that it "may properly be called a Medicinal novel: the precepts are agreeably delivered, the descriptions natural and striking, the examples pertinent, and the excursions of fancy are such as must be felt by all who have feeling." Dr. Hume might have said the same about the accompanying *On Onanism* that he translated.[108]

No one took the idea of fighting fire with fire — the dangers of the imagination with the most imaginative of medical books — further than D.T. de Bienville, the doctor to whose genius we owe "nymphomania." He was a cunning wordsmith, if not a great physician, who understood the joys of masochism. As attractive to the youthful imagination as his book admittedly was, its point is to terrify the young, especially young girls. Novels, he holds, were certainly a major cause of the diseased imagination that led to masturbation, but they were also part of the cure. "The perusal of a novel," he wrote, as well as "a voluptuous picture, a lascivious song, the conversation and caresses of some seducing man," could excite the young maid. But the main problem was that the content of fiction as well as the social world in which it circulated stimulated the very desires that novels were meant to channel. (Bienville did not need Michel Foucault to tell him that desires

326

were created in order to control them.) Reading about unre-
quited love, thwarted marriage, vacillating parents, and evil servants in the context of an overstimulating modern society was
his heroine's downfall. Germs of corruption are strengthened by
reading; it induces her to "improve every occasion of gratifying
her curiosity" regarding the nature of her desires.[109]

And the cure was also the poison. "What a remedy" these
"tender and lascivious" works — novels — would prove to be!
They "were like a burning-glass which collects the rays of the sun
in order to fix them on one particular spot, which they must set
fire." Under these anatomically precise circumstances, it comes as
little surprise that Berton, the maid, teaches her charge to masturbate. (Servants, second perhaps only to school friends, were
the leading teachers of self-abuse for both boys and girls in two
centuries of reporting on masturbation; self-discovery was third.)

Salaciously novelistic as all this might seem, we are invited to
interpret the story benignly. It is a morality tale; things end badly
for our antiheroine. Julie's passions are ever more inflamed by an
erotic imagination that writhes out of control without the coun-
terweight of another's flesh, the physical presence of a real lover.
She becomes seriously ill; a doctor is called in and tells her parents that the only hope is for them to give permission for Julie to
see St. Albin, her would-be beau. They refuse. A new physician is
called in; Julie gets worse; the parents are horrified when they
discover the truth about their daughter's masturbatory adventures
— heightened to a fever pitch by her thwarted love of the ideal
lover her imagination had invented. They banish her. Nymphomania has set in, and we leave this odd little twist on the eighteenth-
century novel with our heroine incurably ill but not yet dead. The
book and the hand, they excite the same spot. The novel gives
birth to impossible love and masturbation and ultimately to the
disease of hypersexuality and proffers a cure for their ill effects.
Bienville's book is, after all, a work of the medical imagination, in
part a self-conscious fiction, that tells a cautionary tale and suggests a remedy for ignoring it.

Anti-masturbatory books, in short, were meant to work like
novels in creating a new morality in the Enlightenment. We are in

the presence of a very literary medical genre that adapted the conventions of the kind of fiction that most clearly exemplified the dangers it sought to counter. In a sense, the anti-masturbatory tract is an example of the novel tamed in the interests of socially appropriate love.

But masturbation was more openly and overtly linked to the novel untamed, and more generally to the problem of delusion in art, religion, and politics. These have their own histories in the eighteenth century that articulate with the cultural history of masturbation in that they share core problems — undisciplined imagination and unsocialized desire. We could point to debates about how to civilize artistic creation: how, for example, to make it more like the work of reason than of a perfervid imagination, less like Bienville's masturbating, nymphomaniacal woman who transformed her lover, Pygmalion-like, into an Adonis ("a Vulcan into an Adonis," to be exact) through her imagination and more like the male artist whose enthusiasm to create was, somehow, of a different order.[110] *Schwärmerei*, the disorder that worried so many eighteenth-century German thinkers in which people mistake "fictions" for real knowledge and delude themselves into falling for a variety of false prophets, secular and profane, was not so far from masturbation. ("Enthusiasm," with all its lunatic revolutionary resonances going back to the seventeenth century, would be the English equivalent.) It was supposedly caused, like onanism, by weak nerves and a repressed sex drive, among other things, and shared a common cultural milieu. The enemies of *Schwärmerei* regarded the mania for novel reading as a sign that the hyperemotional subjectivity that had long plagued Protestantism was not dead in the supposedly more secular Enlightenment. Introversion in one realm easily blurred over into others.[111]

Of course these issues are not new. Fiction as a threat to both reality and morality had had a very long history by 1712: millennia of anti-theatrical rhetoric as well as the anguished confessions of those seduced by art. The problem of aesthetic solipsism — the dangers of self-absorption in fantasy — goes back at least to Plato if not before, and famous examples of such delusion appear continually in Western literature. In his *Confessions*, for example,

Augustine bemoans that he felt sorrow for the fictional Dido, who killed herself for love, but failed to weep over his own very real spiritual death. And perhaps more to the point, he condemns his transports of grief, pity, and pleasure — pernicious pleasure, vile joy — in sharing vicariously the joys and sorrows of characters onstage. It is a self-indulgent emotion with no purpose in the world — "the auditor is not aroused to go to the aid of others" — abject wallowing in one's own objectless emotions: "What sort of mercy is to be shown to these unreal beings upon the stage?"[112]

What was new in or around 1712 was that such imaginative flights lost their old constraints across an enormous swath of economic, social, and cultural life. (In fact, they were of the essence of modern life.) Masturbation was the moral threat of this revolution in its unredeemable form. While some reading is edifying and some credit redounds to the general good and not to empty excess, no kind of rubbing of the genitals produces anything but ill. The secret vice became a scapegoat for its more respectable neighbors, the place bearer of the dangers of the imagination, excess, and privacy on which they could be securely located, condemned, and sent out into the desert beyond civilization.

And by the late eighteenth century, all these themes had come together in the antirevolutionary rhetoric of certain circles. The Swiss conservative zealot Johann Georg Heinzmann, writing in 1795, argued that novels "read in secret" created the same sort of unhappiness that the French Revolution spawned in public. They fostered all manner of illusions about life that not only were politically dangerous but also made their readers — male and female — sick physically and morally. Victims of novel reading, like the votives of the solitary vice, were driven into "all the madness of fantasy"; their nerves were put in a state of high tension; their "inexperienced hearts" were tossed around in storms of anxiety; they ceased living in the real world. And from adventure stories, readers — again male and female — succumbed to even more freethinking and obscene literature, which pushed their already-fragile souls over the edge.[113]

Heinzmann was an exception. By some time in the early nineteenth century, the novel had been domesticated; whether or not the works of Sir Walter Scott are the watershed is less relevant than the fact that it had been successfully policed and assimilated into polite society. One could, as we have seen, still find objections to novels and indeed to reading alone, but both seemed more or less under control. Masturbation, however, remained exemplary of the failure to control both fiction and sexuality; and so did its literary twin, pornography.

"To be anti-pornography is to be anti-masturbation," as some modern wag has it. Conversely, pornography was, and is, made largely to use while masturbating. This is and was, of course, not its only use, and it may not be one that is shared equally by all genders and sexualities all the time. But a visit to the local sex shop or even the neighborhood bookstore, not to speak of a visit to one of the tens if not hundreds of thousands of masturbation Internet sites, will make the connection today transparently clear (A Google search for masturbation yields 1,570,000 hits. A few are about masturbation; many more offer material for doing it.) Historically, the advent of masturbation as a serious moral question for men and women, boys and girls and the spectacular rise of pornography in the West share a social, economic, political, philosophical, and psychological world: urban, commercial, literate, generally antiestablishment, grounded in nature — in the material world — rather than in divine authority, attracted to narrative over mere description. Commercial pornography was born in the generation before *Onania*.

Pornography and masturbation are linked at all levels. The dreamer in Diderot's *Rêve de d'Alembert*, for example, interrupts a lecture on materialism to masturbate, a generally recommended practice in the book, in front of his hostess. And even if it is not entirely clear that he, the character who seems to speak for the author, is actually masturbating, another character in the discussion, Dr. Bordeu, delivers an attack to Mlle de L'Espinasse against the "magnificent praise that the fanatics have lavished on chastity and continence" that ends with an unambiguous endorsement, in some circumstances, of the secret vice. Actions that are pleasant and useful are at the top of the heap, he explains, and those that are neither are at the bottom. No question here of whether plea-

330

sure itself is a good thing. She promises not to draw back "no matter how rough" the conversation gets, and he immediately asks, "How about secret pleasures?" "Doctor!" she exclaims in shocked disbelief as he proceeds to explain that they rank high: certainly pleasurable, and they actually do some good. Then he offers the "if Cato the Elder were alive today" argument that we have already heard: a sensible man would prefer masturbation to either putting himself in the way of disease by having sex with a prostitute or corrupting someone else's virtuous wife or sister. And more generally, why deny oneself a necessary and delicious pleasure just because the greater pleasure of having sex with someone is not available? "But our doctrine shouldn't be taught to children," she declares. "Nor to grownups," the doctor replies.[114]

This was far-out and Diderot knew it; even he did not brief an affirmative case for masturbation. Nor did libertines, who much preferred the unbridled pleasures of sex *with* anyone or any thing. Masturbation in most circumstances was regarded as radically antisocial in a way that even pornography was not. Bad books, so some believed, regularly made good points; much Enlightenment anticlericalism and radical philosophy were articulated through a demimonde print culture that combined elevated argument with stories and pictures of sexual adventure. Masturbation, on the other hand, was at best a meager substitute for something more social. If the anti-philosophes used the incident in Diderot — and much else they could adduce — as evidence that sexual depravity was an essential part of the Enlightenment project, even those who endorsed this depravity could muster little enthusiasm for onanism.

Pornography is not tied specifically to a moment in Western history, nor is it necessarily connected to solitary sex as a terrible secret vice. Alternative modernities produced alternative sexual ethics. We know of societies that enjoyed bad books and prints for purposes of masturbation or stimulation without either the books and pictures or the acts that they sustained coming under any particular moral cloud (figure 5.3). The commercial, urban, sophisticated world of eighteenth-century Japan, for example, produced thousands of *shunga*, whose purpose was acknowledged

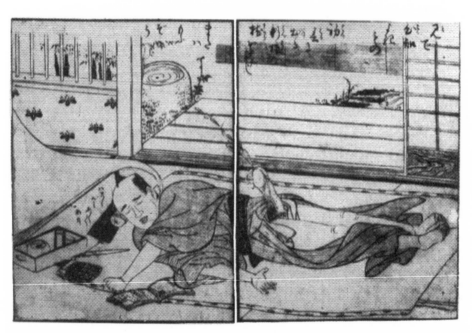

Figure 5.3. Katsukawa Shunshō, *Wet Dream After Using a Pillow Book,* monochrome woodblock illustration for Jinatku Sanjin, *Ukiyo no itoguchi* (1780). This woodblock comes from a Japanese erotic tradition that recognized and profited from the power of reading to produce sexual arousal.

to be masturbation. Males more than females were thought to indulge, but we have pictures of nuns as well as young men masturbating while reading or looking at images in books or scrolls. (See figures 5.1a and 5.1b) No great political import was attached to either image. And though it was assumed that if grown men read porn to masturbate they were lacking the real thing, nothing more seemed to follow. Porn and masturbation thus existed symbiotically in a commercial culture governed more by the sorts of sexual sumptuary laws that regulated masturbation in Antiquity than by the modern sense of an especially dangerous vice.

Not so in the West. Pornography was dangerous knowledge. Even if it was not sold secretly — we know that dirty pictures and bawdy songs were widely available in the streets of eighteenth-century London, as was medical soft-core porn — it was consumed secretly, privately, beyond the reach of authority, of social and religious scrutiny. Pornography, like masturbation, was antiestablishment. Not entirely so, of course. William Gladstone fought long and hard against evil books and what they did to him. He made a resolution, he tells us, to avoid "all books of which the title suggested they might probably offer food to depraved appetites." That night he went into a bookshop in search of something in particular but started browsing. He saw a suspicious book that he looked into; a "vague curiosity so full of danger" led him further afield. After a few desultory passes he opened the poems of Rochester and his resolution collapsed. With "a corrupt sympathy" he read two of them, trying at first to convince himself that he was doing so only to learn about the facts of nature and manners of men but aware that this was but a "wicked delusion." Whether on this occasion he masturbated or flagellated himself, as he would do after subsequent temptations, we do not know. But that pornography attracted him and men of his class is beyond question.[115] Still it was antisocial in the sense that it was openly sustained by suspect social groups — adolescents, unsupervised students, the unrespectable poor, libertines, philosophes and less elevated opponents of the Church, radicals of all sorts, including some unsavory underworld types, and, by the end of the nineteenth century, revolutionaries as well — who threatened good

333

order. Pornography and masturbation were in the shadows of the Enlightenment and modernity more generally, and together they represented weakness of the will, the dangers of privacy, the imagination, and excess beyond the fringes of civilization or in the realms of the Church, which the philosophes routinely portrayed as rife with perverted love and private pleasures. (One thinks, for example, of Diderot's parodic, pornographic litany in which a young nun is brought to confess her solitary pleasures to a lesbian mother superior.)[116]

By pornography I mean not only those dangerous books — the books to be read with one hand, in Rousseau's famous phrase — whose explicit purpose was to spark sexual fantasy and sustain masturbation but a considerable swath of modern imaginative fiction: the "ill books ... love stories, lascivious discourses, and other Provocations to Lust and Wantoness [sic]" that Onania, and all works against masturbation for the next two centuries, identified as a prime cause of the supposed new epidemic of solitary sex. (That pornography did political work as well is beside the point here except to suggest once again that masturbation had always been associated with subversion, if not of the body politic then of the body social and the body private.) Whether more pornography led to more masturbation we cannot say; but the spectacular rise of the genre in the context of the private reading of fiction certainly made the question of solitary sex far more exigent culturally than before.

Some bad books take relatively little imagination to translate into excitement and masturbation. (I speak here of books that seem to be addressed to men; some eighteenth-century ones clearly had both sexes in mind, but we know little about women's use of "bad books.") L'Ecole des filles, the first pornographic bildungsroman, the first full-fledged story of sexual self-discovery, the book that Samuel Pepys took to bed and then burned so as not to have such trash found in his library, leaves very little to chance as one girl tells another how she was initiated into the various pleasures of sex. Unlike the reveries of past pleasures that Pepys conjured in order to get excited as he lay in a boat traveling the Thames, this first great porn "novel" demands relatively little work. One can identify with the voyeuristic author and go from there. But making something erotically exciting out of less promising material was precisely the sort of exercise of the imagination that enemies of the new private vice regarded as so very bad. Porn was where one found it and what one could make of it.

"I got Aristotle's Masterpiece which cost me one shilling," John Cannon, whom we met earlier, tells us, writing about his youth in the 1690s, "which I got to pry into the secretes of nature, especially of the female sex." This would be roughly the equivalent of a twentieth-century adolescent's looking for excitement in Marie Stopes's *Married Love* or Theodoor van de Velde's *Ideal Marriage*, although *Aristotle's Masterpiece* says nothing about adroit lovemaking as the basis for companionate marriage and a lot about how to reproduce successfully. It, like the twentieth-century books, offers little that is salacious and lots that is moralizing — "eager pursuit of sensual gratification disqualifies for the exercise of the loftier powers." But all these books do speak of secret things that could be explored secretly. "Lustful thoughts" ensued from his reading, Cannon says, which led him to bore a hole between the privy and an adjoining room through which he could watch the servant "do her occasions" and "placidly see that parts my lustful thoughts provoked." With all this intense reading and looking, he says that to remedy his arousal "the aforementioned practice of my schoolfellows was sometimes put into practice without a remorse or reflection on the vanity of such folly." That is, Cannon masturbated. He had learned how five years earlier, when he was eleven, from an older boy at a swimming hole.[117]

He made no efforts in the midst of these masturbatory reveries to have "carnal familiarity" with the servant or any other woman, he writes in his memoir, but he did find more bad books. Popular books and health guides — a booming part of publishing, second only to religion since the advent of print — seemed to offer nearly limitless and cheap fantasy fodder. This time it was *The Book of Midwifery* by the herbalist Nicholas Culpepper. (Culpepper was a mid-seventeenth-century revolutionary, enemy of the Royal College of Physicians, and a man whose life's work was to make knowledge more widely available.) Cannon confessed it "served

335

for a further inlett to Youth's forbidden Secrets of nature"; that is, it served as material for more sexual fantasy. But "being bolder than ordinary," he read it at a time when his mother was nearer than he had thought. She confiscated it, and he never "fingered it again." Sexual desire and curiosity were magnified and embedded in reading; masturbation was intensely textual and owed its new sinful status to the bigger problem of regulating a flood tide of overt pornography and an even greater tsunami wave of potentially arousing books and images.

Onania, John Marten's earlier books, Tissot's *Onanism*, and the whole anti-masturbatory mass of print share a problem with earlier confessional literature: they elaborate so lovingly on the very vices they wish to suppress. Like confession, the genre is one big "invitation to discourse," as Michel Foucault put it, which limns an aspect of the psyche in order to police it, to make it the core of new guilts and new moralities. (Unlike confession and confessional literature, the anti-masturbatory stuff was not a once-a-year occasion or a reference guide in the hands of priests but a widely distributed always available body of work.) But the point here is that the new guilty practice becomes exigent not so much *through* as *because of* the moral exigency of a more general cultural phenomenon: new dangers of the imagination whose most irredeemable aspects were pornography and solitary sex.

In his earlier *Gonosologium novum*, Marten lets his male readers know that he realizes that "the parts of women that are calculated for that office [for intercourse and sexual pleasure] are very curious" and that his public will want to know the details. These he provides: women know that they find pleasure only in the clitoris, a word he takes "to signify lasciviously to grope the privities"; girls pleasure themselves if they cannot find men; and so on. Little wonder the book was prosecuted. *Onania* is coyer in the manner of centuries of moral advice and confessional literature. What sounds like a come-on echoes *Holy Living* by the pious Anglican clergyman Jeremy Taylor and hundreds of works before that. Critics may say that masturbation "ought not to be spoke of, or hinted at, because the bare mentioning of it may be dangerous to some, who without it would never have thought of it." Just in case, though,

336

working by reverse, [it might] furnish the Fancies of silly people with
Matter for Impurity.... I beg the reader to stop here, and not proceed any further, unless he has the desire to be chaste, or at least apt
to consider whether he ought to have it or no.

Whether this is intended as advertisement for the soft-core stories
that abound in the book — the school mistress who with tears in
her eyes informs the wife of a local gentleman that she had "surprised and deterred some of her scholars masturbating 'cum digi-
tis,'" the guilt-stricken boys who write that they could not stop
and pray for the medicine to cure them of their acne and shyness,
the clergyman who writes of a young man and a young woman
who died of self-abuse (she specifically of *furor uterinus*, nymphomania *avant la lettre*) — is not something we can know. The author,
in fact, agrees that some of the more far-fetched letters he prints
may be feigned; he publishes other letters which say that he
encourages the very vice he was the first to condemn so extensively; and he offers long extracts from his enemies' pamphlets
that straightforwardly accuse him of obscenity. Some rivals, as we
saw, accuse him of masturbating. All this said, Marten in *Onania*
offers the defense that manifestly serious works like Tissot's
would offer: that "*Onania* is a Book of Morality."[118]

Tissot goes back and forth for three or four apologetic pages
on the same question. His books "stands in the same predicament
as all books of morality" easily condemned for "multiplying a
vice to display its dangers." It is a problem, he says, that he shares
with the Bible. What he hopes to do is especially difficult in vernacular languages, he admits, but in Latin — in which *Onanism* was
originally published — the audience would be small. He is being
so novelistic only because he wants to terrorize his readers into
virtue. The whole project, in short, exemplifies the dangers of
knowledge and enlightenment. Having given up divine authority,
Tissot and his colleagues must rely on "letting the eyes of youth
be opened," letting them see "the dangers as well as the evils"
in order to prevent the further decay of humanity and return us
to "the strength and power of our ancestors." The ideal seems to be
the peasant of whom Tissot writes in his *Essay on the Diseases*

337

Incidental to Literary and Sedentary Persons: "Sheltered from dangerous discourses, far from alluring objects ... his desires have not that impetuosity, which is oftener the effect of imagination than necessity."[119] Little wonder Rousseau found in his countryman such a kindred spirit. But also little wonder that the creators of the new vice shared so much with their enemies, the writers of "ill books ... love stories, lascivious discourses, and other Provocations to Lust and Wantoness [*sic*]" and especially the pornographers.

This is a literature caught up in its literary surroundings. Bienville is utterly conventional in condemning the sexual, and specifically the masturbatory, dangers of the novel: whatever natural vehemence girls might suffer from, it is immeasurably increased "when they read such luxurious novels as begin by preparing the heart for the impression of every tender sentiment, and end by leading it to the knowledge of all the grosser passions and causing it to glow with each lascivious sensation." That something should assuage such fires is scarcely surprising. But he himself spares no novelistic detail. Everyone in his position, he admits, must come to terms with the "real boundaries of decency" and not transgress them. But one must be clear and vivid: "May my pencil be sufficiently expressive, may my colours be sufficiently natural to inspire all that horror, with which so detestable a vice should be surveyed." He promises "striking pictures" of "shocking and incredible miseries" ready to overwhelm girls. This reads like a slasher-film preview. He is back and forth on the problem of readership. On the one hand, *Nymphomania* seems to be addressed to parents and educators. But Bienville admits that copies might fall into the hands of young girls — through lack of parental attention or even the "seductions of libertines, who are never at a loss for an artifice, whereby they can gain a foothold." He as much as admits that his book is porn. Still, if a young girl were to get hold of a copy, the most that would happen is that the premature knowledge thus acquired would make her feel the "fragility of her nature" and the "impending wreck" that she would become if she followed the path of the book's victims. And, yes, Bienville admits, "by this book [*Nymphomania*] the curiosity of young men will be more excited than that of the sex [women]" but they

338

should not be taken in. Lest they think only girls suffer from self-abuse, they should read as an antidote Mr. Tissot, whose "frightful impressions . . . painted with such expressive force" will set them right.[120] Clearly, the masterpieces of eighteenth-century anti-masturbatory literature are very close to the novels and especially to the pornography that they identified as prime suspects for the self-abuse epidemic.

But here is the rub. If masturbation was the evil doppelgänger of the imagination, then pornography was the moral nadir of imaginative fiction, the bad seed of a potentially wholesome family. In the eighteenth century, this whole class of fiction — pornography — which later was so neatly ignored in the family tree, in fact represented in its purest form the power of literature to arouse the imagination and make itself felt on the body. If, as we know, Rousseau's novels shook their readers' bodies deeply, the books we have called pornography since the late eighteenth century produced still more striking effects. And we might make the same claim for the visual arts. Representations have been known since classical Antiquity to be arousing — men masturbated on the cold marble of statues — and the arousing, even explicitly sexual content of much high art is clear as well. Looking at the overtly pornographic image is the bottom line of this kind of looking: arousal without the self-conscious aesthetic disinterestedness that art demands. Perhaps all of this is true only from a masculine perspective: men actively gaze at images of women and make them their own; many literary pornographic confections seem to be about male power over women's bodies. Men look at pictures of women sexually enthralled in reading a romance and create for themselves a voyeuristic viewing place outside the picture; women supposedly only identify passively with the reader.[121]

In fact, we know very little about the relationship of women to images or to pornography either in the eighteenth century or later. (Bienville hints that they may have been salaciously interested in his would-be medical porn.) An argument could be made that the image of the curious girl that is so prominent in straightforward erotic literature and so much discussed in anti-masturbatory tracts can be understood as allowing both objectification (the male view) and identification (the female view). And who knows how different viewers identify with a picture or what sort of position of watching they create for themselves or what sexual pleasures they get from that vantage. We do know that being able to look at images and to make something of them, erotically or not, is an act of the imagination and was understood as such in the eighteenth century. The power to look entails the power to imagine. We also know that today women's claim to create and enjoy pornography is part of a larger claim on sexual and personal autonomy and a contentious issue in feminist politics. But more on this in the next chapter.[122]

We have ample evidence that women were thought by men — and by some women — to be the prototypical absorbed readers, ready to give themselves over to the imaginative flights of fiction. And we know that the limit case was women reading something so arousing that it caused them to masturbate. Whether women were the main readers of novels we do not know for sure, but almost certainly they were not; whether they masturbated as much or as little as men we do not know at all, and neither do we know whether they masturbated while reading more than, less than, or the same as men. But we do know that just as the woman masturbator was the poster girl of dangerous solitary sex — she produced nothing but desire, pure libidinous pleasure — the woman reader was the gold standard of the moral corruption latent in all fiction. She was the misguided reader par excellence, the enthralled reader, the prototypical victim of imaginative excess, the representative of "the literary marketplace rather than the literary public," the perfect onanist.[123] In the erotic and pornographic images of women touching themselves, these threats were combined in one place.

Mandeville, once again, is prescient. He envisages a physically engaged reader, one in less innocent circumstances than those who would write to Rousseau about their tears and heart palpitations after reading his novel. Fiction was seductive, and in the absence of a lover women made do as they could. In one dialogue, Antonia is reading plays and romances; she lets her fancy roam. Lucinda suggests that as she "passionately" throws herself backward, she might

340

clasp her legs one over the other and then tightly clasp her thighs together with all her strength. She should repeat this after fifteen minutes, a technique that Mandeville seems to have learned about from *The School of Love* by his contemporary John Marshall. Male fantasies about women reading, self-absorption, sexual desire, and masturbation — if not these things themselves — have a pedigree that goes back roughly to the age of *Onania*.[124]

Before the late seventeenth century, reading for women — and men as well — is generally represented in art as a relatively safe activity. Sometimes we see men engaged in business; sometimes the book is little more than a prop, a sign of piety or learning: a physician or a scholar is shown with a book; a woman is reading a missal. Sometimes it is part of an allegory, as when the Virgin is shown with the Christ child and a Bible, the Word made flesh and the word on the page, so to speak. And if reading is depicted as absorptive and otherworldly it is the world of the spirit that is in question: a figure is intensely engrossed in reading sacred texts. When, as we rarely do, we see people reading secular books, they are anything but solipsistically involved in the page but look out at us. Sometimes, as in Rembrandt's depictions of his mother reading, the figure is too old to count as sexual by conventional standards and the reading matter is, in any case, clearly safe: a map or diagram. All of this changes in the late seventeenth century.

Seventeenth-century Dutch art begins to offer us an abundance of bourgeois women gazing raptly at a text — often a letter. This is in itself new; in earlier art we saw mostly men reading their correspondence. But with women, "love is in the air in these letter pictures." Gerard Ter Borch's *A Lady Reading a Letter* is exemplary; she is quite lost to the world in the process (figure 5.4). There is a hint of danger in some of these pictures, a sense that more might come of the sentiments conveyed by the letter, the soft features and intense eyes of the readers suggest a melting if restrained passion. Men were rarely depicted in this sort of absorptive reading, although judging by the many condemnations of bad reading, we can assume that they did it; their reading is usually work-related, public, directed outward. By the eighteenth century, women had come to be depicted exclusively as lost to the world in their little

341

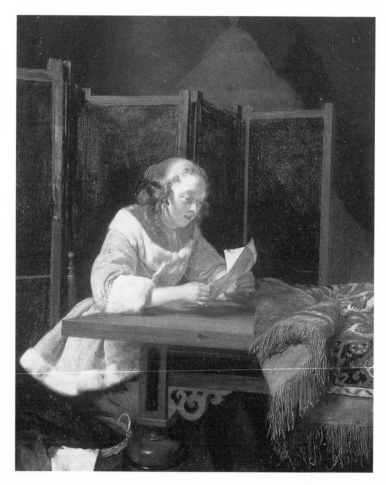

Figure 5.4. Gerard Ter Borch, *A Lady Reading a Letter,* 1660. "Love," as the art historian Svetlana Alpers notes, "is in the air" in this and other letter pictures of the later seventeenth and eighteenth centuries. (Reproduced by permission of the Trustees of the Wallace Collection, London.)

books, lounging in luxurious, sensual surroundings that promised, but did not quite deliver, more explicit displays of sexual pleasure. Fragonard's *Souvenir* serves as an illustration, but his *Love Letter* would do as well (figure 5.5). The idea is the same yet with more explicit voyeuristic pleasure for the viewer of Boucher's *Lady on a Sofa* or Greuze's *Lady Asleep*, where the subject has her arm on a book and a dog in her lap — a commonplace icon of sexual plea- sure in eighteenth-century art (figure 5.6).[125]

This visual tradition is translated into explicit pornography of women rapturously masturbating while reading. (The only depic- tions we have of men engaged in autoeroticism are anticlerical representations of monks or voyeurs who are missing the action. "Real" men are absent from the visual record.) Here, arguably for a male audience, certainly by male artists, are the titillation and the danger of women, aroused and reading alone, reveling in their erotic imaginations. Isaac Cruikshank's *Luxury* could not be more explicit: the excess of goods, the cupids on the mantel, the warmth of a fire heating the woman's exposed backside in a well-appointed room with a softly bolstered sofa to one side; a book open on the table; another book, Matthew Gregory Lewis's *The Monk*, with its gothic pathos and sexual sadism, perhaps a racy passage marked with her thumb, in her left hand, which is positioned so that her arm pulls down on her loose chemise to reveal most of her swelling breast, her right hand under her clothes masturbating (figure 5.7). A somewhat rigid little lapdog is on his back — actu- ally, one cannot tell its sex — and seems to be trying to look up her dress if it is not just tense from the sexual excitement of the whole scene.[126] The engraving *Midday Heat*, based on a gouache by Pierre-Antoine Baudouin, is almost as clear; alternative versions leave no doubt (figures 5.8a and 5.8b). A book has fallen out of the woman's hand, light falls on her hands, one dropped languorously to her side, the other between her legs. She is alone in her rever- ies except for the gaze of the classical bust of an androgynous youth; this is about solitary sex. And if there is any doubt look at the unexpurgated version. (In *The Dangerous Novel*, it is unclear whether the woman reader, oblivious in her dreamy sleep, has already given herself enough pleasure or whether she might be

343

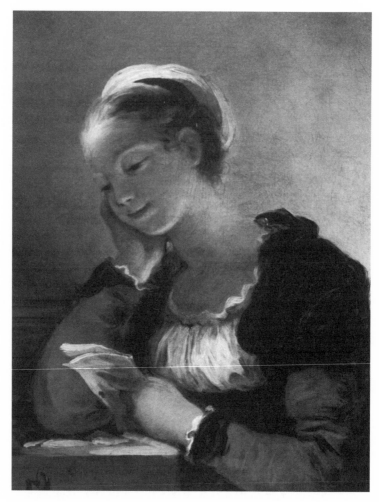

Figure 5.5. Jean-Honoré Fragonard, *Souvenir*, 1776. It is clear that this young woman absorbed in her letter is remembering love.

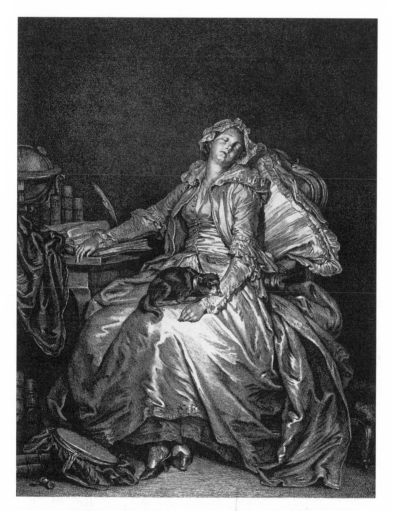

Figure 5.6. Jean-Baptiste Greuze (1725–1805), *Lady Asleep.* Although the globe and pen suggest that this lady might have been occupied with more active, worldly affairs, the languorous look of contentment on her face and the dog in her lap — often a sign of the erotic — suggest literary and sexual self-absorption. (Staatliche Kunsthalle Karlsruhe, Germany.)

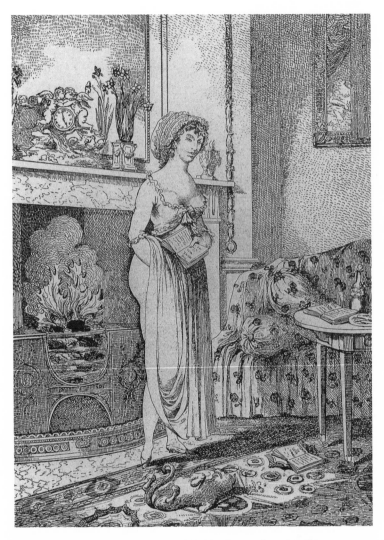

Figure 5.7. Isaac Cruikshank, *Luxury,* 1801. The themes of novel reading, consumption of ever more goods, and masturbation are brought together in this print by one of England's best-known political artists. (From Edward Fuchs, *Geschichte der erotischen Kunst* [Munich: A. Langen, 1922]. Courtesy of the Bancroft Library, UC/Berkeley.)

happy to see the miserable figure of a man crouched near her bed stand; viewers of neither sex will identify with this pitiful creature (figure 5.9). The lover in Laborde's *The Dormeuse* is more promising as he comes upon his mistress in a rapturous swoon, book fallen by her side, but again solitary sex seems to have beaten him there. [(figure 5.10)] There are many variations on the theme, aided sometimes by text. An illustration to Claude Joseph Dorat's poem "Anthem to a Kiss," for example, makes much of the dual meaning of the verb *baiser* — "to kiss" and "to fuck" — and the engraving is meant to give force to the critical seductive energies of literature (figure 5.11). It is what corrupts the young virgin who imagines much and is about to take matters into her own hands. ("Safe, hidden from her mother's eyes / Learn in my songs what kisses mean / As in her bed alone she lies . . . And to her mind reveal the whole / Of pleasure's tempting ecstasy.") This is the stuff of Tissot's worst nightmare.[127]

From here it is a short step to pornography bereft of any artistic pretensions if this is not already it. In *Le Progrès du libertinage*, a nun masturbates as she reads while looking at herself in a mirror (figure 5.12). In one way, this is simply an illustration, albeit a sharply graphic one, of the very old attack on clerical celibacy that had been going on in Protestant circles since the Reformation. Try to enforce unnatural celibacy and this is what you get. But it is also a catalog of the dangers of the Enlightenment that masturbation represented: the capacity of reading to arouse as well as to instruct; the threat that knowledge, and indeed self-knowledge, will corrupt as well as exalt. The liberatory narrative of holding a mirror to the genitals — so powerful in the feminist women's health literature of the late twentieth century — is marshaled at the intersection of libertinage and anticlericalism and modern self-creation. Thomas Rowlandson's 1812 pornographic caricature *Lonesome Pleasures* is onto the same theme without the anticlericalism: A woman is exposing her genitals in preparation, the title of figure 5.13 suggests, for solitary gratification; a dildo rests on the ground as if not really needed but there in reserve. She is manifestly the object of the gaze — ours to be sure, perhaps that of the randy man whom we see behind the open curtain, although

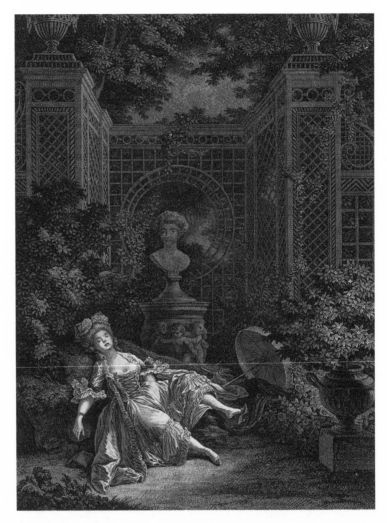

Figure 5.8a. Emmanuel de Ghendt (1738–1815), after a gouache by Pierre-Antoine Baudouin, *Midday Heat*. Everything in this picture — the faraway, rapturous look, the book that has apparently just dropped from her right hand, and, of course, her left hand under her dress and between her legs — suggests that the woman happily collapsed on her chaise longue is engaged in doing what one does with "books to be read with one hand." (Bibliothèque Nationale, Paris.)

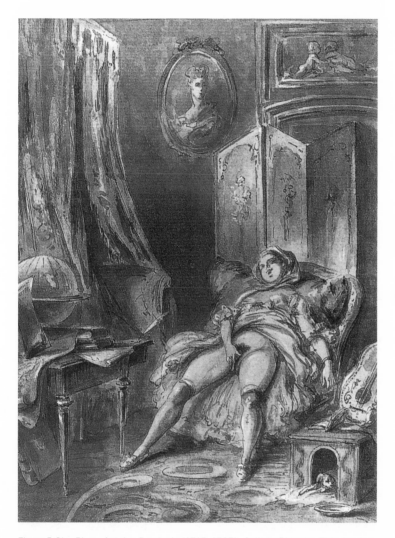

Figure 5.8b. Pierre-Antoine Baudouin (1715–1797), *Solitary Pleasure*. This drawing explores the same themes, leaving little to the imagination and even less for icono-graphic ambiguity. Note, for example, the open book that seems just to have dropped out of her left hand onto a small box, from which peers the little dog that is so common in this representational tradition.

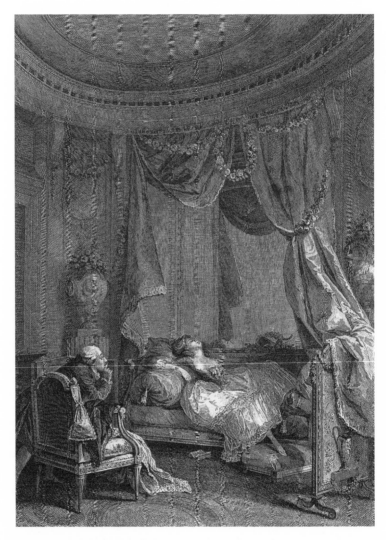

Figure 5.9. Isidore Stanislas Helman, after a design by Nicolas Lavreince, *The Dangerous Novel*, 1781. (Bibliothèque Nationale, Paris.)

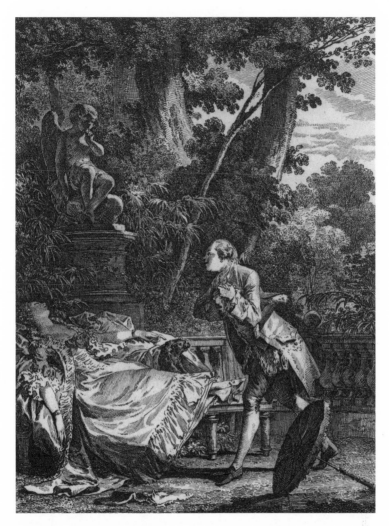

Figure 5.10. J.M. Moreau, *La Dormeuse,* from Jean Benjamin de Laborde, *Choix de chansons* (Paris: Chez de Lormel, 1763), vol. 1, p. 26. The caption, "Her eyes are closed today as her heart is to love," the books fallen by her side, and her pose seem to say that she has found satisfaction alone.

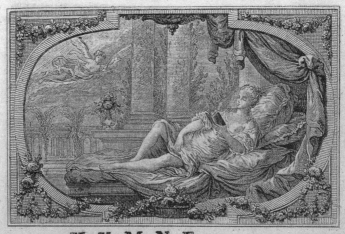

HYMNE
AU BAISER.

Don céleste, volupté pure,
De l'Univers moteur secret,
Doux aiguillon de la Nature,
Et son plus invincible attrait,
Éclair, qui, brûlant ce qu'il touche,
Par l'heureux signal de la bouche,
Avertis tous les autres sens ;
Viens jouer autour de ma lyre ;
Qu'on reconnoisse ton délire
A la chaleur de mes accens.

D iv

Figure 5.11. "Anthem to a Kiss," headpiece from Claude Joseph Dorat, *Les Baisers, précédés du mois de mai* (The Hague and Paris: Delalain, 1770), p. 55. Even if she is not reading a book explicitly "to be read with one hand," there is no question about where literary self-absorption and imagination lead. (Victoria and Albert Museum, London.)

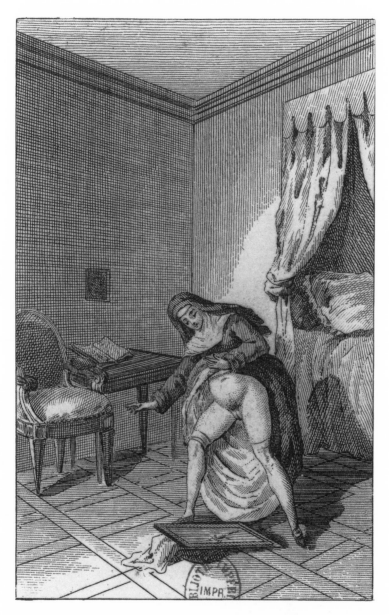

Figure 5.12. *Nun Examining Herself,* from P.J.B. Nougaret, *Le Progrès du libertinage, historiette trouvée dans le porte-feuille d'un carme réformé* (1765–1766). The title of the book from which this is taken makes clear where reading can lead. (Bibliothèque Nationale, Paris.)

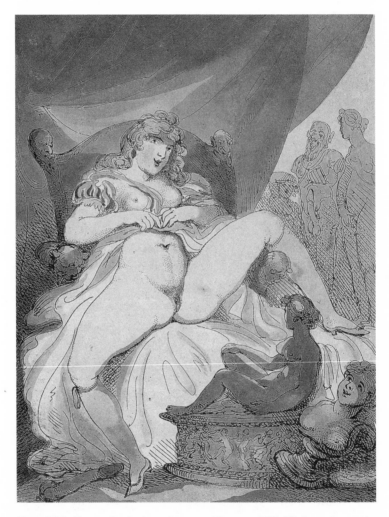

Figure 5.13. Thomas Rowlandson, *Lonesome Pleasures*, 1812. Whatever else may be going on in this drawing from a portfolio of erotic pictures by one of the best-known English artists of the early nineteenth century, we see here a woman making her own sexual destiny. (Victoria and Albert Museum, London.)

he stands so far behind her that not much can be in view and no one expects him to enter the scene, and certainly that of two female statues who look intently at the sights being revealed. However voyeuristic this piece of erotica might be — everyone is looking — it is an image of a woman who is the maker of her own sexual destiny. She is claiming her genitals for herself, a gesture that takes on an entirely different political valence in the dinner-party installation of Judy Chicago. Here it is an image of the very worst possible consequence of individual autonomy from the point of view of those who initiated the attack on private vice. In Andréa de Nerciat's *Le Diable au corps* (The Devil in the Body), one of the biggest-selling works of eighteenth-century erotica — a naked woman gazes toward an open book on her nightstand, one arm resting sensuously behind her head; her finger is posed between her open thighs, though not quite on the pudenda — a hand rests on her poodle, who is doing the job (figure 5.14).

The open book next to, or fallen to the side of, a masturbating woman had become almost an icon of the pleasures and the dangers of literature. She is probably reading some philosophical pornography, but she might as well be reading *Tristram Shandy* or *Pamela* or any of a host of perfectly respectable French, German, or English novels that aroused eros to teach virtue. In those more innocent days, as we saw, even reading Schiller could make an adolescent boy aroused enough to masturbate. Solitary sex and images like these — representative of vast reservoirs in the eighteenth and the early nineteenth century and harbingers of an even vaster supply once photography and new printing processes made dirty pictures truly cheap — are the unassimilable residue of the revolution in consumption, in reading, and in a vast cultural infrastructure of individual moral autonomy. (Still today there is enough energy left in the old image of reading and masturbating to make it work in an altogether different political setting. For example, a poster that was up in the Women's Studies Department of Sydney University in 1991, shows a woman with her hand in her crotch, her eyes absorbed in a book, and a balloon that tells the man she does not need him or his purchasing power.)

The foundations for the fear of masturbation as exposed in

355

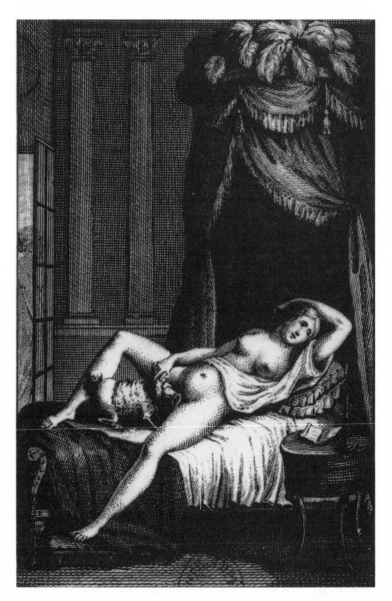

Figure 5.14. Andréa de Nerciat, *Le Diable au corps* (Paris: L'Or du Temps, 1969).
This print comes from one of the most famous eighteenth-century works of erotica.
It expands the theme of reading and masturbation to include what we might call
sexual aids. (Bibliothèque Nationale, Paris.)

Chapter 4 and explained in this one are not quite evident in the most descriptive term used to designate the practice itself: "*solitary* vice." Yes, a sort of reclusive, secret, abject, and miserable isolation awaited the onanist, but the really big problem was that masturbation turned on its head the proper relations between the self and society and created instead a set of horrible alternatives: hordes of autonomous but somehow complicit individuals who do not cooperate because they know they do not need each other. At their most nightmarish, masturbators were the unspeakable expansion of Sade's "society of friends of crime," who support one another based on their common commitment to disregarding the feelings and needs of others.

Two of the eighteenth century's most powerful proponents of solitude — the German Zimmermann, whose work on the subject was immensely popular throughout Europe and the New World, and Rousseau, whose "state of nature" represents a sort of prelapsarian, blissful autonomy — were among the most powerful opponents of the solitary vice. For Rousseau, and less explicitly for Zimmermann, solitude is the place where we long for a lost innocence and independence; it is the place where we realize that there is no going back, that the way forward is social intercourse, exchange with others, and hope for the future; it is the place where we realize what is best for ourselves and how this might be attained through working for the common good; and, finally, it is the place where we come truly to value and enjoy the fruits of our labor. The social world is the place where we practice what we learned in solitude. But for the masturbator the opposite is the case. Onanists learn in the social world that they are autonomous — potentially autarkic — beings, and take this dirty secret back to their solitude, to that place of supposed purity, which they thus pollute. Theirs is the world turned upside down.

The community of novel readers struck contemporaries as a reasonable facsimile of such a world: hundreds of thousands of people taking the dangerous trash of the social world into the solitary sanctum of their inner being.[128] At the dawn of the Enlightenment, the onanist thus became the alter ego, the nasty bad brother or sister, of the modern self and has remained so ever

357

since. But as the threat of death and insanity began to wane at the beginning of the twentieth century, the ethical problem that was always foremost emerged with a new clarity, and the errant sibling became, in some circles at least, a model of virtuous self-sufficiency, moral autonomy, and freedom from the overweening power of patriarchy and heterosexuality. How and why this happened is the story of the next chapter.

CHAPTER SIX

Solitary Sex in the Twentieth Century

A prolific Japanese writer of popular books on sexual matters, himself a gynecologist, returned home in 1913 from two years of study in Germany full of praise for how this Western powerhouse had dealt with the masturbation problem: "not only from the perspective of morality" as did his native country, "but also in a scientific way." This approach, he said, had been brilliantly successful. Because of the "overwhelming number of books" on the subject "there is hardly anyone in Germany over twenty who still masturbates."[1] Little did our Japanese observer know, he was witness to the last hurrah of the effort to treat masturbation as a cause of physical disorders. The public health aspect of our topic — at least in its negative aspects — comes to an end sometime between the late nineteenth century and the third decade of the twentieth. Most doctors and those who looked to them for advice stopped believing that masturbation killed, maimed, or drove insane those who did it. Yes, "wankers' doom" was still current slang in the 1950s, and children were still being told that blindness, paralysis, tiredness, and hair on the palms were among the possible costs of playing with themselves. But in specialist circles by the 1930s, masturbation had once again become medically benign.

With the threat of disease fading into the background, at least in public discussion, the cultural anxieties that had produced modern masturbation came fully into their own. No longer a threat to health, sex with oneself could represent a rejection not only of socially appropriate sexuality, not only of appropriate sociability, but of the social order itself. Masturbation, which had

359

long been construed as the greatest of challenges to moral policing, became an even more catastrophic and atavistic threat. No
longer filling mental hospitals or registering in mortality statistics, it was finally freed from its epiphenomena and could be
revealed, in all its nakedness, for what it had always been suspected of being: the collapse of culture and a return to the most
primitive level of desire and gratification. No longer the cause of
spinal or pulmonary tuberculosis, blindness, deafness, or wasting
away, it became something sublime: that moment when, in the
words of the famous expositors of psychoanalysis Jean Laplanche
and J.B. Pontalis, "sexuality... is constituted qua sexuality," objectless, unmoored, and given over to pure fantasy. It is "the lowest of the sexual strata," according to Freud, not just the earliest
but also the most primitive, the most resolutely antithetical to
the process of civilization, especially for women. It is "the sexual
activity of the narcissistic stage of the allocation of the libido";
even if we imagine something outside our autoerotic activities,
their true end extends no farther than ourselves.[2]

The change from the world of Tissot and Rousseau to that of
Freud and liberal sexology was therefore much less, but also much
more, pronounced than it seemed to participants or might seem
to us. Gone were outlandish claims about disease, but in their
place was a far more developed complex of theories about why
masturbatory guilt was the core guilt and masturbation the foundational sexuality. It became the work of civilization to transform
the narcissistic, autonomous pleasure of autoeroticism into culture. (There is, of course, the opposite view — suggested first by
Havelock Ellis — that autoeroticism represented civilization in its
highest forms; the foundation of the arts and of creativity. This
was decidedly not the view of Freud and his colleagues.) Gone
were efforts to terrorize children and adults into stopping their
masturbatory reveries — the self-avowed aim of Tissot, Rousseau,
and their colleagues — but in their place was a far more elaborate
version of Onania's original insight: the vice that it launched to
undreamed-of success was, in fact, "that trick of childhood, that
first darling sin" from which much else followed.

Masturbation became the frontline encounter of sexual desire with culture, with some purpose beyond pure pleasure; it was the omni-poetic erotic stem cell from which developed all that came after. In the new century, proper nurture, moral suasion, sublimation, and above all education, instead of raw terror, were meant to ensure that it was indeed channeled to produce the social ideal of healthy adulthood. Guilt and its psychic costs replaced death and madness but were no less terrifying or engrossing for being less organically morbid. "Portnoy's Complaint" as the pseudo syndrome that opens Philip Roth's novel could only exist after the 1930s. Masturbation has thus remained crucial to thinking about sexuality and the self but in a new register, a startlingly new register in which the old telos of sex and its pleasures — reproduction — could no longer be taken for granted.

The story does not stop, however, with the demise of the old medical model and the rise of the new psychoanalytic one. There is a coda, an even more radical shift.

Beginning already in avant-garde circles in the 1920s, masturbation since the 1960s has become variously and in combination an act of individual liberation, a proclamation of autonomy, an affirmation of pleasure for its own sake, a way to make money from sex toys, a practice in the cultivation of the self, a gambit and counter gambit in the sexual and more general cultural politics of the era, a subject of painting and performance art, a deeply interesting part of the human erotic experience as a sign of abjection or of triumph. Supposedly sterile, masturbation has given rise to new communities both real and virtual; as of 5:00 P.M. the day I write this, the Web site of the New York Jacks, a gay masturbation network, has had 1,073,006 visits, and there are a score of similar "jacks" sites around the world. Straight and gay, men and women have embraced masturbation as something beyond the immediately pleasurable. True to the spirit of *Onania*, and sponsored by Good Vibration, purveyor of erotic goods, National Masturbation Month (figure 6.1) combines commercial gain with social commentary. Our subject is everywhere: on television, on the Web, in bookshops and art galleries, in feminist and men's liberation settings, in gay and straight contexts, in student health clinics, and presumably in the private thoughts and conversations

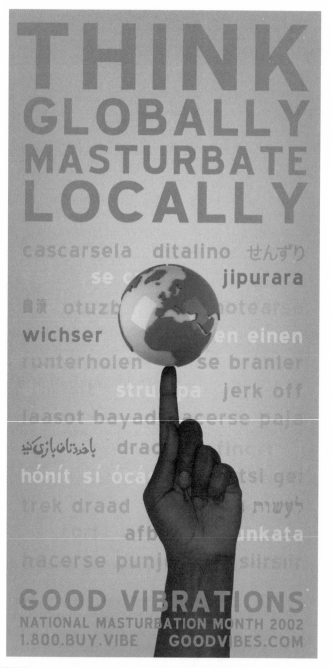

Figure 6.1. National Masturbation Month poster, 2002. Treating masturbation as if it were just another one of the many activities and interests that have months dedicated to them is both an affirmation of the new public place of the formerly secret vice and a shrewd commercial move by a company that sells pornography and sex toys. (Courtesy Good Vibrations.)

of many, many people: those who embrace the practice, those who don't think it is very important, and those hostile to it.

The Persistence and Decline of Masturbatory Disease

It would not seem difficult to account for why masturbation had subsided as a cause of serious disease by the end of the nineteenth century and the beginning of the twentieth. First, specific pathogens came to replace vague social and cultural causes of disease with the triumph of the germ-theory revolution beginning in the 1880s. By 1900, it had become clear that tuberculosis, one of the major diseases that had been attributed to self-abuse, and wasting diseases in general, were caused by bacteria or organic lesions and not by masturbation. Also, fewer people were dying near to the time when they masturbated most or, in any case, were thought to masturbate most. Infant mortality dropped dramatically during the last decades of the nineteenth century. No longer were thousands of five-, six-, and seven-year-olds dead from anything, much less, as Larousse's *Grand Dictionnaire* had claimed, from masturbation. Life expectancy generally rose as well, which reflected the fact that not only did fewer people die young but fewer, per capita, died at any age. Teenagers by the early twentieth century were likely to grow into adulthood and old age. In short, the massive demographic shift of the late nineteenth and the early twentieth century, due primarily to better public-health measures, made the problem of premature death much less exigent.

Medical disciplines also changed their focus in such a way that masturbatory insanity seemed less probable. Neurology was in its ascendancy and localized lesions, specific organic pathologies, were becoming more attractive to explain insanity than behavioral excesses like onanism. The process was not smooth and steady. In fact, the term "masturbatory insanity" was not even coined until 1868, when the English psychologist Henry Maudsley used it to describe the disease caused by the organic damage that masturbation supposedly did to the brain. How this was related to degeneracy — his general concern — is not clear: whether masturbation caused degeneracy, was caused by it, or adversely affected only those youths who were congenitally vulnerable was an open

363

question in this context, as in so much discussion of degeneracy. But however novel this disease entity, attributed by Maudsley to "offensive egotism," psychiatry did not go his way.[3]

Emil Kraepelin, a giant of early-twentieth-century psychiatry, declared that excessive masturbation was possible only in people who were already organically disposed; if it coincided with insanity, it was because both the mental disease and the self-stimulation had the same degenerative cause. Even reluctant, more old-fashioned psychiatrists admitted that rarely was self-abuse the sole cause of full-blown, florid insanity. Hermann Nothnagel regarded it as insignificant in causing epilepsy (although, as we saw, there is a neurological connection); Eduard Hitzig, a pioneer in exploring the electric excitability of the brain, concluded that it did not cause cerebral atrophy; and Albert Eulenburg argued that it did not cause muscular atrophy. No one even bothered to rebut the claims about sudden death or accelerated decay. Masturbators — in any case, those who read the most advanced thinkers — by some time around 1900 no longer had to fear the grave or the wheelchair.

Furthermore, as almost all the forward-looking sexologists and respectable doctors pointed out, the horrors of masturbation had been exaggerated and painted in such lurid hues by unscrupulous quacks in order for them to sell their pseudo medicines and dubious advice. Of course, quacks had been in the masturbation business since *Onania*, but by the late nineteenth century the medical profession had become active everywhere — even in the United States and England, where regulation came late — in distinguishing itself from shady operators. Masturbation, in short, was déclassé, and medicine backed away from the century-old tradition of which Tissot had been the champion well into the late nineteenth century.

Still, for two reasons the association of solitary sex with infirmities of the body died slowly. First, no single discovery or set of discoveries ever destroys a whole way of thinking about a problem until an alternative theory offers a different explanation. There were still plenty of physical symptoms that could not be easily explained and that could be attributed to self-abuse. Freudian psychology and its progeny provided a new model, but it took some time to take hold in an arena where most people's views are set in childhood.

Second, the underlying ethical problem raised so dramatically in the early eighteenth century was still exigent; while masturbation hovered for decades between being the cause of organic disease and being the origin of psychic ill ease, it never became inconsequential. Guilt and neurosis and painful personal failure slowly displaced tuberculosis, wasting, and madness as the consequences of self-abuse and were construed as comparably terrible. A progressive writer on Christian sexual ethics of the early twentieth century who quoted Havelock Ellis and other secular experts with approval and who had little interest either in pathology or in Thomist theories of "naturalness" brought forward his heaviest rhetorical artillery against masturbation: "secret impurity"; "this dire foe of childhood and youth." Parents who fail to guard their children against it are "more reckless than the Moloch worshippers of antiquity" who offered their young to the flames. Habits of impurity will take root and acquire strength, and both "will-power and the nobler developments of the human soul" will be ruined.[4]

If masturbation for those in the know no longer plausibly led to organic disease by 1900, the moral collapse that solitary sex represented still seemed to have dire consequences on the body because of what it did to the mind. Thus masturbatory disease lingered despite all the disavowals. Even Freud was uneasy about giving up on the idea that anything as bad as solitary sex *had* to be bad for you, if not quite as bad as once imagined. It "has been the *bête noire* of the sexual problems," wrote A.A. Brill, a leading American exponent of Freud, after the Great War; it is not yet "settled today." No other subject had been given as much attention; none had been so "confusingly represented or misrepresented." The question has hung like "the sword of Damocles over the head of almost every civilized being." Notwithstanding the work of eminent sexologists, "old medieval views" about masturbation were still rife among the laity and among most physicians. These Brill hoped to set right.[5]

365

The views he condemned were not, as we know, "medieval," but there were good reasons why they persisted despite — or perhaps because of — the eminent experts whom he cited approvingly. Of course, these experts saw themselves as combating darkness; they moved many so-called perversions from the realm of sin and damnation into the more comforting orbit of medicine and nature.[6] And they limited the range of illnesses that might be associated with masturbation. But all of them, including Freud, were adolescents in the age when onanists were being told that they were risking their lives through self-abuse. They came of age professionally in the last decades of the nineteenth century, the years in which, for example, the now-infamous Dr. Daniel Gottlieb Moritz Schreber, father of Freud's famous patient, was a respected educator who devised instruments and regimens to break children of their "dangerous, hidden aberration," the years in which prominent psychology textbooks could still proclaim confidently that 26 percent of neurotic boys who masturbated ended up demented.[7] (Schreber was a major figure in the world of middle-class pedagogy, however insanely cruel he was to his son.)

Outside these circles, the most gruesome of old stories persisted as if none of the distinguished German, French, or English sexologists, psychologists, or neurologists had ever written. As late as 1944, a well-known educator and popular author on matters of race, sex, and biology said that when he was writing his textbook, he came upon John Thompson's *Man and His Sexual Relations* and discovered that the hoary stuff about dry and brittle bones, languid heartbeat, and degeneration was alive and well.[8]

But even leaving such atavisms aside, serious debate on the subject continued well into the 1920s. Even progressives kept coming back to the well-rehearsed argument that fantasy, excess, and secrecy on the one hand and incompleteness, falseness, and lack of sociability on the other were seriously threatening if, perhaps, not in quite the horrific ways described by their opponents. In short, masturbation was caught between two paradigms for decades. Freud could not quite bring himself to go along with the implications of his own work and insisted that masturbation really did cause more than neurosis. In his report on a contentious 1912 meeting of his Vienna colleagues called to discuss onanism, he said that he hoped to avoid the question of the injuriousness of masturbation because it was not of central concern to the group. But avoidance was impossible. He felt compelled to say *something* because "the world seems to feel no other interest in masturbation."

This is perhaps a bit disingenuous; Freud may have wanted to stress the disharmony in his group because he was one of the hold-outs for the more old-fashioned view. In 1895, he had argued that there was a specific *somatic*, depleting quality to masturbation that resulted in neurasthenia — nervous debility — and that this neuro-sis could be distinguished from *Angstneurose*, "anxiety neurosis," which was caused by other incomplete sexual acts like coitus in-terruptus or by sexual abstinence.[9] He reminded his colleagues that an earlier meeting on the subject, in 1908, had been so divi-sive that he, as its recording secretary, had not been able to cobble together even the semblance of a summary. At that meeting, a dis-tinguished pediatrician had wanted the group to tell him "how far is masturbation injurious and why it injures some people but not others." Perhaps Freud was trying again to avoid an answer.

In any case, by the 1912 meeting Freud obviously had decided to salvage something from all his group's talk. No joint "denial of a somatic factor in the effects of masturbation" would be forth-coming. Possibly — here he is clearly speaking for himself — the "pathogenic effects" of masturbation are due to the peculiarities of the act itself and are not to be equated with sexual activity in general: "*Organic* damage may occur by some unknown mecha-nism ... the injury may occur through the laying down of a *psychi-cal* pattern." One simply cannot be sure. In fact, he concluded, no general view on the subject is possible, and one needs to judge the question case by case, rather like — I think the irony is unin-tentional — the Scottish king in a Victor Hugo novel who boasted that the only way to tell whether a woman was a witch was to stew her and then taste the broth: "Yes, that was a witch."[10]

The experts could not let go of the old model. Of course, they had taken on board all the latest work, but it was far from decisive. One French physician, writing when Freud was in medical school, began his book by declaring that masturbation was relatively benign and concluded by offering a list of hundreds of ailments to which women in particular were prone.[11] The structure of the argument around the turn of the century was always the same. "If masturbation is practiced with moderation it can not be considered pathological," declared an American gynecologist. Indeed, he continued, it is universal and ubiquitous: Hottentots and bicyclists, sewing-machine operators and "Kafirs," not to speak of lower primates, all do it. But for something so ordinary, the psychic and physical downside was considerable: "the female masturbator becomes excessively prudish, despises and hates the opposite sex.... [M]asturbation is often the cause of obstruction, painful menstruation, of ovarian neuralgia, of weakness of the legs and of sexual irritation." No, masturbation did not produce blindness in most women who did it, but excessive masturbation did have effects on the optic nerve, reported a distinguished Breslau ophthalmologist. *Onanie* was benign, declared Iwan Bloch, a widely read sexologist of the era, but *onanismus* was not. Unfortunately, he said, "the borderline cannot be easily defined." Indeed, the conflation for two hundred years of ordinary masturbation with genuinely obsessive and publicly inappropriate behavior is a sign of the high cultural stakes of the post-1712 discussion.[12]

Nowhere is this back-and-forth more evident than in the work of G. Stanley Hall, the man who, as president of Clark University, invited Freud to the United States, the man to whom Freud dedicated the five lectures he gave there on psychoanalysis, and, in his own right, one of the greatest figures in American psychology in the early twentieth century. However enlightened he tried to appear on our topic, at the end of the day he could not shake the guilt of a boy who had come of age in the bad old days when Tissot was still the reigning expert. An adolescent in the years before the Civil War, he admitted in his autobiography that he had been "almost petrified" by the slightest physical excitement or "nocturnal experience." He remembered well the story his father had told him of a youth who "had abused himself and sinned with lewd women" and as a result had a disease that ate away his nose and left two holes where it had been and finally turned him into a complete idiot. (Here he conflates tertiary syphilis and masturbation.)

Hall lived in terror of this happening to him and carefully examined his nose to be sure it had not flattened. He taped down his penis to avoid unconsciously produced erections. Later, all the very real sexual brutality of his third-order boarding school was remembered through the filter of masturbation and a host of "perversions" that he, as did many others later in the century, grouped together: every kind of distasteful sexual practice one might find described in Krafft-Ebing, Tarnovski, or Havelock Ellis could be found in his school.[13]

Readers of Hall's canonical two-volume textbook on adolescence knew none of this. (His autobiography appeared only at the end of his career, two decades later in 1924.) Hall himself seems solidly with the moderns at first:

> We must recognize that the immediate and sensational effects often seriously believed in, and often purposely exaggerated for pedagogic reasons, are not so immediate or disastrous as represented in both the popular and the earlier literature.

The brain, he continued, "is not literally drained away; dementia, idiocy, palsy and sudden death are not imminent." Nor is there any infallible sign in a boy or a girl that he or she has masturbated.

But readers could take little comfort from these disclaimers. The list of miseries that flowed from this, the most disastrously prevalent of "perversions," was staggering. First, it was eugenically bad. "Yielding to mere and sensuous pleasure shortens the growth period" of individuals, weakens the race, and speaks for the pathos of our modern age. "The invective of a decadent son upon a sire but for whose private vice he might have been well born, is as haunting and characteristic a note for our culture as was the curse of Atreus's time for ancient Greece." (Atreus's wife commits adultery; he killed his own son whom the wife's lover had brought up; he brought up as his own another's son and given to her lover the golden lamb which represented kingship.) Likewise, masturbation haunts generations to come.

Second, it was bad for the individual. No one today, Hall says with great assurance, could still believe that it was no worse than "excess in the natural way," whatever people might have claimed in the past. The dangers of solitary excess are manifestly far greater: "The act is more brutal and descends far lower in the phylogenic scale"; the imagination is made "morbidly intense and acute" by the "unnatural act." Hall is essentially repeating the jeremiads of the *Encyclopédie* and those in its tradition that the imagination subjects the onanist "to the most excessive strain in order to produce the desired climax" and that therein lies the danger. But worse is to come. The imagination induces not only perversions but also hallucinations. The entire sensory apparatus can be thrown askew. Whatever the unpleasant consequences of sexual intercourse, those of masturbation were worse. Coition makes one sad — this is the old adage — but masturbation makes one much sadder. And sicker. "Pain and traces of epilepsy, palpitation, and photophobia, . . . neurasthenia, cerebrasthenia, spinal neurasthenia, and psychic impotence, . . . subjective light sensations, optical cramps, perhaps Basedow's disease [named for Carl Adolph Basedow, who in a well-known 1840 paper described exophthalmic goiter], intensification of the patellar reflex, purple and dry skin, clammy hands, . . . anemic complexion, dry cough, and many digestive perversions" can often "be directly traced to this scourge of the human race." And Hall had yet to get to the "Masturbator's heart" — the authority for which is six "interesting cases" reported in a major German medical journal of the last decade of the century — and the many other pathologies of "these forbidden joys of youth."[14]

Solitary sex thus stood poised between the moral and the pathological more precariously than it had before. Or, more precisely, now that germ theory and cellular pathology were the bases for thinking about organic diseases, the ills of masturbation were harder to incorporate in a medical model and stood ever more exposed for what they had always been: symptoms of the moral seriousness of the offense, of the profound deviance that masturbation represented in the order of things. As doctors voiced more and more skepticism about actual diseases caused by self-abuse, they made clearer than ever that masturbation was an offense against the process of civilization itself and against all those institutions which made it possible. Ordinary people suffered through this confusion.

It would take a while to be sorted out and the process would push solitary sex deeper and deeper into the psyche. John Meagher, whose study of the psychology of autoeroticism went through many editions and revisions, summarizes the moral and social centrality of masturbation in a world that seemed to have transcended John Marten and Samuel August Tissot but was in fact still engaged with their issues. Physical dangers had been exaggerated; indeed they were negligible. Imbecility and consumption were not caused by self-abuse. Likewise, its psychological consequences were not as bad as had been formerly thought. But that was as far as Meagher would go.

Meagher regarded as the "opposite extreme" Wilhelm Stekel's position that autoeroticism is entirely harmless or even benign. (Freud also took pains to attack this position in 1912.) There were real consequences to masturbation, he insisted; they were mostly moral, but also physical. It was a seriously culpable act after adolescence and not to be taken lightly: ten percent of the cases of adolescent delinquencies were said to be caused by masturbation because, in that proportion of individuals, it had caused "breaking of the moral stamina." Meagher's critical point — one that reflected the progressive secular thinking of his day and shaped the rehabilitation of masturbation in our own — is that the physical act is "relatively unimportant compared with the crippling effect of the autoerotic introversion." *Onania*, Tissot, and the vast tradition constructed on their medical views might no longer be sustainable but the grave moral danger first launched into the world in or around 1712 was all the more evident. The way in which Meagher and his generation condemned solitary sex owed everything to eighteenth-century formulations even if they spoke in the language of Freud.

Masturbation was still the radical other of coitus: it "never satisfies the spiritual value of responsibility as a socialized adult"; it causes ill-being and unrest, whereas legitimate coitus causes well-being and relaxation. Masturbation is about fantasy, Meagher says, and we are back to the old wine in new bottles: "Fantasy replaces reality, which is an infantile attitude." (Fantasy is "the *mise en scène* of desire," as Laplanche and Pontalis put it, and masturbation is its fundamentally regressive staging.) Although Meagher does not make the point, colleagues said, as *Onania* had, that the danger of masturbatory excess arises from the ease with which it can be performed. Act for act, doctors in the twentieth century argued, masturbation was no worse than coition: "The danger is the frequency with which the act can be performed in comparison to sexual congress." As the *Encyclopédie* had pointed out almost two hundred years before, if done only when there is "need," there might be no problem.

Like Tissot, Meagher maintained that onanism was far worse in women than in men not primarily because of its effects on the body but as a rejection of proper sociability: married women, for whom the erotic outweighed the affective and who were not satisfied by their husbands, masturbated; women who feared having children masturbated because they preferred it to coition with birth control, wrongly believing that they would not feel guilty and could thus avoid neurosis; women who thought they were "'victims' of sex which they feel is purely a male attribute" developed the habit as "their relief from coitus." In short, masturbation is *the* act through which women signaled their rejection of the normative sexual order.[15]

Guilt and its consequences — neurosis, tiredness, anxiety, hysteria, physical discomforts of all sorts, failure to achieve what life promised, moral collapse, abjection — replaced death and imbecility as the primary wages of solitary sex, which still carried the ethical burdens of its early modern history. The old hung on as the new emerged in fascinating ways.

We can catch a glimpse of this slow rethinking in an unexpected place: the pages of one of the most progressive suffragist journals of the early twentieth century, where feminist debates swerved weirdly from questions of the double standard and the control of prostitution to the nature and consequences of masturbation. In one series of articles and letter exchanges, E.W. (Edith Watson of the Women's Freedom League, a militant, nonviolent suffragist organization with more than sixty branches and four thousand members) argued that complete freedom in matters sexual was neither possible nor desirable and that, even more dangerous, was the idea that sexual abstinence was either harmful or impossible for men or women. Here she was following the thinking of Elizabeth Blackwell, the first licensed woman doctor in England, whose work we have already noticed in connection with her views on moral purity. The notion that abstinence was "painful and physiologically injurious," Watson argued, had "done more harm to women and more to foster the horrors of prostitution than anything else." (Blackwell had observed in her clinical practice that young men went to whores with their parents' permission so as to avoid the worse horrors of seminal retention on the one hand and masturbation on the other.)[16]

In response to Watson's claims and to letters that supported her, a "new subscriber," who turned out to be Stella Browne, entered the fray. A socialist, sexual radical, and freethinker who noted late in her life that she "had never met a normal woman," Browne accused Watson and her ilk of being "sexually anesthetic." They had, she said, overgeneralized from the trepidations of brutal, ignorant, and demanding men who abused their wives within marriage and prostitutes and lovers outside it. The middle path between excess and abstinence—here she is speaking about women—was masturbation. Turning Watson's argument against the double standard on its head, Browne argued not that men and women were equally capable of abstinence but that they were also equally desirous of sex and equally capable of indulging in it with forms of "auto-eroticism" and "Onanism." She does not distinguish these, but she does show how up-to-date she is in that Havelock Ellis had only coined the term "auto-eroticism" a little over a decade before. She marshals him and Auguste Forel—somewhat self-servingly but no less interesting for that—in support of this middle masturbatory way. And, finally, she accused those women who wrote about the healthiness of the celibate life of being hypocrites, because they no doubt lived by the substitution that they condemned.

Here things get really complicated. Some women wrote in to say that they certainly did not masturbate and were morally supe-

rior to its allure. "Intellect and reason" ruled their "lower instincts and desires," and this was what elevated them "above the
lower animals," including men. Watson, however, responded not
so much to Browne as to the more general argument that men
needed sexual relief. If they did — which she doubted — it still
would not warrant, as many argued, the state's licensing prostitution. (A big argument for state regulation was that because men
by nature needed sexual release and because many men either
were unmarried or had wives who were not willing to meet their
needs, they should have a safe outlet available to them. Hence the
state should see to it that prostitutes did not transmit disease.)
Watson suggested that they masturbate. Her "case for self-abuse"
was that, first, unlike prostitution, it did no harm; at worst, it
harmed only the practitioner and not another. But, more tellingly,
the real truth about male sexuality is most clearly evident when
men masturbate: "it strikes even men as degrading" and reveals
"sexual 'necessity' in all its ugly nudity." But then when a reader
responds that there "are innumerable cases in which self-abuse
has led to insanity" and that we need "medical testimony [of] the
immunity from mental and bodily aberration" before we can
accept Watson's views, she expands her argument in a thoroughly
modern direction. Masturbation is perfectly safe, and word of its
ill effect is a "scarecrow that has been set up"; there is no truth to
the old shibboleths. But this does not detract from her main ethical point. Neither she nor her authorities are recommending self-
abuse — as Browne did — because ethical human beings do not
need to yield to sexual desires. "The highest liberty of man consists in his dominion over himself," and this is clearly what masturbation belies. Even in advanced circles of the early twentieth
century, the eighteenth-century legacy lived on, although now in
its purely moral inflection.[17]

Likewise, for the men and women who wrote asking help from
Marie Stopes, people who came of age in the late nineteenth century and the first years of the twentieth, masturbation still figures
as a cause of physical debility at the same time that it is becoming
ever more the sign that something must be terribly wrong with
their inner selves. Not death or madness but moral failure haunts

374

them. A forty-year-old man born in 1890 wrote that in the past two years he had masturbated about twelve times and that in his later teens he had been addicted. Now, on the eve of his marriage, he is neurasthenic, still strongly sexed, and full of "nervousness, guilt and remorse." Another man wants to marry and worries that the "disease" he contracted when a schoolboy has so "deprecated [him] both physically and morally" that he will not be able to have a normal life. Should he have himself circumcised? Another asks whether he will have unhealthy children; confessing to his wife that he had masturbated until relatively recently almost wrecked his marriage; he had come clean because he had been impotent on his honeymoon. He is ashamed of his lack of manhood.

And then there are those who asked permission to masturbate in the context of worries about whether their sexual lives were "normal." One correspondent reports that she and her husband have sex for about an hour and a half once a week and that she is "relieved" ten or twelve times, but because he practices coitus interruptus, her feelings soon become "severe" and she needs to relieve herself again. Might she use her finger? Yes, Stopes replies, on occasion it is fine, but tell your husband that withdrawal is harmful; use condoms. A man writes in that because of his premature ejaculation he has to "rub her clitoris which we both know is bad." He has never masturbated himself, so that is not the problem.[18]

If this archive were our only source, men would seem more anxious and guilt-ridden about masturbation than women, more convinced that the pernicious habit of youth had ruined any chance of happiness. Perhaps their overrepresentation in Stopes's correspondence is because most people consulted her not about neurasthenia, nervousness, hysteria, anxiety, or depression — although it was about that too — but about functional failure: impotence, premature ejaculation, loss of libido. She was a doctor who dealt with birth control and, secondarily, with sexual dysfunction, which she thought was often the result of fear of pregnancy. Women worried lest they prefer masturbation to what was expected. And this is why, in the clinical casework of Freud and his colleagues, women seemed to suffer the most from solitary sex. For them, it represented a more profound deviance from what society expected, the most painful and dangerous return of the repressed. But for both men and women, masturbation loomed in adulthood or late adolescence as a deeply guilty pleasure that *should* have been left behind or never begun. It is this feeling — this seemingly primordial guilt — that the generation of sexologists, neurologists, and psychiatrists which included Freud sought to bring into theoretical perspective. Masturbation as a medical question disappeared only when a full-blown new psychological understanding came to be accepted. But before we get to this part of the story, we need to pause for a moment and look at the interpretive world from which the new Freudian synthesis emerged.

Early-Twentieth-Century Masturbation in Theoretical Perspective

We already had many glimpses of this interpretive world when we discussed the decline of the medical/organic model of masturbatory disease, but I want to summarize the debate in and out of which Freud forged his new and influential synthesis. The story in its early stages differed little from writer to writer, and Havelock Ellis summed it up well in a work first published in 1897 and often reprinted later. Autoeroticism was the core of sexuality, and masturbation was the form of it that concerned doctors and moralists. It went well beyond humans, and that proved its primitive, elemental nature. Ellis and his colleagues knew, as we have seen, that ferrets, dogs, cats, and horses — "even elephants," chimes in Iwan Bloch — do it. And, of course, monkeys do it too, "freely *coram publico*," Bloch enthused. There is a certain irony in this evidence for the primitiveness of masturbation. One recent study has discovered that gibbons raised by humans use their hands to masturbate, presumably as a sign of identification with their captors, instead of rubbing themselves on something. An expert on bonobos comments that they "behave as if they read the Kama Sutra," masturbating creatively as well as practicing all sorts of positions and variations.[19]

But Ellis and his contemporaries did not think of these possibilities: that is, of animals actually, or in the imagination of the scientists, imitating humans. Humans, they thought, imitated animals. By 1900, a large anthropological literature had developed showing that primitive people did it. So did very young children. Whether boys and girls did it equally was much debated, but by and large everyone agreed that few of either sex escaped. Some quite distinguished scholars split the difference. For example, Elie Metchnikoff, the discoverer of phagocytosis and an early winner of the Nobel Prize, believed there was such a thing as natural physical masturbation, a normal autoeroticism, that was the result of uneven development in humans: sexual sensibility arose before the reproductive organs were mature. But he also thought that women had less sexual sensitivity so they masturbated less naturally.[20]

The masturbation of infancy or early childhood that in the eighteenth century had been understood as the result of some outside physical or human intervention — worms, tight clothes, as one of the most famous and much-reprinted German pedagogues argued (have girls wear dresses, he suggested), wicked servants — had, by 1900, come to be regarded as natural. At the right time in life, autoeroticism was neither wrong nor perverted but simply in the nature of the beast and the human as beast.[21]

The question is what happens next: Under what conditions could this uncivilized behavior of animals, children, and primitive people be brought into the social order of bourgeois Europe and at what cost? The interpretive thread from infants and young children to "primitive people" in Bali or the bush, to soldiers at the front, to women on bicycles or working sewing machines or crouching while doing the laundry, to adolescents of all sorts was much more difficult to follow. Havelock Ellis roundly rejected the view that masturbation after childhood is benign, cited a large literature affirming that it was a, if not *the*, major cause of neurasthenia, and concluded that it was deeply antithetical to civilization. What exactly he meant by "it" is open to interpretation. Sometimes the undefined adjective "excessive" to modify "masturbation" affects how we might understand his pronouncements.

But the topic for him is clearly fraught: "In women I attach considerable importance, as a result of masturbation, to an aversion for normal coition in later life" because at puberty "the claim

377

of passion and the real charm of sex" were "trained into a foreign channel." The "precocious excess of masturbation" in highly intelligent women, he thought, was a "main cause," if not the "sole efficient cause," of divorce. For both sexes, masturbation in adolescence causes morbid self-consciousness and lack of self-esteem, because it fails to deliver on the ego-boosting "sense of pride and elation" that comes from being kissed by a desirable person of the opposite sex.

Then there was the problem that in intelligent young men and women autoerotic excesses during adolescence could produce "a certain degree of psychic perversion" and foster "false and high strung ideals." This, according to the authority Ellis relies on, was the source of Søren Kierkegaard's suffering and of Nikolai Gogol's "dreamy melancholy," which, admittedly, helped him succeed as a novelist. Both were apparently notorious masturbators. How far masturbation in healthy adults without normal sex lives can be considered "normal" was a difficult question, Ellis concluded, that could only be decided on a case-by-case basis. The cases he cites would not offer masturbators much hope. They involved people who compared their struggles with masturbation to those of drunkards "chained to their intemperate habits" and "inveterate smokers." In short, beyond some point — still well within the range of what we would consider ordinary — Ellis construed adult masturbation to be a sign and a cause of social and psychological, if not bodily, pathology. It represented, if not quite a return of the repressed, then a rejection of one's place in the civilized order.[22]

Among the Vienna analysts and students of sexual matters at large, only Wilhelm Stekel held genuinely sanguine, optimistic views on masturbation. Although his book on the subject was not published until after the war, he had clearly been the odd man out in psychoanalytic circles for some time. The "egregious Stekel," as Ernest Jones called him, had a dicey reputation among his colleagues quite apart from his views on autoeroticism. He was far more entertaining than Alfred Adler, thought Jones, and an "extraordinarily fluent writer." But he wrote "with the inaccuracy and bad taste of the worst kind of journalist" and more generally had an "irresponsible attitude toward truth." The discredited

Stekel thought that the domestication of autoeroticism as the child became an adult carried no great moral burden and that continued masturbation might have positive effects, both for society and for the individual. Freud's arguments with him at the raucous "*Onanie* discussion" were clearly only one in a long round of disagreements with colleagues in which Stekel invariably stood alone.[23]

The influential Auguste Forel, a German expert on hypnosis, nervous diseases, and sexuality whose major work on the subject appeared in 1906 and was widely translated, came a close second in the mildness of his views about masturbation in human development. He divided the issue into three parts. First, the problem with so-called compensatory masturbation — that which arises because there is no normal outlet for natural desires — was not the act itself but "the repeated loss of will, and the failure of resolutions made many times to overcome the desire for orgasm." Women were less likely to succumb to this kind, but "once the habit is acquired, repetition is produced by the difficulty of resisting voluptuous desires." In other words, the problem with compensatory masturbation seems primarily to have been trying not to do it. It is as if the problem with smoking were less the nicotine than the anguish of trying to give it up. That said, weakness of the will seems to have had no momentous consequences.

As for the second kind of masturbation, "caused by example and imitation," its dangers had been, he thought, exaggerated. Love and normal sexual intercourse would take care of it. As for the third kind, masturbation born of what Forel understood as "hereditary pathological satyriasis," or "psychological precocity" — corresponding, I think, to the obsessive childhood masturbation or other genuine pathology that one still finds reported in the medical literature — "kindness and confidence," gentle help in growing up will take care of it. What remains is, except in a few cases, not terribly dangerous.[24]

But the world of Freud produced few such relatively benign accounts of what it meant for the core sexuality of youth and barbarism to survive beyond its earliest stages. Hermann Rohleder, who wrote what his colleagues considered a comprehensive survey of the subject, regarded masturbation as a sign of "degeneration," that is, a return to some more primitive form of sexuality. He also thought that fantasy was what distinguished masturbation from coition; although this does not quite fit with the idea of primitivism, it does follow in the long tradition that we have traced and that lived on into the twentieth century.[25]

For Richard von Krafft-Ebing, another great figure of the generation just before Freud, the core problem with masturbation was not that it might lead to impotence in men and thus perverse acts, if not actually to perversion. Krafft-Ebing was quite certain that neither masturbation nor any other external factor led to homosexual feelings or "instincts," which he understood to be deeply rooted in the mind and body. Nor was so-called excessive masturbation a symptom of excessive sexual desire or of hereditary madness and degeneracy. That said, masturbation after childhood was, in Krafft-Ebing's view, clearly pathological. It represented arrested development, moral and sexual: "Nothing," he wrote, "is so prone to contaminate — under certain circumstances even to exhaust — the source of all noble and ideal sentiments." It "despoils the unfolding bud of perfume and beauty'" and leaves in its place "coarse, animal desire for sexual pleasure." For men and women, it threatens to become preferred to "the natural mode of satisfaction." And then comes a point when the masturbator wants to quit and restore him- or herself to a normal sex life. The odds for success are not good, because the psychic resources for such an enterprise are simply not there after years of profligacy; morals, character, fancy, feelings, and instincts are all but ruined. Thus, like Forel, Krafft-Ebing thought that the inevitable failure of trying to give up masturbating was itself demoralizing, and far more harmful than his colleague had believed.[26]

Masturbation in all of this literature was no longer deadly; nor was it primarily a disease. It became, at a certain stage in a person's life, an abnormality, an unnatural substitute for normal adult sexuality and sexual pleasure. This had nothing to do with a backward-looking Thomist/Aristotelian sense of "unnatural," meaning "nonreproductive." As in the early eighteenth century, progressives articulated the new formulation of masturbation. One of the leading early-twentieth-century advocates of birth control, for example, begins with the premise that many earlier writers — his adversary here is clearly the Christian tradition of moral theology on such matters — had committed the "cardinal error" of believing that "sexual pleasure was a mere by-product" or a process in which procreation was the final goal. In reality, he said, "it is often the other way about." And then came his critique of masturbation: "the miserable substitute," infinitely more dangerous in the pubescent than in the very young because then it becomes a habit, a need. The extreme limits of what might be permissible are set by the limits on ordinary intercourse; solitary sex exceeds them. It is "far from exerting the soothing and beneficial effect of normal copulation"; "voluntary and forcible induction" of sexual pleasure is debilitating, and the fact that it can be heightened at will creates "the real danger of the habit." We are back to Tissot's primal addiction — to the problem of artifice — but with a new twist. Masturbation is the battleground of individual psychodynamics: the play of infancy and childhood has to be renounced for the serious, more ordered pleasures of adulthood. This is hard going.[27]

Freud, Masturbation, and the Self

We are close to an answer to the question of why medicine and organic disease lost their centrality for the solitary-sex problem sometime during the late nineteenth and the early twentieth century but why the old ethical problem did not evaporate at the same time. Quite to the contrary, it took on new life in new clothes. The key is Freud. He produced a theory that made sense of the disparate observations we have been discussing. It had two consequences. First, after some years of crisis, the revolution that was psychoanalysis finally made the old views seem "medieval." The new theory could account for why masturbation was so prevalent even in children who had been carefully shielded and not put under the care of evil servants or in the company of bad friends; it accounted for guilt and also for the general feeling of ill ease, even disease, that masturbators reported to doctors. Second, Freud made masturbation part of a more general history of how we become who we are, how civilization works to make us useful

381

members; he and those who followed him made us talk about the question in radically new ways. And they made it more central than it had been before. Freud did not, however, change fundamentally the underlying ethical question — the relationship of the solitary, individualistic self to the social order — that had been behind the advent of modern masturbation. In other words, the early twentieth century was not a watershed of the sort represented by 1712; there was no new problem in the sexual body that mirrored a new social order.

I will not try to explain the roots of the Freudian revolution in the society and culture of his day. But we can catch a glimpse of its milieu. In 1911, the Viennese artist Egon Schiele painted a portrait of himself masturbating (figure 6.2). It was the year before the Vienna psychoanalysts met for their second inconclusive "*Onanie* discussion," after which Freud despaired of bringing order to the subject and could only conclude that "the subject of masturbation is quite inexhaustible." Schiele's painting was done in front of a mirror and is full of angst and haunting self-scrutiny: his eyes are large, as if in a frenzy or passion, and yet they look up furtively at us; from a head that seems poised between self-absorption, its own image in the mirror, and us; his arms are stunted, and though his fingers are distorted, they powerfully engage with his genitals. How much guilt can be read into this self-portrait? To what extent is it part of Schiele's efforts to establish his identity as a man and to incorporate in his work the shame and guilt of his self-pleasuring? These are larger questions in the study of the artist. But there had never been a painting of masturbation so psychologically rich and complex; it would have been unthinkable outside the milieu in which it was painted. Clearly he had happier visions of his own masturbation as in another self-portrait of the same year in which a sweet, gentle golden light suffuses an image of innocent adolescent self-exploration (figure 6.3).[28]

If the question of sexual guilt loomed large in Freud's world, so did sexual power and especially the power of unsocialized sexuality. Look at another Schiele drawing: *Crouching Woman with Thighs Spread* (figure 6.4). Her skirt is pulled up, her knee-length hose still on, and her hand is poised to put its index finger further

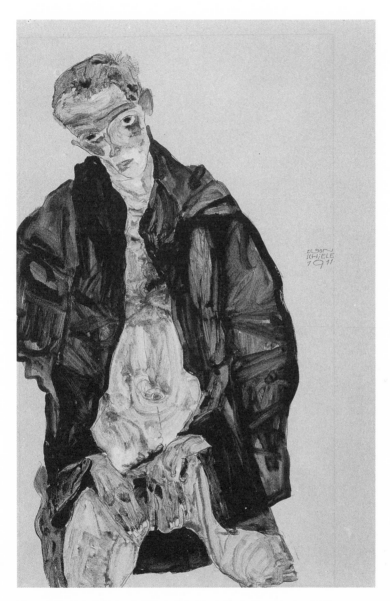

Figure 6.2. Egon Schiele, *Self-Portrait in Black Cloak, Masturbating,* 1911.
Masturbation is at the heart of Schiele's examination of himself as a man and as an
artist. (Albertina, Vienna.)

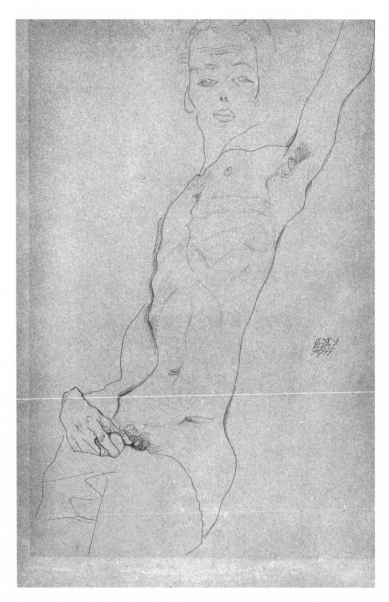

Figure 6.3. Egon Schiele, *Nude Self-Portrait, with Hand on Genitals,* 1911. An altogether more lyrical view of the relationship between autoeroticism and the inner world. (Leopold Museum, Privatstiftung, Vienna.)

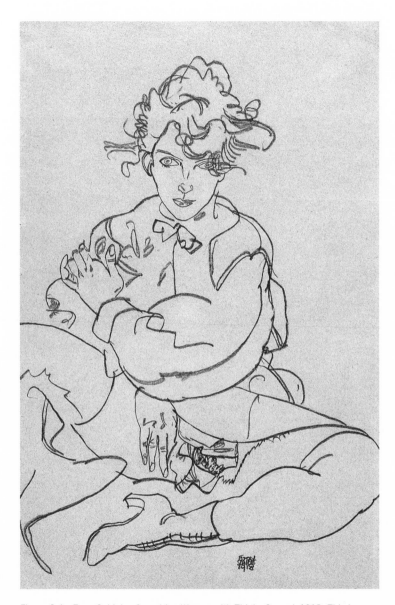

Figure 6.4. Egon Schiele, *Crouching Woman with Thighs Spread*, 1918. This is one of the first visual representations of female masturbation as a gesture of sexual autonomy without offering viewers the simple pleasures of voyeurism to which they had been treated in eighteenth-century pictures. (Leopold Museum, Privatstiftung, Vienna.)

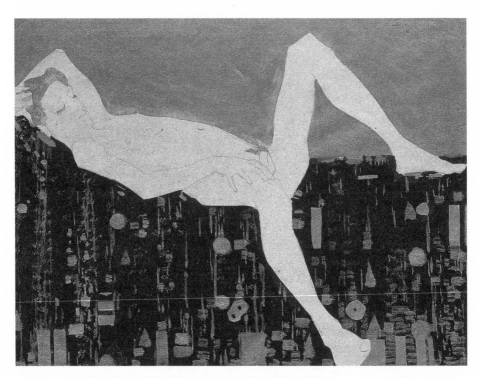

Figure 6.5. Egon Schiele, *Nude Boy Lying on a Patterned Coverlet,* 1909. The viewer does not know precisely what the right hand of this lovely boy has done or is about to do; there is a sense of quiet timelessness about this image of erotic self-absorption. (Leopold Museum, Privatstiftung, Vienna.)

into her bare genitals; she ought perhaps to feel guilty, but we have no hint in the picture that she does. She is not one of the frenzied Bacchae ready to kill and devour the viewer; nor is this a Medusa-like image of the female genitals exposed that threatens men with castration; this is a woman who looks out at us with eyes so intent that they almost dare us to challenge her sexual autonomy and pleasure. However complex the picture, this woman owns her autoerotic powers and will not be made to feel the worse for that. Of course, she is also a model whose role is to make her body public through the artist's gaze; there is no mirror here to reflect a supposedly solitary act; it is Schiele who captures her in a pose that is both defiant and submissive to his professional demands. *Nude Boy Lying on a Patterned Coverlet* (figure 6.5) is, by comparison, a much less assertive image but it does make languidly wasting one's time playing with one's genitals seem not only safe but lyrically attractive. Self-absorption has lost its sting.[29]

Two aspects of these pictures bring us back to Freud and his world: the question of neurosis, anxiety, guilt, and their origins, on the one hand, and the relationship between the driving energy of sexuality — libido — and the use civilization makes of it, on the other. Masturbation plays a central role in Freud's account of both issues. It is absolutely crucial to his story of how the polymorphously perverse, omnivorously pleasure-seeking infant becomes a human being. Once Freud could account for this, masturbation was no longer libido on the edge of the abyss but "the prototype of human sexuality," as a distinguished later analyst put it.[30] More particularly, a new theory of masturbation provided the transition for Freud between the seduction theory he had developed in the mid-1890s and his mature libido theory as alternative ways of explaining neurosis and hysteria. By recognizing the role that fantasy played in autoeroticism, he would make the big breakthrough of his career.[31]

The Freud of the 1890s — and even later — held conventional views about the ill effects of masturbation; I suspect that, deep in his heart, he never overcame his bourgeois adolescence in the late 1860s and early 1870s when it came to this subject. He thought that it was physically harmful and a sign, if not a cause, of

degeneracy; that masturbators were often tired, achy, and neurotic; and that it was generally a very bad, ignoble thing to do. But
this is not what matters. Already in the 1890s, he was interested
less in organic diseases than in neurosis and hysteria, and he was
interested in how external events made themselves felt in the
psyche, where they had, in turn, real corporeal consequences.
Train wrecks and shocks of all sorts made the body act — as was
famously said about hysteria — as if neurology did not matter.
Something was mediating between illness and cause. We have
already seen that he regarded masturbation as debilitating and the
cause of neurasthenia. It was the *act* of masturbation that mattered as the basis of this proposed etiology, but there was already
a purely psychological component — the step in between — that
made the act damaging: the relief provided by sex with oneself
was inadequate because the physical desire that prompted it was
inadequately linked to psychic desire.[32]

In his seduction theory, Freud postulated that some real
trauma, a sexual assault most likely by a girl's father or some other
early sexual awakening, was the main cause of later hysterical
conversions that he claimed to observe in many patients. It was a
real-world, environmental beginning of hysteria, after which psychological energy somehow went from the trauma, through the
psyche, to the body. Masturbation might be the result of this early
sexual trauma and indirectly the cause of symptoms, because
when the too early aroused child's autoeroticism was finally repressed and the sexual energies released through it were bottled
up, they found expression in hysterical symptoms. It was a two-
part process: the trauma of early sexual stimulation and then the
repression of masturbation.

This is not the only way in which masturbation figured in
creating hysteria. It is, Freud said in 1895, "a matter of everyday
experience that conflict ... between irreconcilable ideas has a
pathogenic effect," and he gives as examples a married woman
who suddenly realized she loved another man and a morally sensitive adolescent who masturbated.[33] Hysterical symptoms, obses-
sional behavior, and even delusions — like those of the woman
who accused herself of murder out of a guilt born of masturbation

— could arise from this tension. Freud wavered in the etiologic role he gave in his early work to parental sexual abuse and masturbation, but sometime in 1899 his views took a decided turn to an emphasis on the mental aspect of masturbation, which then took on the role of both an environmental cause of disorders — like real seduction — and an act dangerous primarily because of its place in mental life.

Specifically, Freud read Havelock Ellis and was very much taken with three of his ideas: masturbation is intimately tied to fantasy; autoeroticism is generated from within and, because it is narcissistic, has, or at least needs, no outside stimuli, heterosexual, homosexual, or fetishistic; and, finally, hysterics are those whose autoerotic lives are in conflict. Freud reworked these views: fantasy becomes a later development that is projected back onto very early childhood; nothing happens in early childhood, but there is a germ of the sexual impulse; and this germ is the auto-erotic stage of sexual development upon which fantasy is projected later.[34] As Freud worked through the implications of all this in one case, we can see how masturbation became his transitional object for going from seduction to libido theory.

We know it as the Dora case, and here is Freud's interpretation: the girl had been broken of the habit of sucking her thumb — a form of infantile eroticism — and was thus left in a state of longing; three years later, she had sexual fantasies focusing on her father; at about the same time, she had genital feelings, which, Freud thought, might have been the result *either* of a real seduction or of masturbation but which, in either case, reinforced her Oedipal love; these fantasies stimulated her to masturbate; at the age of eight, she stopped masturbating; she repressed her masturbatory fantasies; and she converted sexual energies into her hysterical symptoms. Dora did not suffer because of her Oedipal love; her trauma was not seduction but masturbation. Or, put differently, trauma may have been what got her started on genital sexuality, but fantasy was crucial in driving her autoerotic reveries, whose abrupt end was the proximal cause of her problem. More likely, Freud thought her fantasies of seduction were a screen for real masturbation. But the main point is that pathogenesis was now increasingly "poised between the inner and the outer, between psyche and soma."[35] And it was masturbation that allowed Freud to connect the unfocused sexual energy and stimulation of early childhood — the autoerotic stage, as he later called it — with fantasy and the sort of inner wishing represented by later Oedipal desires. Fantasy associated with masturbation came to play an enormous role in his later work: though a single and uniform action, he says, it "accomplishes the most various forms of sexual fantasizing."[36] Real environmental trauma still had a place, but it was mediated by the complex relationship between mental life on the one hand and the pure biological pleasures of genital self-stimulation on the other.

One need believe none of Freud's analysis; Dora certainly did not. Nor need we accept the point that his views on masturbation were a way station between his two major theoretical positions. But this story does provide a way of understanding how he got to the position that became so immensely influential — his theory of libido — from a view that was much less innovative. Whether this interpretation of Freud's development is correct or not in every detail, it allows us to see that the vice we are studying was constantly on the mind of the twentieth century's most influential narrator of the inner life from the very beginning of his career.

He would come to tell the whole melancholy tale of how we trade one sort of freedom for another (his reworking of Rousseau), the violent story of how we suppress the instincts so as to progress beyond the beast (his reworking of Nietzsche) as the adventures of autoeroticism. Progressive renunciation is the master narrative of civilization; man — or, more telling, woman — who resists becomes an outlaw (or a hero), someone who does not play their part in cultural creation. The enormous force of the sexual instincts properly sublimated is put "at the disposal of civilized activity"; their course is altered "without materially diminishing in intensity." They cannot be denied, and their redirection can be painful — anxiety, neurosis, hysteria, neurasthenia — but the absolutely essential first step is the sublimation of infantile autoeroticism, the prototypical sublimation.[37]

Freud's general story line is clear: from the pure pleasure of playing to object-directed pleasure. Unrestricted, autoeroticism "makes the sexual instinct uncontrollable and unserviceable later on." Civilization, in short, depends on mastering masturbation: "The forces that can be employed for cultural activities are thus to a great extent obtained through the suppression of what are known as the *perverse* elements of sexual excitement." Autoeroticism is first among these perversions. But in Freudian theory, failure to suppress this particular perversion has other, more specific results as well, which follow from its being so very far from the ideal of civilized sexual morality. It drives young people into conflicts with their education that they had hoped to avoid by just saying no to sex with another. Here is yet another instance of what seems like the deep pessimism of Freud's deployment of autoeroticism for the making of civilization: having said no to premarital sex, they are driven into the arms of something perhaps even more immoral and then are either racked by guilt, or suffering from the consequences of giving up the one form of sexual release available to them, or demoralized by the constant failure to give it up. Masturbation seems to offer something for nothing, to suggest that one can achieve something without taking trouble. And through fantasy, it creates impossible expectations that are culturally dangerous. Freud here cites Karl Kraus's satirical magazine *Die Fackel*: "Copulation is an unsatisfactory substitute for masturbation." There is, of course, much more: masturbation contributes to the substitution of fantasy objects for reality and indeed fixes these objects in the psyche. Taken altogether, this is not a pretty picture.[38]

Much of this language comes straight from the Enlightenment writers we have been considering. But, critically, it became in Freud part of a new master narrative for how we become who we are, not just how we might be derailed. The Freud of *Three Essays on Sexuality* is not the Rousseau of *Emile*. The importance of his new story goes well beyond its influence on those who subscribed to it. For those who disagreed, it became a theory for how we might become something other than what Freud had hoped. If the sublimation of masturbation is the crucial element in Freud's story of how sexuality is redirected to create civilization and "civilized" sex roles, it is also the crux of masturbation's reinvention in alternative accounts of self-creation. Where masturbation need not be repressed, no hysteria need follow; if it was morally rehabilitated, no conflicts with outside standards would arise. Thus Freud offers two scenarios. In one of these, the two-century-long medical attack on masturbation is redirected toward slowly but surely harnessing the sexual energies of autoeroticism, which, in this version, is no longer a deadly vice but the training ground for heterosexuality. Masturbation is a developmental stage, in the senses of both something to go through and something to build on. In the other, less reassuring and less optimistic version, the world is never safe from what masturbation represents; anatomy is destiny only with a great deal of effort, and then not always. This — an interpretation that sees the sexual order as more fragile and hence more malleable than Freud believed — allows openings for the new uses of masturbation imagined in the 1960s and beyond.

Nowhere is the tension between Freud's radicalism — his discovery of a free-floating libidinous energy that queers the neat ascription of difference — and the normative demands of civilization that seem to be predicated on such difference clearer than in his account of how adult female sexuality is constructed. It is women who bear the bodily costs of civilization, who have to give up the most.

We start with pleasures not differentiated by gender. Anal masturbation is common, Freud pointed out, and indeed this is where the infant first discovers an environment hostile to instinctual pleasure. The body is only loosely programmed for genital sexuality; this too has to be coaxed out of it. It is not automatic, although hints are present from the very beginning. Play with the glans penis and the clitoris proclaims that they are, as Freud says, "destined to great things in the future," "the beginnings of what is later to become normal sexual life." How this happens is not clear. I think that, in Freud's view, the *prohibition* against genital masturbation freights these organs with the meaning they would come to acquire. They come into their own because they are the site of prohibition. In any case, he is unambiguous in his view that "the future primacy over sexual activity exercised by this erotogenic

392

zone was established by early infantile masturbation" whether primacy is dictated by destiny or not.[39]

For both boys and girls, infantile masturbation if it continued would "constitute the first great deviation from the course of development laid down by civilized man." The crucial moment for sexual differentiation comes at puberty, when girls have to repress what had been their masculine form of sexuality — that is, abandon clitoral masturbation and clitoral sexuality — and "hand over," as he says in *New Introductory Lectures on Psychoanalysis*, "its sensitivity, and at the same time its importance, to the vagina." Masturbation in little girls resulted in a genital sexuality that is "wholly masculine"; "with the abandonment of clitoral masturbation a certain amount of activity is renounced. Passivity now has the upper hand." Thus masturbation is crucial not only in defining the genital stage of development but also, for girls, in reshaping it so that penis-in-vagina intercourse will be its preferred expression. It is the arena in which a girl becomes a woman, and the failure to undergo this transition in any of its stages has dire consequences. Giving it up is the cardinal sublimation, the redirection of sexual energy in the purported interests of civilization and the social order. The guilt of masturbation for boys and girls, men and women is thus not simply conventional; it is the guilt born of committing an act that "conflicts with the social principle." But this principle demands far more of women than it does of men.[40]

"Normally the center of greatest response should pass with maturity from the clitoris to the vaginal region," writes the author of a 1930s book, very much in the Freudian tradition, on the emotional problems of women. Masturbation, either in adolescence or in adulthood, keeps this from happening as it should, although not irrevocably: "It is possible to educate a region hitherto undeveloped" — the vagina can still be saved — and, in any case, the clitoris does play some part in the pleasure of vaginal orgasm. In other words, the genitals can be retrained if masturbation has spoiled their appropriate development. But masturbating is clearly a big mistake, a doubly regressive act for women that represents a return both to an earlier autoerotic stage and to the

393

erotogenic regions of childhood. For men, the penis remains in-
variant as the source of genital pleasure. If a single woman must
masturbate to relieve tension, advises this doctor, she should do it
only in response "to a definite sense of physical need." No fantasy
at all cost, and "get over it and forget about it."[41]

Freud's argument for the universality of infant masturbation —
its inevitability, moral innocence, and developmental specificity —
had an enormous impact on sexual pedagogy after 1920. Rather
than evil and dangerous *tout court*, it became a part of ontogenesis: we pass through masturbation, we build on it, as we become
sexual adults. Only its survival into a later developmental stage,
like a representative of some primitive people who somehow appears naked and savage amid bourgeois Europeans, suggests that
something is wrong, not with the body but with the mind. Guilt,
neurosis, or hysteria replaces corporeal corruption, but it results
less from the act itself than from its conflict with morality and
civilization. (For some psychoanalytic theorists, in fact, masturbation became the way through which the narcissistic order of shame
was distinguished from the objective order of guilt: "Guilt in relation to masturbation is tied to the fear of castration; shame has an
irrational, primary, absolute character."[42])

These views had an enormous influence. They became the
professional standard that medical textbooks could refer to in
warning against modern quacks and religious teachers — late to
join the anti-masturbation bandwagon in the nineteenth century
but unrelenting once on — who still taught that masturbation
caused horrible physical or mental harm. It did not, they said
quite clearly: "The harm comes from the feeling of guilt that
accompanies the practice," is a standard response. A.A. Brill, the
psychoanalyst we have already discussed, is given as the authority
for this proposition and for the reassurance that "robbing masturbation of its horrors" would not cause it to flourish. On the contrary, adolescents who dread its consequences masturbate twice
as much as those who learn the truth. The problem is psychological; to give up the practice, they need to deal with guilt. But
give it up they must, because adolescent masturbation has to "be
regarded as something different from autoeroticism in children."[43]

394

The new psychology even made its way, slowly and unevenly, into Roman Catholic theology. In the early twentieth century, the Church's teachings were still heavily Thomist. Masturbation was a sin of lust, *luxuria*; it was among the worst of these, the sins against nature; no sin against chastity is venial, and a sin that one wills as actively as one does self-pollution is particularly culpable. This position was rehearsed well into the 1920s. Sometime in the next fifty years, things changed. Looking back from the vantage of 1970, a Catholic writer notes that the Church had become aware of psychology in the last century. The "blanket and sinful gravity of masturbation in the older teaching" was derived from its one-sided emphasis on the physical side of sex and its connection to reproduction. The problem with masturbation in "contemporary approaches" is more nuanced: not always important, easily overcome in most cases, not always grave, a real issue only when it "indicates a failure at a total integration of sexuality in the person." It is wrong because "it fails to integrate sexuality into the service of love." (Marital onanism is another issue and has not been officially redeemed. Of course, Catholic writing on sex did not ignore its psychology; far from it. But in the Church's pastoral teaching about masturbation, there was not much interest in the life of the mind.) Another moral-theology textbook takes up Freud's suggestion that masturbation is, at its core, an addiction. It is the result of morbid compulsive urges; the masturbator is like the compulsive drinker who goes to AA. Yes, he can stop on occasion, but the root of his compulsion goes much deeper, and he is therefore not morally culpable. If, on the contrary, someone makes a conscious decision to masturbate, it is "always psycho-physical infantilism" but still not an occasion of "grave subjective guilt." Basically, masturbation is a problem of "moral pedagogy" for which a dynamic and understanding program has to be created, argues another authoritative force. In other words, masturbation is no longer a sin against nature or a medical threat but a problem of ego psychology. In fact, the Freudian account had spread everywhere by the middle of the twentieth century. And even where it has not yet made inroads, there are those who wish it had. A contemporary writer on Protestant views of our subject worries that his side has been

395

so much slower than the Catholics' to condone masturbation, while still recognizing, as the Church does, the seriousness of anything having to do with sexuality, "personality development... and respect for the sources of human life."[44]

We are now on the verge of the final part of our story. For much of its modern history, masturbation marked the moral boundaries of the self — the far edge of desire, introspection, imagination, secrecy, and sociability. It was the negative capability, the reversal of the proper relationship between public and private. Then Freud and his successors made it the crux of their story of how sublimation and civilization begin.

When exactly the new, third stage begins is difficult to say. At the same time that the high-minded Freudian revision was in full swing, the men who created surrealism took aboard what they wanted from the Master to purportedly liberate their sexuality and creativity from various psychic prisons. There is much that is adolescent, abject, and silly about their investigations of their own sexuality, something of the quality of innocence and touching frankness of a consciousness-raising group. There is also much that is to our ears shockingly homophobic. When Raymond Queneau offered the opinion that onanism had nothing to do with either "consolation or compensation" but "is as absolutely legitimate in itself as homosexuality," André Breton, Pierre Unik, and Benjamin Péret responded violently, we are told, and in unison, "They have nothing in common!" Péret insisted there could be no onanism without images of women. But that said, the surrealists were the first group of sexual radicals to make onanism part of their conversation; eighteenth-century libertines had had little interest in the subject, and nineteenth-century reformers had reviled it. It was of deep interest to the surrealists. They talked about how much each one did it, whether it was a substitute for sex with women, and how it fit into their sexual memories. For many, it was at the beginning: "Pupils masturbating under their portfolios" was Breton's sexual awakening; seeing a boy cover his penis with ink at school and masturbate was Péret's. They talked about what they imagined when they masturbated and whether they felt shame, embarrassment, or satisfaction. (Breton thought it was impossible to masturbate while thinking about a woman he loved.) And they talked about how they felt about women masturbating. None of this amounted to much beyond the conversation of a group of friends and whatever spillover there might have been into their art and writing. (On the periphery of the surrealist circle, Marcel Duchamp's description of frustrated sexual love as "Slow life — Vicious Circle — Onanism," is an altogether more serious claim about desire, but unpacking it — especially in the context of his *The Bride Stripped Bare by her Bachelors, Even*, in which it was made — would take us in other directions.) Certainly the bantering of the surrealists and perhaps the art making of their far greater colleague presaged the new roles that solitary sex would play in the later twentieth century. [45]

By some time in the 1960s or early 1970s, through first the women's movement, and more recently the gay movement, the story that began in 1712 was first roundly rejected and then turned to a radically new use. For the first time in human history, masturbation was embraced as a mode of liberation, a claim to autonomy, to pleasure for its own sake, an escape from the socially prescribed path toward normal adulthood. It went from being the deviant sexuality of the wrong kind of social order to being the foundational sexuality of new sorts of imagined communities, the basis of a new covenant — or lack thereof — between self and other. Far more than free love, free masturbation came to carry new aspirations for alternative constellations "of bodies and pleasures."[46] And, of course, such views elicited their opposite: masturbation as selfish, purposeless, meaningless, destructive of human relations, a representation of commercial excess, and much more. The story continues.

New Directions in the 1960s and Beyond

There are already claims in the work of many of Freud's most distinguished successors that might have suggested to the attentive reader the potential of masturbation to become, someday, the key to radical, sometimes utopian, changes in how we experience ourselves and our sexuality. Normal masturbation, thought Joyce McDougall, was necessary for "finding sexual resolutions to

397

sexual conflict." But more fundamentally, the first autoerotic act
— thumb sucking — recreated through fantasy the infant's first sexual object — the breast — upon which it was dependent; it was thus,
she claimed, the foundation for all independent libidinal pleasure,
all non-biological sexuality. Melanie Kline too thought that autoeroticism was based on an infant's phantasmic creation of "an
inner gratifying good breast," an external breast projected into his
or her own body; it was "a fantasy of an erotic relation with an
internal object" and thus deeply one's own. Bisexual fantasies in
girls, argued Helen Deutsch, were "conquered in the struggle
against masturbation," by implication, they could be freed if the
tides of war changed. However protean these views were, the origin of modern visions of liberation, of alternative sexualities and
alternative communities built through masturbation did not
spring at first from psychoanalysis but from feminist organizations
and pop-cultural translations of sixties alternative culture.[47]

But even in these contexts Freud was still very much present.
Masturbation was political if for no other reason than that his theories had become identified with the master narrative of patriarchy. Feminists got this right away. Martha Shelley in her 1970
account of lesbianism and women's liberation makes much of the
oppressive normalcy that the Freudian narrative imposed: healthy
development means going through a homosexual period, not
being "arrested" at this or any other stage, and emerging to want
exclusively heterosexual intercourse. "All she wants is a good
fuck" is held out by the Freudians as the cure for alternatives. But
the other side understood the political implications of Freud's
masturbation story as well. No less an authority on the subject
than the authors of the Playboy Press nailed it. Masturbation is
used — Morton Hunt means "masturbation by women" — "as the
solution to the real problem of weak ego, low self-esteem and
lack of social skills." The whole clitoral-orgasm brouhaha, a sustained and widely publicized attack on Freud's theories of female
psychogenesis, was, he thought, the work of "extremists of the
women's liberation movement." As long ago as 1922, Freud's colleague Alfred Adler had recognized masturbation for what it was:
a way to avoid "adult gender identity," particularly by women,

who "resent[ed] their own femaleness," "fear[ed] male domination," and sometimes — the clincher — "use[d] masturbation to
help them keep their distance from men." How right Hunt was
that female masturbation was not in keeping with the bunny philosophy. Among the most offensive texts in this regard — attacked
by name — was *The Sensuous Woman* (1969), which "enthusiasti-
cally urged everyone to masturbate freely" and told women that
not only was it a good way to train for lovemaking — that might
not have been so bad — but, worryingly, it was in itself "one of the
most gratifying human experiences."[48]

In fact, *Playboy* need not have worried. *The Sensuous Woman* is
relentlessly heterosexual even if it is critical of men's lovemaking
techniques: "*You must train like an athlete for the act of love,*" "J."
advised women, and the reason you have to do it alone — "to teach
yourself to come alive" (not clear if the pun is intended) — is that
men do not have the patience to do it. ("J.," Americans — and her
mother — learned through a leak in *Time* magazine, was Terry
Garrity, a moderately successful travel and children's book writer
who hit the *New York Times* best-seller list within months of her
book's appearance just before Christmas 1969.) "J." reversed the
moral valences of the eighteenth century with regard to solitary
sex: "Allow your fantasies [all heterosexual, some kinky] to excite
you." She recommends books ranging from *Lady Chatterley's Lover*
and *Gone with the Wind*, particularly the scene where Rhett Butler
carries Scarlett up the stairs, to *The Story of O*, *Fanny Hill*, and *The
Sheik*. She confesses that she is sold on using masturbation —
explicitly clitoral masturbation — as a way of teaching her body to
be responsive, and she recommends — in italics for emphasis —
that readers set aside several hours a week for this project. Never
before had female masturbation made such an unabashed appearance on the stage of middlebrow culture. *The Sensuous Woman*
sold briskly not only in the United States but in much of the rest
of the world as well at least until the mid-1980s. The author then
went into a sad decline — mental illness, bankruptcy, a ruined
marriage — but her book clearly spoke to a moment.[49]

There is no question in *The Sensuous Woman* and in many similar books of the same period that liberating masturbation was

part of the struggle for the human right to sexual happiness; it was like a lunch-counter sit-in of the body.[50] Even Anne Koedt in her foundational "Myth of the Vaginal Orgasm" is more or less of this school, although she does hold out the more radical prospect at the end that if all orgasm is clitoral, women might not need men to be sexually satisfied. Her prolegomena, however, is a call for liberation: if sexual techniques now regarded as "standard" are not satisfying, they should be rejected. The "standard" is simply misguided and inappropriate. "New techniques must be used or devised which transform this particular aspect of our sexual exploitation."[51]

At about the same time that Koedt was writing, feminism and masturbation became more explicitly linked. In 1971, *Our Bodies, Ourselves: A Course by and for Women* was published as an expansion of a somewhat earlier mimeographed booklet — "Women and Their Bodies" — produced by the Boston Women's Health Book Collective. It called for the liberation of masturbation and its transformation into an act that could serve both individual self-creation and community building. As we saw in Chapter 2, it has been enormously successful: by 1995, more than four million copies had been sold and it had been translated into sixteen languages, including Italian, Japanese, Danish, Chinese, Spanish, Greek, Swedish, German, Hebrew, Telugu, Arabic, and Russian.

The section on masturbation is couched both as a critique of Freud's account of guilt and of his rejection of clitoral orgasm and, on the positive side, as an affirmation of autoeroticism. It values fantasy and self-exploration, argues that masturbation "tells us something about the reality we are in" and about "accepting our feelings and then trying to understand them," and concludes with how-to advice and a clarion call for the right to sexual fulfillment. *Our Bodies, Ourselves* is certainly sympathetic to lesbian sexuality; it is fundamentally about a social, if not necessarily a heterosexual, world. Relationships are what count, and masturbation is one way to enrich them.

By the mid-1970s, this way of thinking about masturbation had become widespread. But there were other and more radical, if curiously traditional, claims as well. Betty Dodson's *Liberating*

Masturbation: A Meditation on Self Love, for example, which appeared first in 1974 and most recently in 1996, assumed no such telos: "Masturbation is our primary sexual life. It is our sexual base. Everything we do beyond that is simply how we *choose to socialize our sex life* [my emphasis]." That is, one might choose to go it alone. (This book is now out of print but seems to have been replaced by another of her works — this time from a major commercial publisher — on the same theme: *Sex for One: The Joy of Self Loving*, which Random House issued in 1995. The new title, like the earlier one, suggests both that masturbation is the route to benign narcissism and autarkic pleasure and, by rearranging words from the title of the best-selling *Joy of Sex*, that it has strong links to heterosexual delights.) Dodson shared with other feminists in the tradition of sexual liberation — Lonnie Barbach or Nancy Friday, for example — a commitment to an inner life and self-acceptance for its own sake. "I love you," as Barbach put it, is the message one gives oneself; the imagination is to be cherished, not feared. (Barbach has lots of other things to say about masturbation in heterosexual relations as well. For example, she attributes the problem of premature ejaculation in part to the fact that men learn to masturbate quickly so as to avoid detection. This has created the expectation of rapid orgasm, functional perhaps in furtive circumstances but not in a mutually satisfying sexual life.)[52] But she makes explicit a larger point that others took up: sociability begins with moral autonomy, and one expression of that autonomy is to have control over sexual pleasure.

Dodson's hope for masturbation is not far from Seneca's view of pleasure generally; in fact, she is perhaps the first person to produce a neo-Hellenistic account of solitary sex. "I do not wish you ever to be deprived of gladness," said Seneca. "I would have it born in your house.... [I]f only it is inside you ... it will never fail you," the great Stoic philosopher wrote to his friend Lucilius.[53] He did not have anything as engaging as orgasm in mind, but that does not detract from Dodson's version of the care of the self. Masturbation, she believes, is the ground from which one can safely enter the world; it exists before it and will continue safely after. Her position, and those like it, are the reverse of Rousseau's;

the same problem with the opposite solution. For the philosophe, masturbation represented the pollution of the self by the social world; the private and inner world that each of us carries around was thus no longer serviceable for its social role as a place of refuge and moral reflection. For Dodson, masturbation represents the true self, and we only need to ask for something from the public sphere if it offers a supplement to what we can have alone.

I quote Dodson only because her views are so unambiguous. There are many variants to this new tradition developed in response to particular political challenges: clitoral masturbation as therapy, as the means to a healthy heterosexual love life. Masters and Johnson and the cottage industry they helped create are a good example. There are, as we saw earlier, lots of ways to take their work. Some radical lesbians picked up on what they had to say about the outer one-third of the vagina and used that to argue for dildos. That is, the clitoris was not alone. Alternatively, some people took from Masters and Johnson the view that the clitoris, if one only looked at it differently, was every bit as big and important as the penis. This was the organ that mattered, and it left nothing to envy in the male and nothing to remain passive about. *A New View of a Woman's Body*, for example, offers precise, professionally prepared anatomic illustrations to demonstrate that the clitoris, when its interior is taken into account, is not only bigger than the penis but also more richly endowed with nerves.[54]

There is more than liberation and anti-Freudian polemics at stake here. In the first place, masturbation seemed to some a means to a better and less sexist society. The Furies Action Day Care Manifesto of 1971 ends with the assertion: "The kids should be encouraged to explore their own bodies and the bodies of each other and to masturbate." The not-so-solitary sex that was scorned by nineteenth-century radicals was now center stage in "revolutionary lesbian politics." The enemy was no longer — or at least not exclusively — the church, the family, and conventional morality as it had been for libertines, socialists, neo-Malthusians, and the like but the whole heterosexist order that supported a violent and oppressive masculinity. If, before, masturbation was the evil doppelgänger of ordinary intercourse that had to be repressed,

402

it was now in the company of its enemies whose triumph was to be hoped for.[55] Much of the literature on female masturbation assumed a social setting, although not necessarily a radical one. More often, masturbation built community; women in groups, small circles of pleasure and support, learned to do it together. Here was a project of civil society in America that Tocqueville could not have imagined in his wildest dreams. *The Clitoral Truth: The Secret World at Your Fingertips* by the woman's health writer and activist Rebecca Chalker, for example, is important in this context not only for the political messages it shares with other books on the subject — the claim that masturbation is "a legitimate part of our birthright" and self-pleasure "an essential means of sexual discovery," or the hope that "the male centered heterosexual model of sexuality . . . is undergoing a dramatic transformation" — but for the extensive social networks in which it subsists. It offers its readers the poignant testimonies of women who benefited from communities of masturbation and a long list of organizations that support sexual self-discovery. (The political, liberatory, resonance of this genre is manifest: a *New York Times* review called Chalker's earlier *A Woman's Book of Choices* "a declaration of independence.")

Not all women's communities are so gentle. In response to the tendency within lesbianism that seemed to regard anything other than oral sex as exploitative and sexual pleasure itself as problematic, a pro-pornography and often pro-S/M movement emerged. Or, in any case, it went public. (Women may well have had a continuous history of finding pleasure in pornography that we know nothing about.)[56] A journal like *On Our Backs* makes the claim for lesbian pornography shared by its community of readers explicit: "I love to read *On Our Backs* with my vibrator in hand," says a woman holding her breasts and wearing a baseball cap as she looks out at us from an advertisement. A moral-purity group is parodied with the *reductio ad absurdum* argument that it wants what would amount to "A MASTURBATION FREE ZONE." A survey of a sex shop in Boulder, Colorado, shows that women bought vibrators to pleasure themselves as much as to give pleasure to others. There are lots of ads for porn movies and phone-sex services — "Ruby's Hot Phone Sex: 'I'm wet and juicy ready to turn you on'"

— and for sex stores like For Yourself: The Sensuality Shop. And so on. Finally, masturbation plays an important part in voyeuristic scenes of lesbian S/M that are not so different from the eighteenth-century ones that we assumed had been made for male voyeurs: "Masturbate I said . . . and remember, you beg me to let you come." In other words, the sexual politics of masturbation is not all as restrained and in the tradition of "good taste" as in the earlier sexual liberation movement.[57]

Contemporary artists, in a variety of events and images, have also appropriated masturbation and transformed the stigmatized past of the private vice into a commentary on matters that are very much public. To some degree they use it with relatively little attention to questions of gender, as a way to query the authority of the artist and his or her relationship to viewers. Other works stake out a place in discussions of feminist art practice through comments on masturbation. And some are manifestly about solitary sex and what it signifies, whatever else they may say about art and art making.

Vito Acconci's brilliant, funny, and notorious *Seedbed*, staged in 1972, at first seems to be very much about artistic authority and relatively little about what the artist is purporting to do: masturbating (figure 6.6). But soon the two become not so distinct. But soon the two become not so distinct. For three weeks, Acconci lay in a box under a white ramp on the floor of the Sonnabend Gallery in New York City. When visitors — "viewers" does not quite capture it — walked over his hidden spot, he would begin to masturbate to the accompaniment of fantasies he was having of the unseen guests and broadcasting over speakers in the gallery. So, art making is literally masturbating, and the authority of the artist is confirmed by our having to take him at face value: we do not see him do anything, and for all we know he is drinking tea under the ramp. Mutual voyeurism — and mutually imaginative engagement — seems predicated on no one actually seeing anyone; like a god known only from his work, Acconci contrives the whole business. (In fact, it is now difficult to recapture this innocence, because we know that the artist injured himself through the continuous, weeks-long exercise of his art.)[58] Art making and

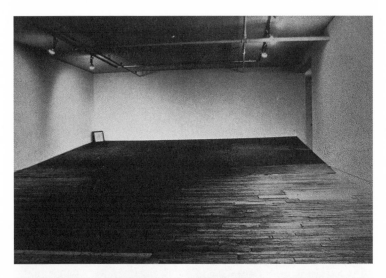
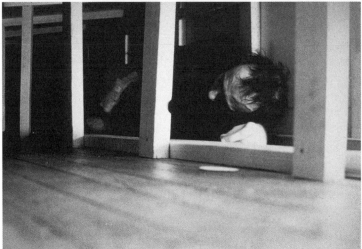

Figure 6.6. Vito Acconci, *Seedbed,* performance, Sonnabend Gallery, New York, 1972. (Courtesy of the artist.)

masturbating, in short, create an architecture of interiority through fantasy, through imaging in the mind's eye.

But if this performance is about art and artist, it is also about masturbation — in all likelihood he was really doing it — and the more Acconci comments on his work, the more it seems so. "You walk across the room, over ramp/under ramp all day," he says. "I hear you, build up fantasies, talk to you/masturbate because of you-for you-with you." If we take this at face value, the relationship of artist and "viewer" is less didactic and more mutual: solitary sex as a communal act and as a way of constituting a self that exists only in the interstices of human interaction. In a more recent interview, he says that in this work he was at first caught up with finding "'self' as if self was a precious jewel," hidden somewhere. But in his three weeks of masturbating to fantasies of unseen strangers, he came to regard "self as part of a social system, a person-to-person space." Whatever the performance might mean about self or masturbation, however, our subject entered resolutely into contemporary art. And it entered as a still unengendered act; the installation would have been understood differently had a woman artist claimed to be masturbating out of sight while "viewers" walked overhead because history has given female masturbation — liberating, ecstatic, dreamy, and lyrical versus abject, humiliating, and decidedly second-rate — its own, gendered resonance. And it would have been different still had the gender of the artist been disguised. But the actual act was disembodied; it was there in its pure form: the ur-sexuality.[59]

Masturbation in the visual art of feminists registers some of these themes but speaks more directly in a conversation about feminist art practice and politics and to the specific history of women. This takes us very quickly to our topic. Judy Chicago's late-1970s work *The Dinner Party*, for example, is one starting point. It was — before its incorporation into a book with the same title — an installation of thirty-nine dinner settings arranged around a large triangular table (48 feet at the base × 43 feet on the sides × 3 feet), each one representing either a real person — Christine de Pisan, Emily Dickinson, Georgia O' Keeffe, Mary Wollstonecraft — or a mythical figure like the primordial goddess.

SOLITARY SEX IN THE TWENTIETH CENTURY

A painted, often highly sculpted, ceramic plate that depicted the folds and crevasses of the female genitals in various styles and degrees of verisimilitude was set on a decoratively embroidered place mat that included the name of the guest. The installation became not only part of a great political controversy — it was kept from being permanently housed in the University of the District of Columbia by an act of Congress after acrimonious hearings — but also the putative beginning of a visual conversation among artists. "There's a lot of vagina in our work, but it's not about vaginas," as one contemporary artist said of her own and her generation's relationship to Chicago. Indeed, their work is about other, ancillary organs as well and much more: "It is about inventing a language radiating of female power." The most important point for now is that these works exist at all. Maybe Anne Walsh's *This Summer I Learned a New Way to Masturbate* is, as one critic notes, "a contemplative and ironic expression of the frustration experienced by a woman artist living and working alone" (see figure 6.7). We are invited to see the cat scratches around the periphery of the page as suggestive of this: just the artist and her cats. On the other hand, the pillow is perhaps not so ironic or the mood so contemplative; in the context of Annie Sprinkle's performance art of the same period, 1992–1993, and indeed of her whole career, a pillow may be a pillow and a new way to masturbate may be a new way to masturbate.

Sprinkle — née Ellen Steinberg — has made herself into a "post-porn modernist" advocate — "celebrant," "high priestess," or "goddess" might be better words — of female eroticism and of masturbation in particular. Her home page shows her as the multi-handed Shiva, spread-legged, surrounded by sex toys, and playing with a dildo. (She is currently offering for sale a limited-edition, signed and numbered polished-black-marble "love handle dildo" — fifty made, forty left — at $200 plus $6 postage and handling.) A picture of herself — one among many that we are invited to download — shows her with her legs apart and the lips of her vulva open, her ring finger playing with her clitoris (figure 6.8). A cigarette is held neatly between her exquisitely manicured index and middle finger. Her other hand plays with her nipple, exposed

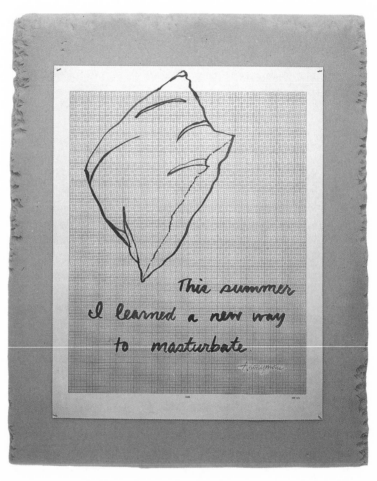

Figure 6.7. Anne Walsh, *This Summer I Learned a New Way to Masturbate,* 1992–1993, ink on graph paper and chewed foam rubber, 20 x 24 x 1½ inches. The subject has entered contemporary feminist art. (Photo courtesy the UCLA Hammer Museum. Photo: Robert Wedemeyer. By permission of the artist.)

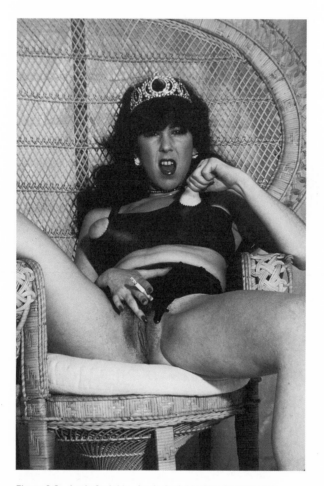

Figure 6.8. Annie Sprinkle, *Annie Sprinkle with Cigarette and Clitoris*, 2001. Sprinkle has made her own masturbation a central part of a wildly funny and brilliant feminist appropriation of pornography. (Courtesy of the artist.)

through an opening in a leather bra. Whatever we might make of this brilliant "prostitute/porn star turned performance artist and sex guru" — her self-description — who is now a regular guest artist at various colleges and universities — Vassar and the University of Oregon are on the calendar as I write — masturbation and the beaver shot will never be the same.[60]

Set beside this twenty-five-year-long career of radical porn and a history of feminist advocacy of masturbation, Zoe Leonard's 1992 installation at the Neue Galerie, Kassel, becomes increasingly complicated. On one side is a painting of a richly attired eighteenth-century matron enveloped in cloth and almost choked by wealth and material possessions. On the other is an equally well-dressed woman being embraced by her young son. Her hands are folded demurely on her lap. In between hangs what appears to be a small reproduction of Courbet's full-frontal painting of a female crotch resplendent with pubic hair, *L'Origine du monde*, which he painted for the boudoir of the Turkish ambassador to Paris. But it is not as Courbet left it; Leonard seems to have added a hand. This juxtaposition may well suggest something about the nature of visual art and how we look at it: "Every art object is a beaver shot in disguise — something to gape at, to possess, something in and through which a sense of the self is derived." But that would be true if there were no added hand and if it were not nestled on the mound of hair and if two fingers were not reaching for the not-quite-visible clitoris. This is no longer the passive woman spread-eagled in the picture that the bey had bought from Courbet but a woman exploring her own genitals, giving herself pleasure quite oblivious of the viewer. If this is voyeurism, it is certainly not of someone we, viewers of whatever sex, are invited to possess or use. If we learn something about ourselves from it, it is that autonomy is the necessary first step to sociability. The point may be not that looking at art generally is like looking at the Courbet beaver shot — or something like it — but that one woman owns herself and the others — the eighteenth-century ones — do not. (The story of this installation is not quite as I have told it, although Leonard's real intention makes it even more on point. At the time of the Kassel show she

410

had, in fact, not seen or heard of Courbet's painting. What we see is therefore not a quotation. She had, however, observed that women in art are "depicted as the catalysts of male heterosexual desire, but that their own desire was never depicted." She asked six friends to pose for photographs to call attention to this state of affairs and remedy it, to "depict women's sexual desire, rather than women's desirability." She invites the full range of possible reactions to what is, after all, our subject in full view.) (Leonard's interest in this installation is less the ubiquity of the male gaze and the power it may or may not convey but the absence from the visual record of women looking: never the artist, always looked at.)[61]

But what a difference a gaze — or perhaps gazer — makes. Sprinkle with her repeated public invitation to viewers to examine her vulva and her cervix — there is a Web page devoted to it — and Leonard with her seemingly historical juxtaposition were not the first to think about what came next for Courbet's model or someone like her. Marcel Duchamp, Hans Bellmer, Auguste Rodin, George Grosz, and most famously Pablo Picasso wondered as well. Nor were they the last: two young Serbian artists in 1997 made a video of what they think she might have done.[62] Picasso's interest is not exclusively or even largely in masturbation; the erotic energy of his art is so overpowering and general that our subject rather pales. It is ostentatiously voyeuristic and not so different from the eighteenth-century images we saw earlier. But Picasso images and many others we could look at make much of women's sexual autonomy. They are not a variant of a joke of Aristophanes but an homage to the erotic power these women possess quite on their own.

Lynda Benglis's notorious advertisement in the November 1974 *Artforum* constitutes another variant on the chameleon-like private vice that John Marten first made public (figure 6.9). It takes masturbation out of the realm of pleasure and erotic autonomy and puts it straight into the domain of power. As many people have pointed out, it endows the female artist with a phallus and mocks the claims of male artists to a monopoly on it. Or, more precisely, it mocks the whole idea of the phallus. But the artist is also fairly obviously engaged in double masturbation: Benglis is

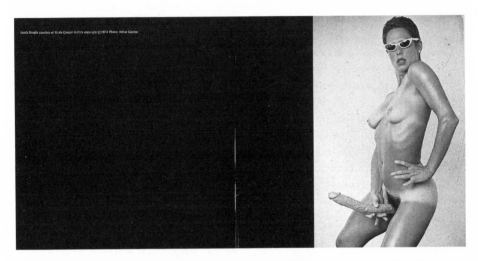

Figure 6.9. Lynda Benglis, advertisement in *Artforum*, 1974. In this startling photograph, the artist is mocking the phallus, masturbating as if she were a man, and using the double-headed dildo to masturbate herself. (©1974 Lynda Benglis. Courtesy Cheim & Read, New York.)

sticking one end of her gigantic, grotesque dildo into herself, and she is stroking its shaft as if it were her penis. Whatever else might be said, the power she speaks of is not only of the phallus but also of playing with its representation. The duality of masturbation is all too evident: it is the source of autonomy and power but also of abjection and pathos. Its pleasures are real and they are illusory.[63]

Perhaps this is why men have been slow to recuperate solitary sex. There might well have been expressions of masturbation as a form of queerness early on: we are all polymorphously perverse, and a self-conscious embrace of autoeroticism — the sexuality before gender, male or female, or sexuality, heterosexuality or homosexuality, divided us — would be a way of expressing this. There might well also have been communal masturbation as part of gay culture before the late 1970s. But I could, however, find no evidence for any of this. The SF Jacks — "a fellowship of men who like to jack-off in the company of like-minded men," as its website announces — started in the late 1970s. The New York Jacks — "an organization of like-minded men who enjoy jacking off together" — began in 1980. All this was before the discovery of HIV and the elucidation of the epidemiology of AIDS that would, in the subsequent decades, make clubs such as these attractive as a safe alternative to bathhouse sex.

But the world wide expansion of such masturbation clubs was based on more than safe sex. The Melbourne Wankers, for example, founded in 1990, define themselves as sexually avant-garde through their enterprise. "Wanking is an Aussie term that means masturbation (that is, jacking-off), and a wanker means a bit of an oddball, someone who believes in, and enjoys, what he is doing, even though he is not mainstream," says their Web site. Male gay porn, intended, like most porn, to facilitate masturbation but also full of solo-masturbation scenes, is a "way of making gay men visible" and "an example of gay male memory." More generally, it is a way of claiming nonreproductive sexuality. Again, Rousseau comes back in reverse: the book that makes these points is called *One-Handed Histories*, the twentieth-century avatar of "books to be read with one hand."[64]

Both gay and straight men have also adopted masturbation as a way of renouncing the old machismo stereotypes and of "getting in touch with their bodies." Sometimes this is expressed functionally, as it was in the feminist literature, as a means toward a better heterosexual relationship: learn new sexual skills, deepen intimacy, enrich lovemaking. Sometimes it is in the neo-Hellenistic terms of Betty Dodson: developing "robust self-love" or finding "authentic power" within is the prelude to social life; "self-touch builds self-esteem"; experiencing pleasure alone "makes it possible to share pleasure with someone." In short, the eighteenth century is turned on its head. Masturbation creates the sort of self that can live ethically in the social world. And, finally, for this kinder, gentler masculinity, masturbation is a way of getting closer to God: "self-loving" is a form of loving God; "the phallus is a *mysterium tremendum*"; "orgasms can be numinous experiences." Various forms of masturbation have also become associated with various spiritual practices: Tantric, vaguely pantheistic, yogic, and more. Joanie Blank's 1996 collection of ninety-five male and female accounts of self-pleasuring constitutes a documentary landmark.[65]

Of course, male artists — gay and straight — also engage with masturbation as self-discovery, self-creation, and a matter of public politics. Others — I am thinking here of Bruce Nauman, self-identified as a heterosexual who lives with artist Susan Rothenberg, and the spare, fleshless neon-light stick figures in his *Masturbating Man* and *Sex and Death/Double 69*, both 1985 — show it, along with other sorts of human sexuality, as mechanical, joyless, and inconceivably distant from any hope of intimacy with oneself or another. But the lyrical tradition of Whitman's homoeroticism lives on in works like Wojnarowicz's *Arthur Rimbaud in New York*, 1978–1979, in which his friend and collaborator, Brian Butterick, assumes the persona (literally, a mask) of one of the artist's culture heroes (figure 6.10); or Robert Mapplethorpe's *Bill* in which we see, in both frames, the soft white pelvis of a man with an erect, darker penis. His braceleted wrist emerges out of an undefined space; he holds his organ in a delicately shaped hand — only the direction in which it points differs between the two — with only a hint of a stroking. Between the images is a quiet black

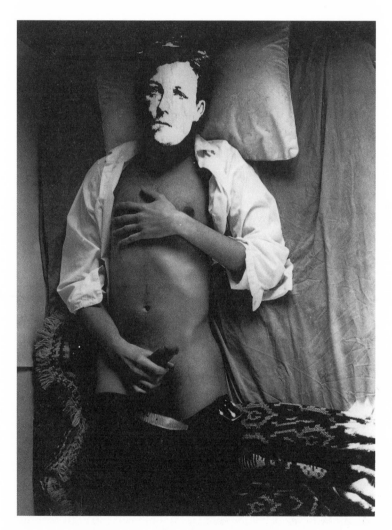

Figure 6.10. David Wojnarowicz, *Arthur Rimbaud in New York*, 1978–1979. Masturbation in the work of this gay artist takes on some of the lyrical qualities of Walt Whitman's *Leaves of Grass*. (Courtesy of the Estate of David Wojnarowicz and PPOW, New York.)

void giving the ensemble — and masturbation — an almost elegiac quality. It is too late in the day to say much more about these images than that they exist and that they incorporate the eighteenth-century insight about the ethical centrality of solitary sex and its translation into nineteenth-century poetic idioms into the very different world of late-twentieth-century gay New York.[66]

These sexual and artistic trends became the lightning rod for conservative criticism of the purported moral decay of America since the 1960s. In the context of what have come to be called "the culture wars" masturbation became overtly and complexly political. Before Americans knew there were White House views on masturbation we learned that Jocelyn Elders, the Surgeon General, did not share them. President Bill Clinton claimed, at a Miami news conference where he announced that he had fired her, that his actions had nothing to do with politics. Her apparent endorsement of the public health benefits of masturbation reflected, he said, "differences with administration policy and my own convictions." Of course, this is not really why he fired her, nor did she say — as the media tended to suggest — that children should be taught to masturbate in sex education classes. As Frank Rich points out, in a *New York Times* column entitled "The Last Taboo," "the President knows that anyone who needs masturbation lessons is unlikely to meet the minimal intelligence requirement for school attendance anyway." Elders had offended many people, especially conservatives, with her outspoken views on AIDS, pre-marital sex, and decriminalization of drug use, and the administration had decided that she was not worth all the trouble she caused. But it is telling that her use of the "M" word in a hastily cobbled together answer to a question at a news conference is what brought her down.[67] Of course the cultural right rejoiced in her demise and in the affirmation that some things could not, in decency, be put on the public agenda. To date no mainstream politician has been willing to publicly defend masturbation as a morally innocent and socially benign sexual practice.

Nonetheless, the culture wars continue to be waged in the mass media and masturbation is at the very heart of the struggle between liberal individualism and those who fear it. On the one hand, the religious right is vehemently anti-masturbatory. The Christian.Answers.Net Web site, for example, gives a purportedly Biblical gloss to the guilt born of the Enlightenment. "I'm a Christian and I have a sort of embarrassing problem," writes a young man, "I need to know if masturbation is wrong in the eyes of God." Admitting that the Bible has nothing explicit to say on the subject, the virtual cleric Dawson McAllister answers that: "Sex was created by God to help prevent man's 'aloneness.'" (Genesis 2:18, which is given as the proof text, does not quite say this; it is where the story of the creation of all beasts and birds begins; it ends 2:21–24 with one version of the creation of Eve and the statement that the two cleave to each other and "become one flesh.") Moreover, McAllister points out, sexual fantasy almost always goes along with masturbation: images, movies, photos provide the material from which people construct their own sexual fantasies. God is explicit on this topic: "He who chases fantasies lacks judgements." And finally, masturbation, he says, can become a substitute for healthy relationships, an emotional crutch. If the good preacher had not in fact read the previous three centuries' views on our subject, he nonetheless knew them in his heart.

American religious fundamentalism finds unlikely company for its views on solitary sex at the pinnacle of contemporary French literary and philosophical culture. Michel Houellebecq's recent, sensational novel, *Elementary Particles*, identifies masturbation as the most abject symptom of the sexual revolution of the sixties and seventies and of the physical and spiritual perils of succumbing to its temptations. One of the two protagonists in this post-modern quest for happiness is an obsessive masturbator who goes mad. The other, his brother, cannot masturbate successfully. This aversion to his own flesh drives his quest to discover in biotechnology a decorporealized solution to the human search for sexual gratification: pure physical bliss liberated from the burdens of intersubjectivity and physical decay. These are old melodies in new times; only the science fiction resolution is different.

On the other hand, network television and Hollywood movies exhibit all the moral irresolution of the commercially driven culture that created *Onania* — titillation artfully blended with fear,

417

embarrassment and abjection. The liberatory, aesthetic, and more generally redemptive impulses we saw elsewhere are rare. In popular American film, men and boys are repeatedly caught "doing it" and are humiliated, mocked, or emotionally pummelled. Jason Briggs in *American Pie* sits with a sock over his erect penis watching a scrambled cable TV porn movie when his parents barge in; the whole movie is one long, sophomoric joke about apple pie as a masturbatory vagina substitute. The eponymous hero of *The Apprenticeship of Duddy Kravitz* wakes up to find his roommate doing it and cracks jokes like "Why don't you use your other hand? It might feel like having sex with someone different"; Kevin Spacey in *American Beauty* is seen masturbating in the shower and, on another occasion in bed, where he awakens his wife who takes umbrage. They fight. Ben Stiller's "cleaning his pipes" scene in *Something About Mary* is grotesque: his semen spurts onto the sink where his would-be girlfriend mistakes it for hair gel and uses it accordingly. The Harvey Keitel character in *Bad Lieutenant* masturbates next to the car with two girls in it that he has stopped. This is not a happy picture.[68]

The cult comedy of the 1990s, *Seinfeld*, is a show "about nothing" and thus the perfect example of the solipsism and self-centeredness that the eighteenth century feared would consume us if masturbation were not stopped. The threats proclaimed by *Onania* live on in the infamous fifty-first episode, "The Contest," that first aired on November 18, 1992. The protagonists make a bet as to who can keep from masturbating the longest. Kramer weakens first after he sees a naked woman in another apartment; Elaine succumbs to fantasies after she gets a glimpse of John F. Kennedy Jr., and Jerry is the third to give in. George wins. And later in the series, when he signs up as a hand model (episode sixty-six, "The Puffy Shirt," September 23, 1993) he assures his new employer that his attractive fingers are safe: he won the not-masturbating contest. The previous incumbent in the modeling job had ended his career in ruin when his precious hands shriveled from we-know-what. And in the last episode George finally confesses that he had lied and so Jerry had won after all. These are not quite the laughs Aristophanes got from this subject. They are jokes born after 1712 by people who have lived through Freud and are steeped in an ironic view of past prejudices and persistent transgressions. But for all their jaded sophistication these gags do not fully exorcise the demons of guilt and obsession that the eighteenth century let loose.

There are signs, however, that the Enlightenment sexual ethics, which made masturbation the evil doppelgänger of modernity, are coming unraveled in the age of the Internet. One finds an extraordinary proliferation of voices on the worldwide Web, a new media that transcends many of the constraints of eighteenth-century print culture. The Web has made it possible for people to exchange stories about their fantasies and desires free from the censorious, disciplining voices of medical, clerical, parental, or pedagogical authority. In the digital world *Onania*, Tissot, Campe, Salzmann, and their kin are multiplying ten thousand fold, shorn, however, of moralizing commentary and the threat of death, disease, or madness. Masturbation has become not only a source of individual self-discovery, but also the basis for a new form of sexual sociability rooted in the celebration of the imagination and its infinite possibilities. (The advent of "National Masturbation Month" to celebrate this new community in the late 1990s is a hilarious carnivalesque reversal of the values espoused in *Onania* [see figure 6.1]).

There are hundreds of thousands of pornographic sites that cater to every masturbatory fantasy imaginable, but what is really new is the proliferation of virtual communities of onanists, an alternative universe of sociability that is created through the public revelation of the not-so-private vice. Over 5000 young men — average age 22.8 — responded to JackinWorld's fifth anniversary survey; one third said that they visited the site to learn more about how their peers feel on the subject. (About one third joined to learn new techniques, and another third because it was a turn on. Each need is amply supplied.) Responses to a "question of the week," at this site (separate for boys and girls), offer a wealth of shared experience far larger than Tissot gathered and almost all cheerily telling about the pleasures of autoeroticism. Exactly who reads these and what they do when so engaged we do not know.[69]

But we do know that cyberspace has vastly enlarged the conversation and made possible an erotic community whose desires are not so easily brought within the bounds of power as they were constituted in or around 1712.

The history of that "trouble and agony of a wounded conscience," launched into the world by the most humble of literary productions — an eighty-eight-page tract, by a profit-seeking quack doctor cum pornographer — is not really in the past. It is not yet really history. Serious men and women, many of the great thinkers and artists of the last three centuries, consider as deeply significant what had once been thought of as a reactively inconsequential ethical sideshow and what to some today seems like simple fun. It remains strange and disturbing that in our century the young Wittgenstein on the eastern front of the Great War was in moral agony because, amidst the death and carnage, he masturbated, just as Rousseau's self-lacerations in more peaceful circumstances are still unsettling. Potentially autarkic solitary sexual pleasure touches the inner lives of modern humanity in ways that we still do not understand. It remains poised between self-discovery and self-absorption, desire and excess, privacy and loneliness, innocence and guilt as does no other sexuality in our era.

Notes

CHAPTER ONE: THE BEGINNING

1. 4th ed., p. 63; 17th ed., pp. 70–71. I cite these two editions because the fourth is the earliest edition that is available in any English or American library:

Onania; or, the heinous sin of self-pollution, and all its frightful consequences, in both sexes, considered, with spiritual and physical advice . . . (London: printed for the author, and sold by N. Crouch; P. Varenne; and J. Isted, [1718?]). The date is unreliable; some library catalogs give 1725 as the date for the fourth ed. while others date the fifth as early as 1720. I discuss the publishing history and dates of various editions on pp. 25–30, 179, and n.132. I suspect that 1718 is about right. I cite the seventeenth edition because it is the one that was in the library of the distinguished Swiss doctor S.A.D. Tissot and that, through his work, made it into the *Encyclopédie. Onania: or, the heinous sin of self-pollution, and all its frightful consequences (in both sexes) considered* (London: printed for, and sold by C. Corbett, 1752). In the rest of this book I have cited page numbers from an easily available reprint edition of both *Onania*, 8th ed. (London: Printed by E. Rumball for T. Crouch, 1723) and its *Supplement* (London: Printed for T. Crouch, 1723) produced by Garland Press (New York: Garland, 1986).

Based on what we know about print runs, two thousand copies is probably about right for eighteenth-century editions. It is not so easy to sort out the authorial personae here. To be sure the dangers-of-masturbation sections are distinct from the medical advertisements, suggesting an alliance between the author and a physician, but the author also says that he — no mention of someone else — will consult with persons for complicated cases if sufferers will leave a time and his fee in a sealed envelope at the specified booksellers. He would also consult by mail upon payment of a fee. This is consistent with my view that the author of *Onania* was the surgeon and pornographer John Marten. See pp. 31–32 above.

2. The place of the medical conscription of masturbation in the making of modern sexuality has been most famously identified by Michel Foucault in *The History of Sexuality*, trans. Robert Hurley (New York: Pantheon Books, 1978),

the first volume in what became his broader treatment of the subject. Dr. Pouil-let, *Essai médico-philosophique sur les formes, les causes, les signes, les conséquences et le traitement de l'onanisme chez la femme* (Paris: Adrien Delahaye, 1876); though specifically about masturbation in women, the book describes many pathologies that strike men as well.

  3. Sir James Paget, *Clinical Lectures and Essays*, 2nd ed., ed. Howard Marsh (London: Longman, Green, 1879), pp. 291–92 and 275–99 passim. The lecture was given in 1870 and stands at the beginning of the end of masturbatory pathol-ogy. (Paget remains famous today as the eponymous discoverer of Paget's dis-ease, a bone dysplasia.)

  4. This formulation is J.B. Schneewind's in *The Invention of Autonomy: A History of Modern Moral Philosophy* (Cambridge, UK: Cambridge University Press, 1998), pp. 6 and 9. Schneewind argues that Kant "invented" the concep-tion of morality as autonomy. But my point here is that Enlightenment theories of morality generally shared its consequences: a rejection of the notion, central to views that morality was obedience, that the capacity among humans for moral judgment differed. This is important for my argument in that it explains why masturbation became for the first time an issue that, like other moral questions, now applied to women.

  5. Charles Taylor, *Sources of the Self: The Making of the Modern Identity* (Cambridge, MA: Harvard University Press, 1989), pp. 305–306. This remark-ably learned and brilliant book has been of great use to me, and so to cite but two pages is to mislead the reader as to its importance in my thinking about the problem of the ethical subject. *Nicomachean Ethics* 1170a5 and the rest of bk. 9, ch. 9, in *The Complete Works of Aristotle*, ed. Jonathan Barnes (Princeton, NJ: Princeton University Press, 1984), pp. 1849–50.

CHAPTER TWO: THE SPREAD OF MASTURBATION FROM *ONANIA* TO THE WEB
  1. On the question of dating, see p. 179 and n.132.

  2. In fact, there were no such prescriptions in any previous literature, and it is odd that the author suggests otherwise, since he makes such a big deal about being the first to bring masturbatory disease to the public's attention. Since anti-masturbation medicines claimed not to stop the practice but only to help recover from its effects, our author might have meant that he would offer gen-eral-purpose strengthening, rejuvenating prescriptions from earlier sources.

  3. See Francis Doherty, "The Anodyne Necklace: A Quack Remedy and Its Promotion," *Medical History* 34 (1990). More generally, see Roy Porter, *Health for Sale: Quackery in England, 1660–1850* (Manchester, UK, and New York: Man-chester University Press, 1989).

  4. Arrangements varied, and it is impossible to sort out how commerce in *Onania* actually worked. Thus, for example, Elizabeth Rumball printed the eighth edition for Thomas Crouch; it cost 2 shillings stitched. The fourth edi-tion, variously dated, does not give a printer but says that it is sold by N. Crouch

at The Bell in the Poultrey; by P. Varenne at the Saracen's Head on the Strand; and by J. Isted at the Golden Ball against Dunstan Church for 1 shilling. It does not give a separate bound price. A sixth edition, purportedly from 1722, says it is printed and sold by T. Crouch, bookseller. All these are well-known printers and booksellers. A 171-page edition of the *Supplement*, not dated and printed by T. Crouch and J. Isted, sold for 1 shilling 6 pence. C. Corbett sold the seventeenth edition of the main text and the eighth of the *Supplement* in 1752 for 3 shillings stitched and 3 shillings 6 pence bound, "Crouch and Isted being dead." The copy of this edition in the British Library (BL) seems — judging from the quality of the signature on the flyleaf — to have belonged to a young girl named Sarah Turk. Pasted on the inside is an advertisement for the ninth edition which claims that fifteen thousand copies had been sold. The last edition in the BL is the twentieth, published in Glasgow by A. MacIntosh, with no date or title page and no advertisements for drugs. Letters that in earlier editions had been addressed to Mr. Crouch are addressed to Mr. ——. Dates have been changed from the 1720s to the 1740s, but otherwise the book has become explicitly soft-core pornography. The BL's copy of this edition once belonged to "Pisiasnus Fraxi," the noted nineteenth-century collector of erotic literature.

5. G.A. Cranfield, *The Development of the Provincial Newspaper, 1700–1760* (Oxford: Clarendon Press, 1962), pp. 222–23, which cites an advertisement from the December 1, 1727, *Brice's Weekly Journal*.

6. For London, see Bryant Lillywhite, *London Coffee Houses: A Reference Book of Coffee Houses of the Seventeenth, Eighteenth, and Nineteenth Centuries* (London: George Allen and Unwin, 1963), pp. 23 and 19 regarding the mail and passim regarding the place of coffeehouses in circulating newspapers and quack medicines. There is no list of provincial coffeehouses but a general account, and for the 1700 London estimate see Aytoun Ellis, *The Penny Universities: A History of the Coffee-Houses* (London: Secker and Warburg, 1956), p. xiv and pp. 129–44 for medicines and coffeehouses.

7. The source for all this, duly acknowledged in the text, is John Quincy, *Dr. Carr's Medicinal Epistles Uppon Several Occasions Done into English, as a supplement to the explanation of Sanctorius's Aphorism* (London, 1714). The nuns' story is the theme of the most salacious of forty-one epistles and is framed in a conventional, sexually loaded anti-Catholicism: Why would the pope give such a task to cardinals who are "in no way conversant in the Differences of Sexes"? But other epistles refer tangentially to matters of generation, and Quincy assures his readers that he will not "omit anything material upon account of modesty." Quincy also translated Albert the Great's *Mysteries of Human Generation Fully revealed with explanatory notes*, which became a staple of the medical soft-core porn market and was published by the "notorious" Edward Curll.

8. [Thomas Stretzer], *A New Description of Merryland: Containing a Topographical, Geographical, and Natural History of That Country*, 7th ed. (Bath, UK, 1741), p. 15.

9. J. Isted was the publisher of at least sixty-eight separate titles or editions, including four editions of *Onania* and such popular standards as *A History of the Remarkable Life of Jack Sheppard* (the most famous of the period's highwaymen, noted for daring prison escapes), a compendium titled *The Lives of the Most Remarkable Criminals*, a play about a cuckolded husband, and a number of learned books on the law. These books, in turn, spread the word about *Onania*. Generally, masturbation did not figure much in works on venereal disease, although it joins the long list of possible causes for impotence, infertility, gleets (discharges), and other infirmities of the genitals: for example, "natural coldness, strains, excessive coition, *or* Self Pollution, which latter in young people forces Nature," in *The Modern Siphylis [sic]; or, The True Method of Curing Every Stage and Symptom collected and digested by I.F. Nicholson of New College Oxford and the University of Glasgow* (London, 1718). On self-pollution in other advertising contexts, see Doherty, "Anodyne Necklace," n.56, citing an advertisement from 1732.

10. John Marten, *A Treatise of All the Degrees and Symptoms of the Venereal Disease in Both Sexes*, 6th ed. enl. (London: S. Crouch, N. Crouch, P. Varenne, C. King, J. Isted, n.d.). The BL gives 1708 as the date; a letter putatively written in 1703 is printed as part of the text. The word "masturbation" occurs in Edward Baynard, *The History of Cold Bathing, Both Ancient and Modern* (London, 1706), which may in fact be the first use. On this text, see above pp. 84–85; I am not counting here the Latin title of a translated epigram: "Frig not thyself with thy lascivious fist," in "Paediconem masturbatem," epig. 23 (*Ex otio Negotium*), 1656. John Marten, *Gonosologium novum; or, A new system of all the secret infirmities and diseases natural, accidental, and venereal in men and women* (London: S. Crouch, N. Crouch, P. Varenne, C. King, J. Isted, 1709). On Marten's prosecution, see David Foxon, *Libertine Literature in England, 1660–1745* (New Hyde Park, NY: University Books, 1965), p. 13. The indictment claims that *Gonosologium novum* was printed as an appendix to the sixth edition of Marten's book on venereal disease. It is bound together with it in the BL edition, although it has a separate title page and pagination. If the lost first edition of *Onania* was indeed published in 1708 and not 1710, then the word "masturbation" and the first, most famous sustained attack on it were born together. And if I am right about the identity of *Onania*'s anonymous author, soon to be revealed, they were the inventions of the same man.

11. Marten, *Gonosologium novum*, pp. 86–87.

12. The tract in question is *Onania Examined, and detected; or, The ignorance, error, impertinence, and contradiction of a book called Onania discovered and exposed... By Philo-Castitatis*, 2nd ed. (London, 1724). The first edition appeared in 1723. We do not know when *Onania* first picked up on its attacker. The fifteenth edition, from which I quote, appeared in 1730.

13. [Math. Rothos], *A Whip for the Quack; or, Some remarks on M—n's Supplement to his Onania. With a full answer and confutation of his boasted-of, and long-promised curious piece from Sckmeider, and of all their arguments for the seeds*

[sic] return into the blood after its secretion (London, 1727). Rothos is almost certainly a pseudonym. The English Short Title Catalogue (ESTC) identifies M——n
as John Marten.

14. The publishers were Joseph Marshall and J. Roberts. Among their other
joint ventures were a life of the highwayman Jack Sheppard and a treatise on
Calvin's and Luther's views on the Trinity. Marshall mostly published virulently
anti-Catholic books—an account of a miraculous conversion from Rome—and
other polemical religious tracts. The tone of the attack on *Onania* is not so
different from that of attacks on Arminianism as neo-Pelagian heresy. Marshall
also published a shorthand manual with N. Crouch, one of *Onania*'s publishers.
There are 106 entries for Joseph Marshall in the ESTC and 9 for Marshall and
Roberts.

15. Michael Stolberg, who has compared Marten's works with *Onania*, says
that H.J.M. Symons at the Wellcome Library had come to suspect Marten years
ago but never published on the matter. In fact, the *Catalogue of Printed Books* 4
(London, 1995), ed. Symons and H.R. Denham, in the Wellcome Historical
Medical Library, gives Marten as the author. The current on-line catalog does
not. Stolberg is dubious that Marten wrote *Onania* both because the moral tone
is supposedly so different from the tone of his other works and because other
evidence is not convincing. No one has noted the connection with "Mathew
Rothos," which, together with internal evidence, clinches the case, I think. See
Michael Stolberg, "Self Pollution," *Journal of the History of Sexuality* 9.1–2
(Jan.–April 2000), n.79 and p. 54.

16. The fifteenth edition, from 1730, announced that it was "printed and sold
only by J. Isted at the Golden Ball between St. Dunstan's Church and Chancery
Lane, Mr. Crouch, bookseller who used also to sell it being dead"; Varenne had
died in 1724. The anodyne-necklace business also distributed free copies of a
perfectly decent shorthand manual for anyone who bought its medicines.

17. For this prehistory, see Doherty, "Anodyne Necklace." *The Crime of Onan*
gives no date; *Eronania* is dated 1724. The distinction between these two tracts
is minimal, with pages from one appearing in the other.

18. The publishing worlds of *Onania* and of the anodyne-necklace crowd
were, however, intertwined. Thus, for example, *Felium Ariadnum; or, The Way to
get rid of the Labyrinth of Venus* by Paul Chamberlen—the necklace's inventor
and big-name endorser who was wrongly associated with the famous family of
accoucheurs who invented the obstetrical forceps—was sold by J. Isted, one
of *Onania*'s publishers. The "Secret Disease" in question seems to be some
old-fashioned venereal ailment in men caused by fermenting seed in "common
women." I do not give the page numbers of these quotations because it is impossible to distinguish the various editions and because page numbers are neither
consistent nor reliable.

19. *Onania; or, The Heinous Sin of Self-Pollution* (London Printed; repr. at
Boston, for John Phillips and sold at his shop on the south side of the town

house, 1724). There is a 1742 edition, which is announced as "Printed and sold by S. Kneeland and T. Green, in Queen Str." Cotton Mather, "The Pure Nazarite: Advice to a young man, concerning an impiety and impurity (not easily to be spoken of) which many young men are to their perpetual sorrow, too easily drawn into. A letter forced into the press, by the discoveries which are made, that sad occasions multiply, for the communication of it" (Boston: Printed by T. Fleet for John Phillips, at his shop on the south side of the Town-House, 1723). Mather and *Onania* thus shared a publisher if this tract is indeed genuine. Thomas James Holmes, *Cotton Mather, a Bibliography of His Works* (Cambridge, MA: Harvard University Press, 1940), claims that it is. My colleague Robert Middlekauf, who has written extensively on Mather, tells me that he was obsessed with the problem of masturbation, which would lend credence to the authenticity of this tract.

20. Ephraim Chambers, "Onania, and Le Onanisme," "Pollution," "Emission," and "Seed," in *Cyclopaedia; or, An universal dictionary of arts and sciences: containing the definitions of the terms, and accounts of the things signify'd thereby, in the several arts, both liberal and mechanical, and the several . . .* (London, 1728), pp. 301, 662, 848. Six more editions had been published by 1751. Chambers is fairly traditional in acceptance of older medical lore. The encyclopedia supports the notion of Galenic humors, recommends phlebotomy for almost everything, and is not skeptical of medical wonders of the old school — girls vomiting up toads, kittens bred in the stomach and vomited up, and such. Perhaps *Onania* raised suspicion in the freethinker Chambers because it does occasionally wax religious, the rantings of "a canting preacher," as "Philo-Castitatis" put it. Or perhaps the "empiric" roots stand in contrast to the high, if not modern, medical tradition that figures prominently in the encyclopedia. On eighteenth-century encyclopedias before the famous French *Encyclopédie*, see Philip Shorr, *Science and Superstition in the Eighteenth Century: A Study of Science in Two Encyclopedias of 1725–1750* (New York: AMS Press, 1967).

21. Chambers distinguishes self-pollution from nocturnal pollution, which arises from too much or too sharp semen or too weak vessels — that is, from natural, as opposed to artful, causes. This is again regarded as a special worry of the Roman Church, which "puts up prayers in the close of evening office to be preserved from nocturnal pollutions."

22. Johann Heinrich Zedler, *Grosses vollständiges Universal-Lexicon*, 64 vols., ed. Johann Peter von Ludwig and P.D. Longolius; *Onania; oder, Die Sünde der Selbst-Befleckung, mit allen ihren entsetzlichen Folgen . . .* (Leipzig, 1736). This edition has 439 pages and thus encompasses both the enlarged *Onania* and its *Supplement*. Later editions in Leipzig and Frankfurt appeared in 1751 ("A new and enlarged edition"), 1757, 1758, and 1765. At some point, the word *Sünde* was dropped from the title and *Krankheit*, "disease," took its place. We have a 1761 book by Philipp Friedrich Sicherer titled *Kurzer und nötige unterricht von den schädlichen folgen der selbstbefleckung in absicht auf die gesundheit: Als ein höchst*

nützlicheranhang zu dem englischen buch Onania... (Short and necessary instructions regarding the damaging effects on health of self-pollution as a highly useful
adjunct to the English book Onania...), which claims to be a newly enlarged
and improved edition of an earlier version and was published — with an "imperial privilege" — by Friedrich Gotthold Jacobäern in Leipzig in 1761. Sicherer
announces himself to be an apothecary in Heilbronn from whom cures can be
purchased; the publisher and "Factor" Wild in Frankfurt am Main also has them
for sale. The same Leipzig printer published a sixth edition of this book in 1773.
I have gathered this bibliographic information from various printed and on-line
catalogs, with additions from colleagues who have found copies here and there.
WorldCat and Deutsche Gesamtverzeichnis (DV) were particularly useful; the
1736 edition, which is not in the DV, is given at the library site www.swbv.
uni-konstanz, title identification 5533962. I am grateful to James H. Spohrer,
the German-collection bibliographer at Berkeley, for his sustained help on this
and other matters throughout this project. For Sarganeck, see Karl Braun, *Die
Krankheit Onania: Körperangst und die Anfänge moderner Sexualität im 18. Jahrhundert* (Frankfurt: Campus Verlag, 1995), p. 207. The book is *Überzeugende und
bewegliche Warnung vor allen Sünden der Unreinigkeit und heimlichen Unzucht*...
(Züllichau, 1740).

  23. I am referring here to what seems to be a translation of the 1773 Leipzig
edition of Sicherer's book cited in the previous note: *Instructions courte... sur les
suites facheuses auxquelles on expose la santé par la pollution volontaire de soi même:
en forme de supplement... au livre anglois intitulé Onania*... (Leipzig, 1775).

  24. Antoinette Emch-Dériaz, *Tissot: Physician of the Enlightenment* (New
York and San Francisco: Peter Lang, 1992), p. 43.

  25. Robert James, *A Medicinal Dictionary* (London, 1743–1745), vol. 2. Dr.
Johnson was among the distinguished contributors to James's work; the novelist
Samuel Richardson, as editor and printer, helped bring it out. On Richardson's
role in bringing it to market, see T.C. Duncan and Ben D. Kimpel, *Samuel
Richardson: A Biography* (Oxford: Clarendon Press, 1971), p. 84. (This is the first
of many accounts of masturbation leading to blindness. "Emission" is the key
missing term here: according to Chambers, it is "the act of throwing or driving a
thing, particular a fluid, from within outwards chiefly applied among us to the
expulsion or ejaculation of seed." The definition of "emission" is from Chambers,
Cyclopaedia. If, as had been thought by many since Antiquity, seeing entailed
emitting rays from the eyes, then excess emission in one corporeal realm — masturbation — could well have an impact on the workings of another — vision. The
entry in James argued that there was something "preposterous" about onanism,
something literally back to front, something that the late nineteenth century
would call a perversion, which resulted in ever weaker emissions — genital and
ocular.) Cases of this sort continue for a century and a half: for example, the
cases in *Annalist* (New York, 1847), p. 193, and in *Journal d'Ophtalmologie* (Paris,
1872), pp. 188–90.

26. The attribution is convincingly made in John Lough, *Essays on the Ency-clopédie of Diderot and D'Alembert* (London: Oxford University Press, 1968), p. 482. Menuret de Chambaud also wrote the article on *mariage*.

27. I quote throughout from the following English translation, which is widely available in reprint: *Onanism; or, A Treatise upon the Disorders Produced by Masturbation; or, The Dangerous Effects of Secret and Excessive Venery*, trans. A. Hume (London, 1761). It is an extremely accurate version of the French that dif-fers from it primarily by translating into the vernacular material that Tissot had left in Latin in his own French translation.

28. This might have been true, but at least one edition did have an imperial privilege, and in any case each city in the Holy Roman Empire issued privileges of its own.

29. Hoffman is presumably the physician Friedrich Hoffmann the Younger, whose views on the debilitating aspects of seminal loss Tissot quotes later in the book. It is here where one Dr. Bekker of London is identified as the author of *Onania*. Many modern historians cite said Bekker as the author, but since we know absolutely nothing more about him other than the one-sentence attribu-tion in Tissot and the possibility that he may be Balthasar Bekker who wrote a treatise on vulgar errors in 1695, he may as well be anonymous. Since this Bekker died in 1698 he is not a likely candidate. No other Bekker appears in ESTC. Tissot reports on one of his Swiss patients' acquiring *Onania* in Frankfurt (*Onanism*, pp. x and 20–24). The only other extant work by the translator Hume is *Every Woman Her Own Physician; or, Lady's Medical Assistant* (London, 1776). There is no hint in this book that its author is the man who translated Tissot into English. On topics where onanism might have come up – hysteria, for example – he is thoroughly Hippocratic. Marriage is the real answer. Like Galen, he rec-ommends massage but, unlike him, does not specify of what parts.

30. The Venice edition claimed to be the third. The Philadelphia edition is more of an adaptation than most. Most translations used the expanded French text as a base and then added – often extensive – local material in footnotes. John Sparhawk, *A table of the several chapters and principal contents of the late famous treatise, called Dr. Tissot's . . .* (Philadelphia, 1771). Dr. Sparhawk, as he was known, sold a specific remedy for weakness of the eyes – perhaps a connec-tion to masturbation – but he is also listed in *Early American Imprints* for a book catalog issued by his London bookstore.

31. For the period up to 1789, I rely on Jo-Ann McEachern, *Bibliography of Jean-Jacques Rousseau* (Oxford: Voltaire Foundation, 1989), vol. 2; I take 1789 from an unpublished paper by Carla Hesse presented at the Ecole des Hautes Etudes, June 16, 2000. It seems likely that we have a more complete bib-liographic record of Rousseau than of Tissot; no proper bibliography of Tissot's works exists, and I take my data from the list in Emch-Dériaz, *Tissot*, pp. 324–26. I am quite certain that at least ten editions I have found in various libraries are not on her list, but without examining copies, it is hard to tell. The

numbers I give constitute a low estimate. Regarding Tissot rip-offs, see, for example, Duncan Gordon, *A Letter to John Hunter respecting His Treatise on the Venereal Disease... pointing out the absurdity and immorality of His Doctrine in Favour of Onanism or Masturbation* (London, 1786). Tissot is acknowledged and directly quoted, but most of this tract is stolen without acknowledgment. The context is Hunter's claim that masturbation is no more — indeed is less — threatening than sexual intercourse. On Hunter, see pp. 217–19 above. On Tissot in Russia, see Laura Engelstein, *The Keys to Happiness: Sex and the Search for Modernity in Fin-de-siècle Russia* (Ithaca, NY: Cornell University Press), p. 226. There are also Russian Tissot rip-offs.

32. Mary Hyde (ed.), *The Thrales of Streatham Park* (Cambridge, MA: Harvard University Press, 1977), p. 160; I quote from the seventh edition corrected of *The Family Physician; or, Advice with Respect to Health... extracted from Dr. Tissot* (London, 1801), p. 3; the sixth edition was published in 1797. Moise Marcuze's *Seyfer Refues* (Book of remedies) clearly relied heavily on the German translation and probably knew the Hebrew, which was undertaken at the behest of Moses Mendelssohn, the leader of the Haskalah, or Jewish Enlightenment. See John M. Efron, *Medicine and the German Jews* (New Haven, CT: Yale University Press, 2001), p. 77.

33. James Boswell, *In Search of a Wife, 1766–1769*, ed. Frank Brady and Frederick A. Pottle, in *The Private Papers of James Boswell* (New York: McGraw-Hill, 1956), p. 214. "Swear with drawn sword never *pleasure* but with a woman's aid." Frederick A. Pottle (ed.), *Boswell on the Grand Tour: Germany and Switzerland, 1764* (New York: McGraw-Hill, 1953), p. 278; Boswell claims that guilt about masturbation is more or less coterminous with his discovery of sexual pleasure, about which he felt little guilt. Writing in 1764 during his tour of Holland, he says: "I saw then that irregular coition was not commendable but that it was no dreadful crime, and that as society is now constituted I did little or no harm in taking a girl, especially as my health required it. Bless me!" Frederick A. Pottle (ed.), *Boswell in Holland, 1763–1764* (New York: McGraw-Hill, 1952), p. 258.

34. S.A.D. Tissot, *The Life of J.G. Zimmerman* (London, 1797), p. 16. The context is the claim that Zimmermann did not renounce novels — the assumption being that he would — but that rather he embraced the "good works... of this species" for what they reveal about the human heart. See pp. 302ff. on the connection between masturbation and the novel. J.G. Zimmermann, "Warnung an Eltern, Erzieher under Kinderfreunde wegen der Selbst-befleckung, zumal bein ganz jungen madchen," *Deutsches Museum* (Leipzig) 1 (1778), p. 460.

35. "Onan, Onanisme," in *Dictionnaire philosophique* (II), vol. 8 of *Oeuvres complètes de Voltaire* (1765; Paris: Chez Firmin Didot Frères, 1862), pp. 94–95. No such article appears in the edition of the *Dictionnaire* published before Tissot's work.

36. Tissot to Rousseau, July 8, 1762, in *Correspondance complète de Jean*

Jacques Rousseau (Geneva: Madison, 1970), vol. 11. Rousseau, *Emile*, vol. 4 of *Oeuvres complètes*, ed. Bernard Gagnebin and Marcel Raymond (Paris: Gallimard, Pléiade, 1969), p. 663.

37. I have calculated the numbers of books in circulation by multiplying numbers of editions in French times two thousand, the usual size of a print run in this period; Christa Kersting, *Die Genese der Pädagogik im 18. Jahrhundert: Campes "Allgemeine Revision" im Kontext der neuzeitlichen Wissenschaft* (Weinheim: Deutscher Studien Verlag, 1992), p. 86.

38. Rousseau to Tissot, July 22, 1762, in *Correspondance*, p. 12.

39. The *Confessions* was published posthumously in the 1780s. This work, so central to how we construct the history of our own sense of ourselves, went through at least eleven editions during the last decade of the century, and thus it, too, played a part in the diffusion of what had begun in 1712.

40. It had been widely rumored that Ruskin was physically impotent and that this was the cause for the annulment of his marriage to "Effie" Chalmers Gray Ruskin. When it became known that he was courting the young Rosie, these rumors reappeared. Mrs. La Touche may have hinted as much to her daughter, and he wrote to her that he was worried about "sure knowledge of some fatal obstacle to our marriage." It was in this context that he wrote to his confidante Mrs. Cowper, Lady Mount-Temple, reminding her that he had often told her about his being "another Rousseau," in the hopes that she would convey this news to Effie and her family. For the context, see Van Akin Burd, introduction to *John Ruskin and Rose La Touche: Her Unpublished Diaries of 1861 and 1867* (Oxford: Clarendon Press, 1979), p. 116, and the commentary in *The Letters of John Ruskin to Lord and Lady Mount-Temple*, ed. and intro. John Lewis Bradley (Columbus: Ohio State University Press, 1964), pp. 123–24. The letter itself is no. 85, June 2, 1868, p. 167. Eugene Rastignac, whose development from a newly arrived but ambitious young man from the provinces into a sophisticated, worldly, and increasingly unprincipled Parisian is the main theme of *Père Goriot*, might not have been speaking of masturbation. He might have been alluding to Rousseau's penchant for being whipped or something else bad. But in the context of two young men talking about such matters, Rastignac's confession of having read Rousseau, and, most importantly, the "Body Bildung" in the novel, our vice seems to be the topic. Eugene's body goes from being, as D.A. Miller puts it, that of a beautiful young man – a "polymorphous range of erotic sites" – to that of a man fit for capitalism, created out of the "renunciation of anything that might interfere with desire in motivating an endless exchange of commodities." The sin of Rousseau represents the opposite of such renunciation. (*Père Goriot* is the first installment of *La Comédie humaine*, *The Human Comedy*, in which Rastignac keeps appearing.) See on this D.A. Miller, "Body Bildung and Textual Liberation" in Denis Hollier (ed.), *A New History of French Literature* (Cambridge, MA: Harvard University Press, 1989, 1994), pp. 681–87 and 681, 683 in particular. The conversation between Rastignac and his friend, the virtuous medical

student Bianchon, reads: "Je suis tourmente par de mauvaises idées. — En quel genre? — Ça se guerit, les idées. — Comment? — En y succombant. — Tu ris sans savoir de dont il s'agit. As-tu lu Rousseau? — Oui." in Honoré de Balzac, *Human Comedy of Balzac, (Père Goriot)* (Paris: Pléiade, 1951), vol. 2, p. 960.

41. Samuel Solomon, *A Guide to Good Health.* The sixty-fourth edition seems to be from around 1814, judging from the date of the latest testimonial letters, the fifty-second from around 1800. While the largest single section of the book is about masturbation, other sections offer advice for healthy living more generally. For Solomon's advertisements, see Irvine Loudon, "The Vile Race of Quacks with Which This Country Is Infested," in W.F. Bynum and Roy Porter (ed.), *Medical Fringe and Medical Orthodoxy, 1750–1850* (London: Croom Helm, 1987). Of the 312 pages of this 3-shilling *Guide,* pages 189–242 are devoted to masturbation. But in fact many of these pages deal with the impor-tance of a healthy life — good companions, fresh air, good food. Tissot earns a long citation. On Samuel Solomon and his empire more generally, see William H. Helfand, "Samuel Solomon and the Cordial Balm of Gilead," *Pharmacy in His-tory* 31.4 (1989), pp. 151–59; I take this from James Hodson, *Medical Facts and Advertisements Submitted to the Consideration of the Afflicted* (London, 1799). His attack on other physicians and his self-promotion are on the inside cover and on p. 1; the quotation is from p. 8 in the context of the doctor offering consulta-tions by mail. I am perhaps being a little cavalier with the names of drops. Per-sian Restorative Drops are for the "enervating practice of boyish folly." Persian Vegetable Syrup is for, among other things, temporary blindness, a sequela of masturbation; Persian Drops, to which a separate ad is devoted, is for youth of both sexes and adults who have indulged in youthful errors. Hodson says also to check out his *School Boy's Monitor and Parents Guardian*, whose title at least con-nects it to an altogether more elevated pedagogical literature in England and abroad. All these works are connected, so that in 1794 the thirteenth edition of a compilation that began in 1789 appeared. In 1799, these texts were being auto-pirated for the specialized onanism market. James Hodson, *Nature's assistant to the restoration of health ... To which is added, an address to parents, tutors, and schoolmasters*, 13th ed. (London, 1794).

42. Alex Comfort, *The Anxiety Makers: Some Curious Preoccupations of the Medical Profession* (London: Nelson, 1967); Vern L. Bullough, "Technology for the Prevention of 'Les Malades produites par la masturbation,'" *Technology and Culture* 28.4 (Oct. 1987), p. 832.

43. O.S. Fowler, *Amativeness; or, Evils and remedies of excessive and perverted sexuality: including warning and advice to the married and single: being a supple-ment to "Love and parentage,"* 13th ed. (New York: Fowlers and Wells, 1848); the estimate of numbers for Fowler is from W.J. Hunter, *Manhood Wrecked and Res-cued* (New York, 1894), p. 109; J.H. Kellogg, *Natural History and Hygiene of Organic Life,* new rev. ed. (Burlington, Iowa: I.F. Segner, 1895), pp. 231 and 231–60 passim; Sylvester Graham, *Graham's lectures on chastity; specially intended*

for the serious consideration of young men and parents (Glasgow: Royalty Buildings, 1837).

44. The 1908 edition of Lt. Gen. R.S.S. (Robert) Baden-Powell's *Scouting for Boys* (London: Horace Cox, 1908) condemns self-abuse in the context of eugenics and empire. It, along with drink, venereal disease, and lack of self-restraint, is destroying the race and explains why half the men called up for the Boer War were found unfit. A promised section specifically on self-abuse is not in the BL copy, although some of the most virulent nineteenth-century anti-masturbatory tracts are recommended: Sylvanus Stall's *What a Young Boy Ought to Know*, for example. I quote from the tenth edition (London: C. Arthur Pearson, 1922), pp. 209–10. The 1946 edition reprints these same pages.

45. Irving David Steinhardt, *Ten Sex Talks to Boys* (Philadelphia: J.B. Lippincott, 1914), p. 120; Irving David Steinhardt, *Ten Sex Talks to Girls* (Philadelphia: J.B. Lippincott, 1914), p. 59; *Child Care* (1918) quoted in Peter Lewis Allen, *The Wages of Sin* (Chicago: University of Chicago Press, 2000), p. 111.

46. Carl Capellmann, "*Usus Matrimonii*, 1. Onanism: *Peccatum Onan*," in *Pastoral Medicine*, trans. William Dassel (New York: Pustet, 1879). This is a translation of a German work that was widely and continually reprinted in the original and in French, Latin, and Spanish translations for at least fifty years. The fifth German edition is in 1881. The nineteenth German edition, from 1923, is the same on the subject of onanism as the one I cite. Capellmann in turn quotes the definition from Jean Pierre Gury (1801–1866), *Compendium theologiae moralis*. I translate from the Latin because the German and English texts leave particularly sensitive material in the original; the books, we are told, are in any case intended only for professionals, for whom this will not be a problem. Capellmann is hard-line on the subject of masturbation, which he considers in a separate section.

47. This was an especial project of Jean Baptiste Desiré Demeaux, who was on the medical faculty of the Sorbonne and vice president of the Anatomical Society. He wrote at least three books on the surgical care of hernias and wrote extensively on the dangers of masturbation and how to stop it in public schools. For his views on this proposal and on masturbation as a question of population policy, see Vernon A. Rosario II, "Phantastical Pollutions," in Paula Bennett and Vernon A. Rosario II (eds.), *Solitary Pleasures: The Historical, Literary, and Artistic Discourses of Autoeroticism* (New York: Routledge, 1995), p. 121.

48. Perhaps there has been an enduring cultural tension between the pro-creative and the pleasurable aspects of human sexual behavior, but that is not what, historically, caused masturbation to be regarded as so threatening. This is the view of P.R. Abrahamson and S.D. Pinkerton, *With Pleasure: Thoughts on the Nature of Human Sexuality* (New York: Oxford University Press, 1995).

49. Elizabeth Blackwell, *Medical Address on the Benevolence of Malthus Contrasted with the Corruptions of Neo-Malthusianism* (London, 1888), pp. 24–26.

50. Charles Knowlton, *Fruits of Philosophy: An Essay on the Population Ques-*

tion, 3rd ed. (London, 1878; repr., Arno Press, 1972). In fact, this version of Knowlton's widely circulated pamphlet was signed by Charles Bradlaugh and Annie Besant to test the right of publication after an earlier edition had been prosecuted under Lord Campbell's Act (the 1857 Obscene Publications Act under which *Ulysses* was prosecuted almost fifty years later). It had first been published by the radical printer James Watson some forty years earlier, which links it intimately with the history of free thought in nineteenth-century Britain. Watson was a colleague of Richard Carlile, the republican, freethinking printer whose *Every Woman's Book* was the first of a series of popular guides to birth control. It was also virulently opposed to onanism. Anti-masturbatory fervor was to be found on all sides of the political and religious spectrum. On "sex starvation," see C.V. Drysdale, *The Malthusian Doctrine and Its Modern Aspects* (London: Malthusian League, 1917?), p. 21. Drysdale, unlike the authors of earlier books in this tradition, does not mention the unacceptability of masturbation in particular, but he does sum up what might be called the "pro-sex" tradition of birth-control advocacy.

51. I cite the professional medical literature throughout this book. The Catalogue of the Surgeon General's Library, the precursor to *Index Medicus* and the modern MEDLINE, gives a reasonably complete list, although I have found articles not listed there. One gets a good sense of the state of play in the high medical tradition from "Onanisme," in *Dictionnaire encyclopédique des sciences medicales* (Paris, 1881), 2nd ser., vol. 15. Daniel Clark, M.D., Medical Superintendent of the Toronto Asylum, *Tenth Annual Report*, Sept. 30, 1877, p. 6, where he repeats what his predecessor, Joseph Workman, had said in earlier reports. One gets a real sense of the elaboration of these themes and their repetition in various forms through these internal references. See *Annual Reports of the Provincial Lunatic Society of Ontario* (Toronto, 1865, 1866–1867), pp. 6–13 and 85–88.

52. Havelock Ellis summarizes this literature in *Studies in the Psychology of Sex*, 3rd ed. (Philadelphia: F.A. Davis, 1920), vol. 1, pp. 177–79.

53. Washiyama Yayoi, quoted in Sabine Frühstück, *Colonizing Sex: Sexology and Social Control in Modern Japan* (Berkeley: University of California Press, forthcoming 2003), pp. 104–105. I am grateful to her for allowing me to read her work before publication.

54. G. Stanley Hall, *Adolescence: Its Psychology and Its Relations to Physiology, Anthropology, Sociology, Sex, Crime, Religion, and Education* (1904; New York: D. Appleton, 1924), vol. 1, pp. 452 and 432. Hall's learning on this topic was great, and I take him to be exemplary of a new social-scientific, post-Darwinian consensus. W. Grant Hague, *The Eugenic Marriage: A Personal Guide to the New Science of Better Living and Better Babies* (New York: Review of Reviews Company, 1916), vol. 2, pp. 155–57. Hague taught at Columbia University's College of Physicians and Surgeons.

55. *Onania*, 8th ed., p. 200.

56. Vicesimus Knox, *Liberal Education*, 5th ed. (London, 1783), pp. 329–30; Samuel Gottlieb Vogel, *Unterricht für Eltern* (1786).

57. Mary Wollstonecraft, *A Vindication of the Rights of Women*, ed. D.L. Macdonald and Kathleen Scherf (Orchard Park, NY: Broadview, 1997), pp. 306–307. Presumably, the vices in question could be various homosexual acts, but in light of Wollstonecraft's engagement with Rousseau and her explicit allusion to Mandeville — private vices and public pest — the referent is quite clearly masturbation.

58. Christian Gotthilf Salzmann, *Über die heimlichen Sünden der Jugend* (Frankfurt and Leipzig, 1786).

59. *Ibid.*, pp. 13–14.

60. *Ibid.*

61. Jean-Jacques Rousseau, *Bekenntnisse* (Berlin, 1782), is the earliest edition I could find.

62. Salzmann, *Heimlichen Sünden*, 16–18. For Freud, the sublimation of infantile sexuality into adult heterosexuality constituted the normative story of the self. (But, we are getting ahead of the story.)

63. "Masturbation," in *Dictionnaire des sciences medicales* (Paris, 1819); David Hunt, *Parents and Children in History: The Psychology of Life in Early Modern France* (New York: Harper and Row, 1972), pp. 162 and 159–79 passim. Fallopius is extensively cited on this point in Winfried Schleiner, *Medical Ethics in the Renaissance* (Washington, DC: Georgetown University Press, 1995), pp. 135–36.

64. Immanuel Kant, *The Doctrine of Virtue: Part II of the Metaphysics of Morals*, trans. with intro. and notes by Mary J. Gregor (Philadelphia: University of Pennsylvania Press, 1971), art. 2; I have slightly modified Gregor's translation. See "Von der Wohlustigen Selbstschandung," in *Metaphysische Anfangsgründe der Tugendlehre*, vol. 6 of *Kant's gesammelte Schriften* (Berlin: G. Reimer, 1907), pp. 424–27.

65. Campe was one of the lights of a group called the Philantropen, literally "the philanthropists" but more generally "the friends of humanity," who, like Kant, believed that morality had to be put on a new footing. One had to begin as early as possible, which is what made education so central an undertaking. On the German pedagogical project and the *Berliner Monatsschrift*'s relationship to it, see Kersting, *Die Genese der Pädagogik im 18. Jahrhundert,* pp. 71–113 passim and pp. 80–81 and 85 on the essay contest in particular. There were contributions by twenty-seven writers in Campe's massive sixteen-volume encyclopedia; three were about masturbation; the third-place winner's piece was, because of its great length, incorporated into the essays of the other three prizewinners. For the essays themselves, see Joachim Heinrich Campe (ed.), *Allgemeine Revision des gesammten Schul- und Erziehungswesens* (Hamburg, 1785–1792), vol. 6, p. 7. A ducat was about 5 guilders, or half a pound sterling; thus 60 would be worth something over 300 guilders, or 30 pounds, a laborer's annual wage. I thank my colleague the economic historian Jan de Vries for this information.

This discussion of masturbation in German medicine and pedagogy offers the merest hint of an extensive and long-lived discussion that continued in more or less the same terms until the late nineteenth century. For an excellent, rich commentary on this literature with ample quotations from the sources, see Karl Heinz Bloch, *Die Bekämpfung der Jugendmasturbation im 18. Jahrhundert: Ursachen-Verlauf-Nachwirkungen* (Frankfurt am Main: Peter Lang, 1998) which I came upon only while revising my copyedited manuscript. Bloch is especially good in showing how long the old tradition survived: the major German ency- clopedia's — the *Grosse Brockhaus'* — article on masturbation, for example, con- tinued the old story unabated until 1898 and only then slowly moderated its presentation. Only in 1932 did a psychoanalytical interpretation take over. See esp. pp. 532–79.

66. P.J.C. Debreyne, *Essai sur la théologie morale* (Paris, 1844). The fron- tispiece advertises another of his books, a précis of human physiology especially for the clergy and for seminarians.

67. Cited in Margery Levinson, *Keats's Life of Allegory: The Origins of a Style* (Oxford: Basil Blackwell, 1988), pp. 16–18 and 22. Perhaps this image subsisted through the generations. Yeats, in one of his dialogue poems, counters the claim that Keats was happy with the observation that he sees him as "a schoolboy with his face pressed to a candy store window"; this is a poet regarded as almost sick from excessive longing, perhaps sick from the vice of schoolboys. On Whitman, see Robert S. Fredrickson, "Public Onanism: Whitman's Song of Himself," *Mod- ern Language Quarterly* 46.2 (June 1985), and Harold Bloom, "The Real Me," *New York Review of Books* (April 26, 1984), p. 4.

68. V. Sazhin, "The Victor's Hand: Selections from the Correspondence between V. Belinsky and M. Bakunin," *Erotica in Russian Literature from Barkov to the Present* [*Erotika v russkoi literature ot Barkova do nashikh dnei*], a special issue of *Literary Review* [*Literaturnoe obozrenie*], (Moscow, 1992), p. 39. I am grateful to Hilda Hoogenbloom for bringing this to my attention and for translating the texts. On Belinsky and Bakunin more generally, see the remarkable book by Lydia Ginzburg, *On Psychological Prose*, trans. and ed. Judson Rosengrant (Princeton, NJ: Princeton University Press, 1991), pp. 59–60 and 84–85.

69. Wagner quoted in Marc A. Weiner, *Richard Wagner and the Anti-Semitic Imagination* (Lincoln: University of Nebraska Press, 1995), p. 341. There is also the long-standing association of Jews and prostitutes, both of whom produce nothing, both of whom turn sex not into offspring but into money. This "use- lessness" was then the basis for the association of Jews with that other useless practice, masturbation. In a British comic book of the 1980s in which anthropo- morphized phalluses are among the main actors, the Jewish phallus is shown masturbating, whereas the others are shown as having at least the option of female partners. On this, see Sander Gilman, *The Jew's Body* (New York: Rout- ledge, 1991), p. 123.

70. Gérard Walter (ed.), *Actes du Tribunal révolutionnaire* (Paris: Mercure de

France, 1968), p. 96, quoted in Chantal Thomas, *The Wicked Queen*, trans. Julie Rose (New York: Zone Books, 1999), p. 146.

71. J.H. Fussell, "Mrs. Annie Besant and the Moral Code: A Protest" (1907). The point of this privately printed pamphlet, as we learn from the typescript letter addressed to librarians that accompanied some theosophical material, was to distance the movement from suspect sexual practices and religious claims. (Letters attached to the University of California at Berkeley copy.)

72. Papers printed in the *British Weekly* (Oct. 1877–April 1888), which are reprinted in *Tempted London: Young Men* (London: Hodder and Stoughton, 1888), pp. 246–48.

73. These are the insights of William A. Cohen, *Sex Scandal: The Private Parts of Victorian Fiction* (Durham and New York: Duke University Press, 1996), pp. 26–72 and esp. 26–38.

74. Ludger Lutkehaus, "O Wollust, O Holle: Onanie, Phantasie und Literatur," *Die Zeit* 47–15 (Nov. 1991), pp. 76–77, which provides references to other secondary works; Heinrich von Kleist, *Sämtliche Werke und Briefe*, vol. 2, pp. 559–62, trans. and cited in Sander Gilman, *Disease and Representation* (Ithaca, NY: Cornell University Press, 1988), p. 68. Braun, *Krankheit Onania*, offers extensive evidence for the wide distribution of worries about masturbation in Germany.

75. Elizabeth Blackwell, *The Human Element in Sex: Being a Medical Enquiry into the Relation of Sexual Physiology to Christian Morality* (London, 1885), p. 29 and passim. The best treatment of the political context is Judith R. Walkowitz, *Prostitution and Victorian Society: Women, Class, and the State* (New York: Cambridge University Press, 1980). For the more general context of Blackwell, see Margaret Jackson, *The Real Facts of Life: Feminism and the Politics of Sexuality, c. 1850–1940* (Bristol, PA: Taylor and Francis, 1994), pp. 71–77.

76. The evidence for the universality of masturbation comes from a remarkable range of sources. Havelock Ellis offers an excellent review of the literature in *Studies in the Psychology of Sex*, vol. 1, pp. 161–82; on the sociology of the use of dildos, see p. 169. Kinsey also surveys the late-nineteenth- and early-twentieth-century literature in both his major works: Alfred C. Kinsey and Institute for Sex Research, *Sexual Behavior in the Human Female* (Philadelphia: Saunders, 1953), pp. 132–90, and Alfred C. Kinsey, Wardell B. Pomeroy, and Clyde E. Martin, *Sexual Behavior in the Human Male* (Philadelphia, W.B. Saunders Co., 1948), pp. 497–516; Elie Metchnikoff, *The Nature of Man: Studies in Optimistic Philosophy*, ed. P. Chalmers Mitchell (New York: G.P. Putnam's Sons, 1903), pp. 95–99; on degeneration and masturbation, see for the case of women Bram Dijkstra, *Idols of Perversity: Fantasies of Feminine Evil in Fin-de-siècle Culture* (New York: Oxford University Press, 1986), pp. 64–82 and esp. pp. 74–75, 79–80, and, more specifically, Charles Feré, "Le Surmenage scolaire" [literally, "The mental strain of schoolboys" but, by extension, of all school-age children]), *Le Progrès médical* (Feb. 5–12, 1887), pp. 111 and 132, where Feré argues that

masturbation is only dangerous in those who are congenitally disposed to be weakened by the mental stress of doing it. His specific concern is for students, but he says the problem is far more general. Slightly older than Freud, Feré was a close disciple of Jean-Martin Charcot's. Iwan Bloch, *The Sexual Life of Our Times in Its Relations to Modern Civilization*, trans. M. Eden Paul (New York: Allied Book Co., 1926), pp. 409–11. This book was first published in German in 1908 and seems to have been something of a best-seller. The sixth reprinting, in 1910, from which the first English translation was made, claims that it begins with the forty-thousandth copy of the work. The view of the distinguished English gynecologist J. Matthews Duncan in his Gulstonian Lectures of 1883 that "masturbation in females is an unnatural and generally excessive indulgence in artificial sexual pleasure" was simply no longer tenable. "Sterility in Women," lecture 2, pt. 4, *Lancet* (March 31, 1883), p. 529.

77. Freud first used the term "autoeroticism" in a letter to Wilhelm Fliess, Dec. 9, 1899, where he acknowledges Ellis. See on this Jean Laplanche and J.B. Pontalis, *The Language of Psycho-analysis* (1967; London: Karnac Books, 1988), pp. 45–47; Havelock Ellis, *Studies in the Psychology of Sex*, vol. 1, pp. 161–63 and 161–283, "Auto-Eroticism," more generally. The first edition was in 1900.

78. Moravia quoted in Lutkehaus, "O Wollust, O Holle"; Ellis, *Studies in the Psychology of Sex*, vol. 1, pp. 161–63.

79. D.H. Lawrence, "Pornography and Obscenity," in H.T. Moore (ed.), *Sex, Literature, and Censorship* (New York: Twayne, 1953), pp. 79–82.

80. Gore Vidal, "Pornography," in *Homage to Daniel Shays: Collected Essays, 1952–1972* (New York: Random House, 1973), pp. 219–20; on Gide, see Naomi Segal, *André Gide: Pederasty and Pedagogy* (Oxford: Clarendon Press, 1998), pp. 41–47 and 70–73.

81. Richard von Krafft-Ebing, *Psychopathia Sexualis*, 7th ed., trans. Charles Gilbert Chaddock (Philadelphia: F.A. Davis, 1908), pp. 188–89.

82. On this point, see George J. Makari, "Between Seduction and Libido: Sigmund Freud's Masturbation Hypotheses and the Realignment of His Etiologic Thinking, 1897–1905," *Bulletin of the History of Medicine* 72.4 (1998), and also pp. 387–94 above.

83. *The Complete Letters of Sigmund Freud to Wilhelm Fliess, 1887–1904*, trans. and ed. Jeffrey Masson (Cambridge, MA: Belknap Press of Harvard University Press, 1985); *Dostoevsky and Parricide* (1928), in *The Standard Edition of the Complete Psychological Works of Sigmund Freud* (London: Hogarth Press, 1975; repr. of 1961 ed.), vol. 23, p. 193.

84. Sigmund Freud, *Three Essays on Sexuality* (1905), in *Complete Works*, vol. 7, p. 187 and n.1 and p. 188 and nn.1 and 2.

85. Marie Bonaparte, *Female Sexuality* (New York: International Universities Press, 1953), p. 74.

86. Wilhelm Stekel, *Auto-erotism: A Psychiatric Study of Onanism and Neurosis*, trans. James S. Van Teslaar (New York: Grove Press, 1950), p. 63.

87. Joyce McDougall, *Theatres of the Mind: Illusion and Truth on the Psycho-analytic Stage* (London: Free Association Books, 1986), p. 250. Luce Irigaray, *Speculum of the Other Woman*, trans. Gillian Gill (Ithaca, NY: Cornell University Press, 1985), pp. 28–31 and 60; and Luce Irigaray, *The Sex Which Is Not One*, trans. Catherine Porter with Carolyn Burke (Ithaca, NY: Cornell University Press, 1986), p. 24.

88. Max Hodann, *Onanie: weder Laster noch Krankheit* (Berlin, 1929).

89. A.A. Brill, *Psychoanalysis: Its Theories and Practical Application* (Philadel-phia: W.B. Saunders, 1922), pp. 153 and 158–59; John F.W. Meagher, *A Study of Masturbation and Psychosexual Life*, 3rd rev. ed. (Baltimore: William Wood, 1936), p. 105.

90. William H. Masters and Virginia Johnson, *Human Sexual Response* (Boston: Little, Brown and Co., 1966), pp. 63–65 and passim. The French trans-lation appeared in 1977 and various Spanish versions beginning in 1967. Bantam produced the mass-market paperback. Masters and Johnson also published well over a dozen books with the same theme. Jill Johnson, selections from *Les-bian Nation* (1973), in Barbara A. Crow (ed.), *Radical Feminism: A Documentary Reader* (New York: New York University Press, 2000), pp. 349–50, in a section called "The Myth of the Myth of the Vaginal Orgasm."

91. I base this both on searches of library catalogs and on a printed list titled "Other Versions of *Our Bodies, Ourselves*, Including Books 'Inspired by' *Our Bodies, Ourselves*," that my research assistant Arianne Chernock acquired from a member of the collective. There are also audiotapes and electronic-text versions.

92. Boston Women's Health Book Collective, *Our Bodies, Our Selves* (Boston: New England Free Press, 1971), pp. 13–14; this was the last printing by the NEFP before the book was taken over by Simon and Schuster.

93. Laura Hutton, *The Single Woman and Her Emotional Problems* (London: Baillière, Tindall and Cox, 1937), p. 83.

94. Boston Women's Health Book Collective, *Our Bodies, Our Selves*, pp. 13–14 and 15–19.

95. Anne Koedt, *The Myth of the Vaginal Orgasm* (Boston: New England Free Press, 1970), repr. in Crow, *Radical Feminism*.

96. This information comes from a summary of the company's financial statement at www.Hoover.com; on Rotermund, see the *New York Times* obituary, July 22, 2001, sec. 1, p. 34.

97. I have these figures from Cory Silverberg, the owner of Come as You Are, a sex shop in Toronto, and producer of a range of films on questions of sex-uality for the Canadian SexTV; http://www.divine-interventions.com.

98. Lonnie Garfield Barbach, *For Yourself: The Fulfillment of Female Sexuality* (Garden City, NY: Doubleday, 1975). The title says it all.

99. The "secret garden" image comes, I assume, from the early-twentieth-century children's story *The Secret Garden* by Frances Hodgson Burnett, in which a ten-year-old girl goes to live in a lonely house on the Yorkshire moors and

discovers an invalid cousin and a mysterious locked garden. *Women on Top: How Real Life Has Changed Women's Sexual Fantasies* (New York: Simon and Schuster, 1991) is yet another follow-up. *Men in Love: Men's Sexual Fantasies: The Triumph of Love over Rage* (New York: Delacorte Press, 1980) broadens the appeal of the original concept but does not argue affirmatively for masturbation as the path to self-realization. *My Mother/My Self: The Daughter's Search for Identity* (New York: Delacorte Press, 1977) followed successfully on the heels of the book on sexual fantasy.

100. Catharine MacKinnon, *Only Words* (Cambridge, MA: Harvard University Press, 1993), excerpted in Drucilla Cornell (ed.), *Feminism and Pornography* (New York: Oxford University Press, 2000), p. 101. *Sunday Times*, June 2, 1997, quoted in David Stevenson, *The Beggar's Benison* (East Lothian: Tuckwell Press, 2001), p. 23.

101. Norman Mailer, *The Prisoner of Sex* (Boston: Little, Brown, 1971), pp. 188 and 187–204 passim. For Millett, see *Sexual Politics* (Garden City, NY: Doubleday, 1970), pp. 322–24 and 180–87 passim.

102. See, for example, http://www.nyjacks.com and the many associated links.

103. Joseph Kramer's school of erotic touch (including self-touch): http://www.eroticmassage.com/cgi-bin/shop.cgi and the comments at http://www.salon.com/people/lunch/1999/05/28/kramer/; for a brief introduction to the print media, see Joanie Blank (ed.), *First Person Sexual* (San Francisco: Down There Press, 1996). On masturbation and queerness — and a brilliant analysis of Austen to boot — see Eve Kosofsky Sedgwick, "Jane Austen and the Masturbating Girl," in Bennett and Rosario, *Solitary Pleasures*, p. 137.

Chapter Three: Masturbation Before *Onania*

1. "Onanisme," in *Dictionnaire encyclopédique des sciences medicales* (Paris, 1881), 2nd ser., vol. 15, pp. 359–60. The article is wrong about many of the historical particulars. We have no evidence that someone named Bekker wrote *Onania* (see Chapter 2, n.29, above). The author's claim that *Onania* had reached its eightieth edition by the time Voltaire took up the subject is based on an unsupported assertion in the *Philosophical Dictionary*. But in the big picture, if *Onania* had predecessors, the author, or someone since, would have found them.

2. Balthasar Bekker, *The world bewitch'd; or, An examination of the common opinions concerning spirits: their nature, power, administration, and operations. As also, the effects men are able to produce by their communication. Divided into IV parts. By Balthazar Bekker, D.D. and Pastor at Amsterdam. Vol 1. Translated from a French copy, approved of and subscribed by the author's own hand. Betoverde weereld. English* ([London]: Printed for R. Baldwin in Warwick-Lane, 1695).

3. Lucinda McCray Beier, *Sufferers and Healers: The Experience of Illness in Seventeenth-Century England* (New York: Routledge), p. 92.

4. I am referring to Karl Braun's scholarly and magisterial *Die Krankheit*

Onania (Frankfurt: Campus Verlag, 1995), which cites recent German studies supporting this view.

5. *Onania*, 4th ed., p. 17.

6. Edward Baynard, *The History of Cold Bathing, Both Ancient and Modern* (London, 1706), p. 68. Baynard was a member of the College of Physicians. His only other works are a pamphlet of advice to claret drinkers that does not seem to have met with public approval and two short papers in the *Transactions of the Royal Society*. He was also the father of Ann Baynard, a well-known learned — and pious — woman. One of his pieces in the *TRS* is about a boy who swallowed two copper farthings. Masturbation, in short, was not much on his mind. The paragraph in question is offered as an afterthought — "I had almost forgotten..." — in a postscript from Baynard to his co-author, Sir John Floyer. I am assuming that the "Ettmüller" of *Onania* is Michael Ettmüller (1644–1683), a prolific doctor whose works began to appear in England, in both translation and Latin, at the very end of the seventeenth century. Marten may well have read *Etmullerus abridg'd* (London, 1699), p. 567.

7. Francis Schiller, "Venery, the Spinal Cord, and Tabes Dorsalis Before Romberg: The Contribution of Ernest Horn," *Journal of Nervous and Mental Disease* 163.1 (July 1976). Tissot's citation is on p. 4, pt. 1, sec. 1 of *Onanism*. His reference is slightly off: the correct citation is not Hippocrates, *De morbis* 2.49 but 2.51. See *Hippocrates*, trans. Paul Potter, Loeb Classical Library (Cambridge, MA: Harvard University Press, 1995), p. 285. *Nouveau Dictionnaire de médecine ...* (Paris, 1826), vol. 2, p. 179.

8. I say "male" because women were usually not the subjects of serious ethical consideration. The exquisitely developed classical ethics of the self was devoted to the behavior of aristocratic men.

9. Aline Rousselle, *Porneia: On Desire and the Body in Antiquity* (Oxford: Basil Blackwell, 1988), pp. 32, 38, 67–77.

10. Aristotle, *History of Animals*, ed. and trans. D.M. Balme (Cambridge, MA: Harvard University Press, 1991). 7.1.581a26 and 581b17–20; I also consulted the translation in *The Complete Works of Aristotle: The Revised Oxford Translation*, ed. Jonathan Barnes (Princeton, NJ; Princeton University Press, 1984).

11. Because serious ethical engagement was generally thought to be reserved for men, the bulk of this medical literature was directed to them. In any case, since the male body was the archetypal human body, little more was required. For an excellent discussion of the complicated regimen ancient doctors offered their patients, both men and women, for balancing the draining and the health-giving effects of orgasm and ejaculation, and indeed for managing desire, see Rousselle, *Porneia*, pp. 14–77. Rousselle supports the view that masturbation as such figured not at all in their discussions. See also Michel Foucault, *The Uses of Pleasure: The History of Sexuality, Volume 2*, trans. Robert Hurley (New York: Vintage, 1990), esp. pp. 1–94. Although he cites a text of the Hellenistic physician Arateus that purportedly refers to masturbation (pp. 15–16),

Foucault's footnote is to the commentary to the nineteenth-century French translation. In fact, there are only two references to masturbation in Foucault's entire book and only one that might be regarded as condemning it. Foucault may well have changed his mind on the subject. In a brief introduction to an excerpt, published in 1982, to what would be volume 3 of the *History of Sexuality: The Care of the Self* (New York: Pantheon, 1986), he says that both he and Philippe Ariès think that "the highly significant question of masturbation goes back a lot further than the doctors of the eighteenth and nineteenth century," meaning to classical Antiquity. See Philippe Ariès and André Béjin, eds., *Western Sexuality: Practice and Precept in Past and Present Times*, trans. Anthony Forster (Oxford: Basil Blackwell, 1985), p. 14. In volume 3, however, he says, "We note in passing the very modest place that masturbation and the solitary pleasures occupied in medical regimes — as was generally the case in all moral reflections of the Greeks and the Romans concerning sexual activity" (p. 140). "Body and City," the opening chapter of Peter Brown's *The Body and Society: Men, Women, and Renunciation in Early Christianity* (New York: Columbia University Press, 1988), is the best introduction to the fundamental ethical stake of the late ancient world in the economy of the body. My discussion is manifestly indebted to his.

12. Galen, *De locis affectis* 8.419–20, in K.G. Kuhn, ed.

13. Diogenes Laertius, *Lives of the Eminent Philosophers* 6.69, trans. R.D. Hicks, Loeb Classical Library (Cambridge, MA: Harvard University Press, 1950), vol. 2, pp. 70–71. Hicks decorously translates *cheirougerein* as "behaving indecently," but the word means "using one's hands unceasingly, continuously."

14. Thomas Cogan (1545?–1607), *The hauen of health, chiefly made for the comfort of students, and consequently for all those that haue a care of their health, amplified vpon fiue wordes of Hippocrates, written Epid. 6. Labour, meat, drinke, sleepe, Venus: Hereunto is added a preseruation from the pestilence: with a short ... censure of the late sicknesse at Oxford* (London, 1612). The Italian translator of *L'Onanisme* thought that Tissot had got Diogenes all wrong and that the whole episode was meant as a joke. He, in turn, cites authorities for this view; see *L'onanismo; ovvero, Dissertazione sopra le malattie cagionate dalle polluzioni volontarie de Signor Tissot*, 3rd ed. (Venice, 1785). Bernard Mandeville, *A Modest Defense of Public Stews*, Clark Memorial Library Publication 162 (1724; Los Angeles: Augustan Reprint Society, 1973), pp. vi–vii.

15. As Winfried Schleiner, *Medical Ethics in the Renaissance* (Washington, DC: Georgetown University Press, 1995), pp. 133–52, points out, many Renaissance commentators use such ambiguous terms to talk about the subject — "unlawful discharges" — that it is not always possible to tell what they are talking about. *Purgatio* and *vacuatio* could mean many things. Whether this vagueness is because masturbation is so controversial, as he claims, or because it simply was not considered independently of other forms of evacuation is another question. In any case, Schleiner offers no evidence that anyone cared about masturbation in particular. Schleiner himself follows his discussion of the unnamed masturba-

SOLITARY SEX

tion with a section discussing Renaissance views of the medical uses of flogging. The question is what conclusions we can draw from silence. Danielle Jacquart and Claude Thomasset, *Sexuality and Medicine in the Middle Ages*, trans. Matthew Adamson (Princeton, NJ: Princeton University Press, 1988), offer a long section on the medical treatment of "guilty imaginings" and conflate this with masturbation. In fact, none of the texts they cite regarding men actually mentions the practice. At stake are the problems of priapism, wet dreams, and "gonorrhea" — seminal loss generally — which were indeed regarded to be in some measure the fault of an inflamed imagination whose heat could be assuaged medically, mostly through dietary restrictions. But nowhere is the problem diagnosed as masturbation or the cure as not doing it.

16. On this, see Ruth Mazo Karras, "Sex and the Singlewoman," in Judith M. Bennett and Amy Froide (eds.), *Singlewomen in the European Past, 1250–1800* (Philadelphia: University of Pennsylvania Press, 1999), pp. 128–35.

17. Galen, *De locis affectis*, 6.2.39. I adapted this translation from that by Rudolph Siegel (New York: S. Karger, 1976). On simulation of intercourse in Galen, see Ann Ellis Hanson, "The Medical Writers' Woman," in David M. Halperin, John J. Winkler, and Froma Zeitlin (eds.), *Before Sexuality: The Construction of Erotic Experience in the Ancient Greek World* (Princeton, NJ: Princeton University Press, 1990), pp. 318–20. Aetius of Amida, five centuries later, tells the same story. Aetius of Amida, *The Gynaecology and Obstetrics of the VIth Century A.D.* (Philadelphia: Blakiston, 1950).

18. Albert the Great quoted in Jacquart and Thomasset, *Sexuality and Medicine in the Middle Ages*, p. 152; see also pp. 152–55. A fuller account, with the Latin text included, is in Dyan Elliott, *Fallen Bodies: Pollution, Sexuality, and Demonology in the Middle Ages* (Philadelphia: University of Pennsylvania Press, 1999), pp. 45–46 and nn.54–56. Albert in fact says that coition does the same thing as rubbing and that a girl who rubs is not a virgin.

19. On Galen and late-nineteenth- and early-twentieth-century use of vibrators, water treatment, and other forms of massage, see Rachel Maines, *The Technology of Orgasm: "Hysteria," the Vibrator, and Women's Sexual Satisfaction* (Baltimore: Johns Hopkins University Press, 1998), who resurrects this previously lost history of sexual pleasure. By the 1930s, the Galenic treatment had run its course as vibrators shifted from self-help to pornography. In the 1960s, new ideologies of self-help would bring them back, but under a different star.

20. Carl Capellmann, *Pastoral Medicine*, trans. William Dassel (New York: Pustet, 1879), pp. 76–77. The author does not say explicitly how women discover this source of relief.

21. François Lissarrague, "The Sexual Life of Satyrs," in Halperin, Winkler, and Zeitlin, *Before Sexuality*. See also Andrew Stewart, *Art, Desire, and the Body in Ancient Greece* (Cambridge, UK: Cambridge University Press, 1997), p. 225, fig. 155, "Masturbating hunchback," c. 200 B.C.E.

22. See the introduction to Martial, *Epigrams*, ed. and trans. Walter C.A.

442

Ker (Cambridge, MA: Harvard University Press, 1979), vol. 1, pp. viii–x. *Masturbatio[n]* is a form not found in any Latin text.

23. The place to start with *masturbor* and its synonyms is J.N. Adams, *The Latin Sexual Vocabulary* (Baltimore: Johns Hopkins University Press, 1982), pp. 208–11. The alternative view is from Oscar Bloch with the cooperation of Walther von Wartburg, "Mastubari, Onanie treiben," *Dictionnaire étymologique de la langue française* (Paris: Presses Universitaires de France, 1932), vol. 2.

24. Martial, *Epigrams* 11.73.3–4, ed. and trans. D.R. Shackleton Bailey, Loeb Classical Library (Cambridge, MA: Harvard University Press, 1993), vol. 3, pp. 62–63. "Cum frustra iacui longa prurigene tentus, succurrit pro te saepe sinistra mihi"; Priapea 33, "fiet amica manus." Whether we are to make much of the mention of the left hand remains an open question. To that hand, to the "unclean hand," are assigned dishonorable tasks, as Adams points out. But the term "amica manus" seems fairly specific — "a hand job" — without specifying which hand or whose. And Martial elsewhere does not specify which hand he uses when he has no boy: "My hand comes to my assistance in lieu of Ganymede" (*at mihi succurrit pro Ganymede manus*) *Epigrams* 2.43, vol. 1, pp. 166–67. Catullus, in lampooning the *cinaedus* Vibennius, says that his father uses his *right* hand in the bathhouses while he offers his asshole. Plautus may have called the right hand *pullaria* because it is used by men to masturbate their boyfriends, *pulli*. So, dishonor does not seem to be so clearly apportioned. On Catullus and the Vibenni and also on Plautus, see Craig Williams, *Roman Homosexuality: Ideologies of Masculinity in Classical Antiquity* (New York: Oxford University Press, 1999), pp. 176, 270, n.61. Satyrs who on vases are shown masturbating with one hand use the right one.

25. Gary P. Leupp, *Male Colors: The Construction of Homosexuality in Tokugawa Japan* (Berkeley: University of California Press, 1994), p. 45. Masturbation was also connected with the erotics of anal penetration in other complex ways; it seems to have been acceptable for a man to be penetrated if he enjoyed the pleasure on a purely physical and not emotional basis, that is, if there was no loss of status. The text advises that the pleasure of masturbation can be increased if while doing it the left hand penetrates the anus. But again, the ethical focus of this is far from what it would be in around 1712. See Leupp, *Male Colors*, p. 179.

26. Herodotus, *The Persian Wars*, trans. George Rawlinson (New York: Modern Library, 1942), II, para. 64, p. 148; Robert Parker, *Miasma: Pollution and Purification in Early Greek Religion* (Oxford: Oxford University Press, 1983), pp. 76–77 and 74–106 passim. Parker also doubts whether the payment of a tithe for "pollution" involves, as at least one scholar thinks, the distinction between an involuntary pollution and masturbation or indeed that semen is the problem at all. See his app. 2, p. 342.

27. Nicole Loraux, *The Children of Athena: Athenian Ideas about Citizenship and the Division Between the Sexes*, trans. Caroline Levine (Princeton, NJ: Princeton University Press, 1993), p. 64.

28. Hugh Northcote, *Christianity and Sex Problems* (1908; Philadelphia: F.A. Davis, 1916), p. 422; Aeschines, *Contra Ctesiphon*, p. 174. Ctesiphon, Demosthenes's friend, made the motion, and Aeschines, his bitter enemy, opposed it.

29. H.C. [Henry Cockerham], *The English Dictionary; or, An Interpreter of Hard English Words* (London, 1623; repr. New York: Huntington Press, 1930). The word remains in the dictionary through many editions. I checked the eleventh enlarged edition (London, 1658), where the early definition is repeated exactly.

30. On satyrs and masturbation, see Lissarrague, "Sexual Life of Satyrs," p. 57. Jeffrey Henderson, *The Maculate Muse: Obscene Language in Attic Comedy* (New Haven, CT: Yale University Press, 1975), p. 200. Dio Chrysostom, *Works*, trans. J.W. Cohoon (Cambridge, MA: Harvard University Press, 1949), vol. 1, pp. 259–61; Philippe Borgeaud, *The Cult of Pan in Ancient Greece*, trans. Kathleen Atlass and James Redfield (Chicago: University of Chicago Press, 1988), p. 77. Not all versions of the story are so innocent. In one, Pan drove the shepherds mad; they tore Echo limb from limb so that only her voice survived.

31. For access to women as a sign of status, especially when women were in short supply, see Carol Clover, "The Politics of Scarcity: Notes on the Sex Ratio in Early Scandinavia," in Helen Damico and Alexandra Hennessey Olsen (eds.), *New Readings on Women in Old English Literature* (Bloomington: Indiana University Press, 1990), p. 119 and passim.

32. Cicero, *Tusculan Disputations*, ed. and trans. J.E. King, Loeb Classical Library (Cambridge, MA: Harvard University Press, 1945), bk. 4, vol. 32, para. 68, pp. 406–407; for Musonius, see Cora E. Lutz, "Musonius Rufus: The Roman Socrates," *Yale Classical Studies* 10 (1947), pp. 4–14. On both Cicero and Musonius, see Williams, *Roman Homosexuality*, pp. 239–41.

33. Martial, *Epigrams* 14.203; *Epigrams* 2.43: "At mihi succurrit pro Ganymede manus." On Martial's general success with boys in the *Epigrams*, see Williams, *Roman Homosexuality*.

34. Juvenal, *Satire* 10.196–208. I have filled in the translation in ed. and trans. G.G. Ramsay, *Juvenal and Persius*, Loeb Classical Library (Cambridge, MA: Harvard University Press, 1979), pp. 208–209.

35. I am grateful to Katherine Zieman for putting me on the track of this reference. The scene in Ovid is from Ovid, *Fasti* 1.423–38, ed. and trans. James George Frazer, Loeb Classical Library (Cambridge, MA: Harvard University Press, 1976), pp. 31–33. Geoffrey Chaucer, *The Parliament of Fowls*, l. 256, in *The Riverside Chaucer*, ed. Larry D. Benson (Boston: Houghton Mifflin, 1987), p. 388.

36. Heinrich Wittenwiler, *Der Ring*, trans. into modern German, with medieval German facing text, by Horst Brunner (Stuttgart: Reclam, 1991), pt. 1, ll. 1564-1606. The only existing manuscript is from 1395. I have given a free translation of the German; as in all such parodies, the humor comes from the piling on of obscenities; it is difficult to find equivalents for everything she does

to various aspects of her genital anatomy. The section in full reads: "Mätzli sas allaine, / Sei schawt ir weiseen paine. / Do sach sei ir vil praunen mutzen: Solich zuchen, rupfen, smutzen / Huob sich auf den rauchen fleken, / Reissen, chlenken und ainzweken, / Dar zuo fluochen, trewen, schelten, / Das des jamers ghort man selten. Mätzel zuo der futzen sparch / Got geb dir laid und ungemach / Und dar zuo allen smertzen, / Den ich an meinem hertzen / So pitterleichen dulde / Nur von deiner schulde!" (1564–1575). The word *mutzen* seems to have transformed itself into the nineteenth-century *mietze*, which meant cat, the rough equivalent of the English slang "pussy." I am grateful to Stephen Casey, my former student at Washington University, St. Louis, for sending me the material on which this is based.

37. Joseph V. Guerinot, *Pamphlet Attacks on Alexander Pope, 1711–1744: A Descriptive Bibliography* (London: Methuen, 1969), pp. 254–56. "Prologue and Epilogue to the Wild Gallant," in *The Poetical Works of Dryden*, new rev. enl. ed., ed. George Noyes (Boston: Houghton Mifflin, 1950), pp. 52–53. Dryden also equates writing naive plays with lack of real sexual experience. I am grateful to James Winn for these references.

38. Rochester, John Wilmot, Earl of, *The Complete Poems of John Wilmot, Earl of Rochester*, ed. David M. Vieth (New Haven: Yale University Press, 1968), "A Ramble in St. James Park," p. 40, ll. 15–20; "Song," p. 28, ll. 36–40; "On Cary Frazier," p. 137; "Signor Dildo," p. 59, l. 74. I am grateful to Holger Schott, a graduate student in the English department at Harvard University, for reminding me of the relevance of Rochester and sharing his interpretations with me.

39. I am grateful to Carol Clover and Karin Saunders of the Department of Scandinavian at Berkeley and to Thomas Bredsdorf of the University of Copenhagen for this poem and their learned commentaries and translation of its heavily Germanic Danish. The allusion seems to be to playing the cello.

40. Martial, *Epigrams* 9.41. The verb I translate as "fuck" is *futuo, future*, the basic Latin obscenity for the purpose.

41. On this, see Maud W. Gleason, *Making Men* (Princeton, NJ: Princeton University Press, 1995).

42. Daniel Boyarin's remarkably learned *Carnal Israel: Reading Sex in Talmudic Culture* (Berkeley: University of California Press, 1993), which is devoted to understanding what the rabbis thought about sexuality, does not, for example, discuss Genesis 38.8–10 at all nor masturbation in any other context.

43. On the absence of any commentary on female masturbation, see the old but still useful book by Julius Preuss, *Biblical and Talmudic Medicine*, trans. and ed. Fred Rosner (New York: Sanhedrin Press, 1978), pp. 489–90. None of the literature that claims to be about masturbation in the Jewish tradition deals with the subject. In one account, "all the women of the house of Rabbi who exercise friction are designated Tamar." See Babylonian Talmud (hereafter BT), Yabamoth 34b, where the point is also made that no woman conceives from her first contact. To know carnally means to know carnally naturally.

44. For how the Onan story fits into the structure of Genesis, see Gerhard von Rad, *Genesis: A Commentary*, trans. John H. Marks (Philadelphia: Westminster Press, 1961), pp. 343–57. Zerah's scarlet thread appears often as an element in priestly garments or as a veil for the tabernacle. For more on it, see Francis Brown, with the cooperation of S.R. Driver and Charles A. Briggs, *Hebrew and English Lexicon of the Old Testament: The Brown-Driver-Briggs Hebrew and English Lexicon: with an appendix containing the Biblical Aramaic: coded with the numbering system from Strong's Exhaustive concordance of the Bible* (Peabody, MA: Hendrickson Publishers, [1996]).

45. Calum M. Carmichael, *The Laws of Deuteronomy* (Ithaca, NY: Cornell University Press, 1974), pp. 232–38. On the heels of this account comes the law that a woman who interferes in a fight between her husband and another man by grabbing the other man's balls shall have her hand cut off. This is not the world of the solitary vice. On Ruth's marital vicissitudes, see Jack M. Sasson, *Ruth: A New Translation with a Philological Commentary and a Formalist-Folklorist Interpretation* (Baltimore: Johns Hopkins University Press, 1979), pp. 144–45 and 229–30.

46. On these issues, see Jeremy Cohen, *Be Fertile and Increase, Fill the Earth and Master It: The Ancient and Medieval Career of a Biblical Text* (Ithaca, NY: Cornell University Press, 1989).

47. For this version and its sources, see Louis Ginzberg, *The Legends of the Jews*, trans. Henrietta Szold (Philadelphia: Jewish Publications Society of America, c. 1909–1932), vol. 5, p. 334.

48. Esther Marie Menn, *Judah and Tamar (Genesis 38) in Ancient Jewish Exegesis: Studies in Literary Form and Hermeneutics* (New York and Leiden: Brill, 1997), pp. 1–3, 19–23, 143–51. Menn offers a wonderful analysis of how this dysfunctional family's crisis was variously interpreted, and I cannot begin to do it justice. The point is simply that none of the elaborations of the story is about masturbation in any sense. Jubilees 41.1–6 can be found in James Charlesworth (ed.), *Old Testament Pseudepigrapha* (Garden City, NY: Doubleday, 1983), vol. 1, p. 130. A much later interpretation of the standard biblical version by the eleventh-century French rabbi Rashi holds that Onan and Er committed the same sin — "Like the death of Er (so was) the death of Onan" — and that Er destroyed his seed "so that [Tamar] would not conceive and mar her beauty." See Abraham Ben-Isaiah and Benjamin Sharfman, *The Pentateuch and Rashi's Commentary: A Linear Translation into English* (Brooklyn: SSR Publishing, 1949), p. 383. Rabbi Samuel Ben Meir (1249–1316) notes that Er and Onan died for the same crime — coitus interruptus — but committed for different motives. See his commentary and the editorial notes in Martin I. Lockshin, *Rabbi Samuel Ben Meir's Commentary on Genesis: An Annotated Translation*, Jewish Studies, vol. 5 (Lewiston, NY: Edwin Mellen Press, 1989), pp. 262–63. *Midrash Rabbah*, trans. H. Freed (1939; London: Soncino Press, 1987), vol. 2, p. 797.

49. Pollution in the Jewish tradition is an enormous topic, but Hyam Mac-

coby in his *Ritual and Morality: The Ritual Purity System and Its Place in Judaism* (Cambridge, UK: Cambridge University Press, 1999), pp. 31–66, offers an economical survey of texts and modern commentary. Without committing myself to his views on how questions of pollution became questions of morality, I have found Jacob Milgrom's *Leviticus 1–16: A New Translation with Introduction and Commentary* (New York: Doubleday, 1991), especially on ch. 15, thrilling and informative. On the Deuteronomy passage, I have relied on Carmichael, *Laws of Deuteronomy*.

50. BT, Yabamoth 34b; Rabbi Eliezer's views regarding holding the penis are in BT, Niddah 13a. The Spanish poet, grammarian, and rabbi Ibn Ezra (1089–1164) says he is shocked that the Iraqi sage Rabbi Ben Tamin Ha-Mizrachi would read this as *schichet artzah*, meaning "corrupted her ground," that is, the place with which she sat on the ground, her anus. Alternative readings include "dealt corruptly with the ground." See Ibn Ezra, *Commentary on the Pentateuch*, trans. and annotated by H. Norman Strickman and Arthur M. Silver (New York: Menorah Publishing, 1988–) ch. 38, p. 357; *Midrash Rabbah*, vol. 2, pp. 791–92; and Cohen, *Be Fertile and Increase*, pp. 137–38.

51. I take this interpretation from the careful source criticism in Michael L. Satlow, "'Wasted Seed': The History of a Rabbinic Idea," *Hebrew Union College Annual* (1994).

52. All references are to BT, Niddah 13a. I have consulted translations in *The Babylonian Talmud*, trans. and ed. I. Epstein (London: Soncino Press, 1935–1952), and also that offered by Satlow, "'Wasted Seed,'" app. 2, pp. 172–75. I am also grateful to Daniel Boyarin, Jack Levinson, and Naomi Janowitz for help with the Hebrew original.

53. BT, Niddah 13a–b; Berakoth 12b; Yoma 29a.

54. *Midrash Rabbah*, vol. 2, pp. 791–92; Zohar 2.221b and 188a. Cohen, *Be Fertile and Increase*, pp. 194–95 and 205–10.

55. For "destruction of seed" in this sense, see David Biale, *Eros and the Jews* (New York: Basic Books, 1992), pp. 106–108.

56. On this, see John Noonan, *Contraception: A History of Its Treatment by Catholic Theologians and Canonists*, enl. ed. (Cambridge, MA: Harvard University Press, 1986), p. 161, and more generally on the subject, pp. 10–11, 35–36, 52–53, 96–103, 120–21, 138–39, 160–61, 174–75, 216–35. Noonan argues that Gratian and Lombard in the twelfth century moved the discussion of Onan from the allegorical realm into an attack on contraception. He also suggests that the long silence may have been because the method was so little used, although he offers no evidence for this.

57. Geoffroy La Tour Landry, *The book of the knight of La Tour-Landry compiled for the instruction of his daughters*, with intro. and notes by Thomas Wright (London: Published for the Early English Text Society by Kegan Paul, Trench, Trübner, 1906). William Caxton — printer of the first English Bible — translated, as well as printed, this book in 1483.

58. St. Ephraem the Syrian, *Commentary on Genesis* sec. 34.1, in *Selected Prose Works*, trans. Edward G. Mathews Jr.; David Winston and John Dillon, *Two Treatises of Philo of Alexandria: A Commentary on "De gigantibus" and "Quod Deus sit immutabilis,"* Brown Judaic Studies, no. 25 (Chico, CA: Scholars Press), pp. 274–75. On Bede, Augustine, and the early Christian tradition generally, see Noonan, *Contraception*, pp. 120 ff. Venerable Bede, *Expositio in Primum Librum Mosis*, in *In Pentateuchum Commentarii* (*Exposition of the First Book of Moses in Commentaries on the Pentateuch*, in J.P. Migne (ed.), *Patrologia Latina* (hereafter PL) (Paris: Migne, 1844–91), vol. 91, col. 266C–D for Bede's argument. Noonan's striking point is that when, in the context of the Manichean use of coitus interruptus on religious grounds, Augustine condemns the practice – the first such attack in the Catholic tradition – he does not cite Onan. A few pages later when he does mention Onan it is as one "who does not do the good he is capable of." Er, a name that Augustine derives etymologically from a word meaning "active evil," is the villain of the passage. Onan does appear fleetingly in a passage about marriage that Noonan does not discuss but that identifies him as one who was struck down for violating the purpose of marriage: procreation. The general context is an explication of the dictum, *Si non se continent, nubant,* "if they cannot control themselves, let them marry" but there is no reference here to how precisely Onan failed to propagate. See Augustine, *De Conjugi Adulterinis* (Migne, PL 40), col. 479 or a translation in Augustine, Saint, Bishop of Hippo, *Treatises on marriage and other subjects*, ed. Roy J. Deferrari, trans. Charles T. Wilcox (New York: Fathers of the Church, 1955), p. 117.

59. Martin Luther, *Lectures on Genesis Chapters 38–44*, trans. Paul D. Pahl, in *Luther's Works* (Saint Louis: Concordia, 1955–86), vol. 7, pp. 17–21; on his views of how colleagues have made inappropriate use of these passages in much-welcome attacks on Catholic doctrines of celibacy, see the letter to Georg Spalatin, Aug. 15, 1521, in *Letters*, ed. and trans. Gottfried G. Krodel, in *Luther's Works*, vol. 48, pp. 293–94.

60. John Calvin, *Commentaries upon the First Book of Moses*, trans. Thomas Tymme (London, 1578), pp. 53 and 10.

61. Gervase Babington, *Certaine Plaine, brief, and Comfortable Notes, Upon every Chapter of Genesis* (London, 1596), p. 278; [Patrick] Simon, Lord Bishop of Ely, *A commentary upon the First Book of Moses Called Genesis* (London, 1695), pp. 502–504; Henry Ainsworth, *Annotations upon the Bookes of Moses* (London, 1627); George Hughes (1603–1667), *An Analytical Exposition of the Whole First Book of Moses called Genesis* (1672), p. 473. (The book was published posthumously; Hughes lost his parish in 1664 as a consequence of the Restoration.)

62. For Ramban (Nachmanides) on this and other aspects of the Onan story, see *Commentary on the Torah: Genesis*, trans. and annotated by Charles B. Chavel (New York: Shilo, 1971–76), pp. 472 and 466–72 passim.

63. John Cassian, *The Conferences*, trans. and annotated by Boniface Ramsey (New York: Paulist Press, 1997), Conference 5 ("On the Eight Principal Vices"),

sec. 11, para. 4, pp. 190–91. The editor, note 23, identifies Ephesians 5.5 as the textual authority of the avaricious person, and by association the fornicator and impure person are idolaters. Because of biblical authority, he calls this second form of fornication "impurity of the Holy Scripture." 1 Corinthians advises these categories of people to remain chaste but if that is not possible to marry, "for it is better to marry than to burn." I have checked the Latin in the bilingual French-Latin edition of the *Conferences* by E. Pichery (Paris: Les Editions du Cerf, 1955–1959). Conference 5 is in vol. 1, Conference 12 in vol. 2, Conference 22 in vol. 3.

64. William Langland, *The Ancrene Riwle* (Guide to anchoresses), trans. into modern English from "semi-Saxon" by M.B. Salu with an intro. by Gerard Sitwell (London: Burns and Oates, 1955), p. 91.

65. John Cassian, *Institutions cénobitiques*, Latin text with French trans. by Jean-Claude Guy (Paris: Editions du Cerf, 1965), bk. 6, ch. 18, pp. 284–85: "et mulierem, inquit, ignoro, et virgo non sum."

66. Cassian, Conference 22.3.

67. There is a seventh, higher state of chastity still that can be had by divine gift but cannot be "posed as a kind of general precept." That is, it is conceivable that one reach the state of the blessed Sirenus, in whom "even the natural movement of the flesh would have died and one would not produce any disgusting fluid at all" (Cassian, Conference 12, sec. 7, para. 6, p. 444).

68. I am not sure why Foucault in vol. 3 of *The History of Sexuality* or Aline Rousselle in *Porneia* would think that so very refined a discussion would suggest the importance of masturbation in late Antiquity. Generally, and not just in Christian moral writing, it was of minor significance.

69. The history of thinking about nocturnal emissions in the early Church offers a fascinating way of understanding the meaning of individual, male impurity in relation to the purity of the Church and of the soul. But again, masturbation simply does not figure into the discussion; nocturnal emissions in third-century Syria or fifth-century Gaul are not the spermatorrhea of the eighteenth and nineteenth centuries. On the early Church, see David Brakke, "The Problematization of Nocturnal Emissions in Early Christian Syria, Egypt, and Gaul," *Journal of Early Christian Studies* 3.4 (1995).

70. Michel de Montaigne, *The Complete Essays of Montaigne*, trans. Donald M. Frame (Stanford, CA: Stanford University Press, 1976), bk. 3, essay 5.

71. This and the preceding paragraph are manifestly indebted to Brown's *Body and Society*; further evidence for the fundamental irrelevance of masturbation to the making of the early Christian ethos is that major recent treatments of sexuality and the body discuss it not at all or only tangentially with reference to classical medico-ethical views on how to get rid of surplus fluids. For their silence and for a sense of what does matter, see Susannah Elm, *Virgins of God: The Making of Asceticism in Late Antiquity* (New York: Oxford University Press, 1994), and Teresa M. Shaw, *The Burden of the Flesh: Fasting and Sexuality in Early*

Christianity (Minneapolis: Fortress Press, 1998); St. Jerome, *Ad Eustachium*, Epis. 22 (Migne, PL 22), para. 2, col. 395.

72. For this discussion of the question of pleasure and marital intercourse in relation to sin and guilt, I have relied on Jean Delumeau, *Sin and Fear: The Emergence of a Western Guilt Culture, 13th–18th Centuries*, trans. Eric Nicholson (New York: St. Martin's, 1990), esp. pp. 214–21, and on Thomas Tentler, *Sin and Confession on the Eve of the Reformation* (Princeton, NJ: Princeton University Press, 1977).

73. Huggucio is cited in Tentler, *Sin and Confession*, pp. 174–75; Bernardino of Siena is cited as having over-read Gratian in Henry Ansgar Kelly, "Bishop, Prioress, and Bawd in the Stews of Southwark," *Speculum* 75 (2000), p. 344, n.9. Burchard is cited in Jacques Rossiaud, *Medieval Prostitution*, trans. Lydia G. Cochrane (Oxford: Basil Blackwell, 1988), pp. 75–76.

74. The Dominican William of Rennes makes this statement in a commentary on the penitential of St. Raymond of Peñafort (1175/80–1275). Raymond was enormously influential; his was one of the most widely circulated — over one hundred manuscript copies are known — of medieval penitentials; William is quoted in Delumeau, *Sin and Fear*, p. 216. For the Latin, see Raymond of Peñafort, *Seu summa . . . de poenitentia et matrimonio cum glossis* (Franborough, Hants: Gregg, 1967; repr. of 1603 ed.), vol. 4, p. 520; lower left gloss reads, "Provocat eam minibus, vel cogitatione, vel utendo caldis, & incentiuis, ut pluries posit cum uxore coire"; Gregory, cited in Delumeau, says plainly, "This pleasure [of sex within marriage] cannot be without fault" (p. 215).

75. Raymond, *Seu summa*; Delumeau, *Sin and Fear*, pp. 216–20.

76. Rossiaud, *Medieval Prostitution*, pp. 94–96; for the pro-natalist argument, see pp. 86–103.

77. For a summary of the discussion about prostitution, see Kelly, "Bishop, Prioress, and Bawd," pp. 340–49; for the demise of prostitution as a widely accepted practice in the context of increasing regulation of marriage and the sexual activities of unmarried youth, see Leah Lydia Otis, *Prostitution in Medieval Society: The History of an Urban Institution in Languedoc* (Chicago: University of Chicago Press, 1985), pp. 108–109 and passim.

78. The best recent study of these penitentials for our purposes is Pierre J. Payer, *Sex and the Penitentials: The Development of a Sexual Code, 550–1150* (Toronto: University of Toronto Press, 1984). Payer gives what I think are convincing arguments for this sort of moral backward projection. I have also profited from John T. McNeill and Helena M. Gamer, *Medieval Handbooks of Penance* (New York: Columbia University Press, 1938), pp. 1–75, and from Ludwig Bieler, *The Irish Penitentials*, with an app. by D.A. Binchy (Dublin: Dublin Institute for Advanced Studies, 1963). The introduction in Hermann Joseph Schmitz, *Die Bussbücher und die Bussdisciplin der Kirche* (Graz: Akademische Druck — U. Verlagsanstalt, 1958), is excellent; I have also used his Latin texts as my source.

79. See Payer, *Sex and the Penitentials*, pp. 14 and 46–47.

80. See note 87 below on Theodore.

81. The verb *quoinquinaverit* is from *inquino, inquinavi*, to pollute.

82. I have used the text reprinted in Payer, *Sex and the Penitentials*, p. 177, n.12.

83. *Immunditia* comes from *immundus*, "unclean" or "impure." Theodulf carefully distinguished illicit sex involving married people (*adulterium*) and that involving single people (*fornicari*). In other words, he could be precise when something was really at stake.

84. *A commentarie vpon S. Paules epistles to the Corinthians. Written by M. John Calvin: and translated out of Latine into Englishe, by Thomas Tymme minister* (London, 1577).

85. There is some question as to whether one can generally correlate the amount of penance with the severity of the lapse. Payer in *Sex and the Penitentials* thought so but was less sanguine in a later study, "Confession and the Study of Sex in the Middle Ages," in Vern L. Bullough and James A. Brundage (eds.), *Handbook of Medieval Sexuality* (New York: Garland, 1996), pp. 3–31, where he argues that the complicated textual traditions of these texts make it difficult to produce an index of sinfulness from ranking of punishments. At the very least, one can say that what seems to have been masturbation was not severely punished.

86. Schmitz, *Bussbücher*, pp. 619–20.

87. "Das Bussbuch Theodore's von Canterbury," in *ibid.*, vol. 1, sec. 2.8.14. sec. 1, on fornication. I will not engage with the thorny question of how good Schmitz's edition is. His editorial choices, however arguable, will not change the basic point. The strictures against fornication discussed above, sec. 2, p. 526, read: "9. Si se ipsum coinquinate, XL dies poeniteat." The subject is clearly male. "12. Si mulier cum mulier fornicaverit, III annos poeniteat. 13. Si sola cum se ipsa coitum habet, sic poeniteat." The diverse lapses of the servants of God, "De diverso lapso servorum Dei," that I discuss are all in sec. 8, pp. 531–32: "1. Sacerdos si tangendo mulierem aut osculando coinquinabitur, XL dies poeniteat. 2. Presbyter si osculatus est feminam per desiderium XX dies poeniteat. 3. Presbyter quoque si per cogitationem semen fuderit ebdomada, jejunet. 4. Si tangit manu III ebdomadas jejunet.... 6. Monachus vel sacr virgo fornicationem faciens VII annos poeniteat. 7. Qui saepe per violentiam cogitationis semen fuderit, poeniteat XX dies. 8. Qui semen dormiens in ecclesia fuderit, VII dies poeniteat. 9. Si excitat ipse, primo XX dies, iterans XL dies poeniteat.... 11. Qui se ipsum coinquinat, XL dies poeniteat," which is distinguished from the one before, which presumably refers to the much more serious pollution through intercrural intercourse: "10. Si in femoribus, I annum." These are translated in McNeill and Gamer, *Medieval Handbooks of Penance*, pp. 184–85 and 191–92, but without any effort to distinguish the various ways in which pollution takes place; penances are also inaccurately described.

88. Burchard as cited and discussed in Mark D. Jordan, *The Invention of Sodomy in Christian Theology* (Chicago: University of Chicago Press, 1997), pp.

52–53; the original can be found in Burchard of Worms, *Decretum Libri Viginti* 19.5 (Migne, PL 140), p. 968, cols. 967D–968A.

89. Peter Damian, *Book of Gomorrah: An Eleventh Century Treatise Against Clerical Homosexual Practices*, trans. with an intro. and notes by Pierre J. Payer (Waterloo, Canada: Wilfrid Laurier University Press, 1982). This book is a translation of Peter Damian's *Liber Gomorrhianus* (Migne, PL 145), p. 29; Burchard seems to have been a source for Damian's classification; p. 29 and n.3. Damian's classification of the four sorts of ways to commit this iniquity in Latin reads "Alii siquidem secum, alli aliorum minibus, allis inter femora, alii denique consummato actu contra natura delinquunt."

90. This comes as a warning that those who do not "fall together with another" are no less guilty. The hermit on his deathbed in the desert "who fell to the contaminations of lustful attractions" polluted no one but ruined himself with impurity. This would seem to be an instance not of masturbation — an unlikely deathbed activity — but of involuntary emission, nocturnal or otherwise, occasioned by surrender to the demons. I know of no case in which these demons proffered sex with men. Damian, *Book of Gomorrah*, p. 78.

91. *Ibid.*, p. 78.

92. See *ibid.*, the twenty-six chapter headings; p. 41. On the vexed question of the medieval Church's position on sodomy, before and after the twelfth century, see the judicious account by Warren Johansson and William A. Percy, "Homosexuality," in Bullough and Brundage, *Handbook of Medieval Sexuality*.

93. On the reception of Damian's disputation, see Jordan, *Invention of Sodomy*, ch. 5, and L.K. Little, "The Personal Development of Peter Damian," William C. Jordan, Bruce McNab, and Teofilo F. Ruiz (eds.), in *Order and Innovation in the Middle Ages* (Princeton, NJ: Princeton University Press, 1976).

94. For this and the succeeding paragraph, see Thomas Aquinas, *Summa theologiae* 2a2ae and 12, Latin text and English translation (New York: McGraw-Hill, 1964–1976), pp. 154 and 244–47. The translator renders *peccatum immunditiae* as "self-abuse," but this is clearly an anachronistic rendering. He gives for *mollitiem* "unchaste softness," but we have already seen how problematic this word is.

95. Tentler, *Sin and Confessions*, pp. 186–89; *Jean Gerson: Early Works,* trans. and ed. Brian Patrick McGuire (New York: Paulist Press, 1998), p. 188.

96. Obviously, this discussion of marital adultery follows not only from classical traditions about the unseemliness of such things but more directly from the Church's abhorrence of contraception. This colored thinking not only about permitted positions but also about masturbation. Religious traditions such as Islam that held that legitimate intercourse need not always be for procreative purposes also explicitly condoned masturbation. It was held to be licit in the absence of a legitimate partner; the traveler, the lonely, the poor, the woman whose husband was absent were better off satisfying their lusts alone than in some illegal heterosexual way. And the jurists also agreed with the doctors that

too much accumulated semen was dangerous, so that self-stimulation was allowed even during the fast of Ramadan, lest the surplus result in serious illness. B.F. Musallam, *Sex and Society in Islam: Birth Control Before the Nineteenth Century* (Cambridge, UK: Cambridge University Press, 1983), pp. 32–34.

97. Jean-Louis Flandrin, *Sex in the Western World: The Development of Attitudes and Behaviour*, trans. Sue Collins (Chur, Switzerland: Harwood Academic Publishers, 1991), pp. 103–106, 247–50, esp. 248; see also the notes pp. 323–33. Flandrin thinks that the Church was trying to eliminate masturbation or reduce its frequency after the fourteenth century — Gerson is his main evidence for this, although as we saw it is not strong — but that it was in practice distinguished from sodomy as a sin so bad that prescribing penance was left to the bishop. Payer, "Confession and the Study of Sex in the Middle Ages," pp. 12–14; see also James Brundage, "Sex and the Canon Law," in Bullough and Brundage, *Handbook of Medieval Sexuality*, p. 41, who says that most writers treated masturbation as a "minor peccadillo."

98. On Florence, see the remarkable excavation of municipal records on sodomy by Michael Rocke, *Forbidden Friendships: Homosexuality and Male Culture in Renaissance Florence* (New York: Oxford University Press, 1996); Gregory XI is quoted on p. 3; the statistics I cite come from p. 47. On prostitution as an alternative to sodomy, see Ruth Mazo Karras, *Common Women: Prostitution and Sexuality in Medieval England* (Oxford: Oxford University Press, 1996), pp. 32 and 137; on masturbation as a way station to sodomy, see Rossiaud, *Medieval Prostitution*, p. 94.

99. The two confessionals between Aquinas and the fourteenth century that ask about masturbation are specifically those of the Canon of St. Victor Peter of Poitiers, *Summa de confessione*, and the grand master of the Dominican order, Humbert of Romans, *Instructions de officis ordinis*. I am grateful to Yaron Toren, a graduate student at St. John's College, Oxford, for this material, and, more generally, for his invaluable help in guiding me through the medieval discussion of masturbation in relation both to sodomy and to questions of sexual morality generally. See on this point also Jordan, *Invention*, p. 105.

100. Peter of Poitiers derived *mollities* from mollifying the mind/spirit, which seems pretty specific.

101. Caesarius of Heisterbach, *Dialogus miraculorum*, ed. J. Strange, 2 vols. (Cologne, Bonn, and Brussels, 1851), vol. 3, p. 47.

102. Langland, *Ancrene Riwle*, p. 91. Elsewhere he warns nuns that the devil is strong in the hindquarters and weak in the head and proceeds with a long riff on how an old woman set a house on fire with straw — much comes from little — and that sparks fly upward, that flames start below, and soon everything is aflame (pp. 131–32).

103. Thomas de Cantimpré, *Bonum universale de apibus* (Douai, 1627), ch. 30. I owe the reference and translation to Yaron Toren. Elliott, *Fallen Bodies*, p. 47, discusses three of these in the context of his claim that autoeroticism is

regarded as a problem of women. I do not think that in the medieval and early modern period this is the case; he leaves out the story of the male masturbator.

104. James A. Brundage, *Law, Sex, and Christian Society in Medieval Europe* (1987; Chicago: University of Chicago Press, 1990). See also his "Playing by the Rules: Sexual Behaviour and Legal Norms in Medieval Europe," in Jacqueline Murray and Konrad Eisenbichler (eds.), *Desire and Discipline: Sex and Sexuality in the Premodern West* (Toronto: University of Toronto Press, 1996). On heresy being public, see Gratian, *Decretum* II 124 Qiii, cols. 27–31, ed. E. Friedberg, in *Corpus juris canonici* (Leipzig, 1881), vol. 1, pp. 997–98, cited in R.I. Moore, *The Formation of a Persecuting Society* (Oxford: Basil Blackwell, 1987), p. 68, which also makes the point that heresy and its representation in the body — leprosy — are by nature public. There is perhaps a parallel here to traditional Muslim jurisprudence on matters sexual. Deviance per se, what we would think of as homosexuality, was not condoned, but neither was it much discussed. What mattered were heterosexual relations that could have public consequences — rape and consensual sex between unmarried people. And even here, the more infamous — the more disruptive of public order — the more likely to be prosecuted, because such serious crimes required witnesses to prove. See Judith E. Tucker, *In the House of the Law: Gender and Islamic Law in Ottoman Syria and Palestine* (Berkeley: University of California Press, 1998), pp. 159 and 148–78 passim.

105. On this and on the deep imbrication of prostitution with medieval and early modern society, see Karras, *Common Women*, pp. 30, 45, and passim. There may have been something disingenuous — deeply misogynist — about the preaching against such women; the priest usually got off; his "whore" was free game for rape among the town's young men.

106. Rossiaud, *Medieval Prostitution*, p. 106.

107. In this case, it is unambiguous that *mollitiei* means "masturbation." Large parts of this tract are available in Tentler, *Sin and Confession*, but I quote from the translation by Yaron Toren, which he has kindly made available to me.

108. For Gerson's view on confession generally, see his "On Hearing Confession," in *Jean Gerson: Early Works*, pp. 365–77; and for the confessions of the young in particular, see Brian Patrick McGuire, "Education, Confession, and Pious Fraud: Jean Gerson and Late Medieval Change," *American Benedictine Review* 47.3 (Sept. 1996), esp. pp. 316–38.

109. *Ibid.*

110. The claim that "On the Confession of Masturbation" is out of character for Gerson is in Tentler, *Sin and Confession*; the counterclaim is in McGuire, "Education, Confession, and Pious Fraud," esp. pp. 322–23. I base what I say on the manuscript here and below entirely on the unpublished work of Yaron Toren.

111. With regard to copies of "On the Confession of Masturbation," Toren writes, in a personal communication, that there are two in addition to the one

he used in making his translation (BN lat. 1492), "although neither was copied in St. Victor: Erfurt Ampl. Qu. 146 (ff. 125–36) and Wien Nat. Ser. n. 3887 (ff. 25–28), both from the first half of the fifteenth century." In the first manuscript, the work is euphemistically titled *De informacione confessorum* and ascribed to Gerson. The manuscript contains twenty-seven different works, mainly of devotional character, and *De informacione confessorum* is the only text ascribed to Gerson. The second manuscript is part of a two-volume set dedicated to works ascribed to Gerson (some wrongly). The first volume (3886) consists mostly of letters, while the greater part of the forty-six works contained in the second volume are related to the administration of the confessional. All of Gerson's principal works on the topic appear in it. Toren thinks that there may be another copy in the Vatican, but four copies in three hundred years does not constitute popularity and is extremely small for an author of Gerson's stature.

112. This is the view of Robert de Sorbon, *De confessione secreta sacerdoti facta de peccato luxuria*, in William of Auvergne, *Opera omnia* (Paris, 1674), vol. 2, supp., pp. 231–32.

113. See Rocke, *Forbidden Friendships*, pp. 19–44; Nicholas Davidson, "Theology, Nature, and the Law: Sexual Sin and Sexual Crime in Italy from the Fourteenth to the Seventeenth Century," in Trevor Dean and K.J.P. Lowe (eds.), *Crime, Society, and the Law in Renaissance Italy* (Cambridge, UK: Cambridge University Press, 1994), pp. 74–77 and 88–90. Sodomy seems to have been more openly discussed and prosecuted in Italy than elsewhere.

114. Robert de Sorbon, *De confessione*.

115. The whole notion of private interrogation and interior discipline in the Church is novel in the sixteenth century; it had made little progress in rural areas even by the middle of the seventeenth century; and where it was used, private failings, especially private sexual failings, were not its focus. See John Bossy, "The Social History of Confession in the Age of the Reformation," *Transactions of the Royal Historical Society*, 5th ser., 25 (1975), pp. 36–38.

116. Robert Burton, *Anatomy of Melancholy*, ed. Thomas C. Faulkner, Nicolas K. Kiessling, and Rhonda L. Blair (Oxford: Oxford University Press, 1989), 1.3.2.4, vol. 1 (417–18), and J.B. Bamborough with Martin Dodsworth, *Commentary* (Oxford: Clarendon Press, 2000), vol. 5, p. 58. Burton was following established medical opinion when he argued that "Immoderate Venus in excesse, as it is a cause, or in defect; so moderately used, to some parties an only helpe, a present remedies." He cites a case of mad maids cured by coition; "wrestlers, dicthers, and laboring men" who are likely to use up semen in their labors are cautioned to be moderate; really excessive creatures like sparrows live short lives (2.2.2.1, vol. 2, p. 32).

117. I use here Mary Douglas's famous formulation "Dirt is matter out of place" from her *Purity and Danger: An Analysis of Concepts of Pollution and Taboo* (Harmondsworth, UK: Penguin, 1970); J.F. Ostervald, *The Nature of Uncleanness Consider'd: to which is added a discourse concerning the nature of Chastity* (London,

1708). The earliest edition of this work of Ostervald's I could find in the original is the 1706 *Traité contre l'impureté* published in Amsterdam. There is an enlarged second edition printed in Neuchâtel in 1708 by Jean Pistorius. Ostervald (1663–1747) was a prominent writer whose writings on the Bible and on the question of corruption were widely translated. He was a member of the Royal Society. Parker, one of the publishers of the English edition of *The Nature of Uncleanness*, was already into sexual matters before he latched on to masturbation. His edition of Ostervald on uncleanness lets it be known that readers can buy his *Pharmacopeia veneria* at his "sign."

118. Ostervald, *Nature of Uncleanness Consider'd*, pp. 177 and 180.

119. *The life of the Reverend Mr. Geo. Trosse late minister of the gospel in the city of Exon, who died January 11th, 1712/13..., Written by himself, and publish'd according to his order...* (1714). The autobiography deals with events up to 1689 and was written in 1692–1693. It was published posthumously by his wife. After this early life of sin, Trosse became a famous nonconformist clergyman.

120. Samuel Clarke (1599–1682), *A Mirrour or Looking-Glasse both for Saints and Sinners, held forth in thousands of Examples*, 3rd. enl. ed. (London, 1657), pp. 7–11; "Examples of God's Judgments upon Whoremongers, and adulterers," pp. 67–70; "Examples of Chastity and Modesty" and throughout. Clarke was a moderate Puritan who opposed the trial of the king; he became a nonconformist after 1662 and spent the rest of his life writing popular books. He is a paradigmatic example of Puritan "warmth" toward marriage. In his memoir of his wife, he says that "she was a spur and never a bridle to him in those things which were good." Jeremy Taylor, *The rule and exercises of holy living, in which are described the means and instruments of obtaining every virtue, and the remedies against every vice, and considerations serving to the resisting all temptations. Together with prayers, containing the whole duty of a Christian, and the parts of devotion fitted to all occasions, and furnished for all necessities* (London, 1651), pp. 83–84 and 80–100 passim. Although not as popular as his *Holy Dying*, this work went through fifteen editions in London and the provinces between 1651 and 1700. It is thus all the more telling that so widely read a book specifically on "every vice" should remain silent on the solitary one.

121. William Byrd, *The London Diary (1717–1721) and Other Writings*, ed. Louis B. Wright and Marion Tinling (New York: Oxford University Press, 1958), pp. 263, 68, 72; Bernard Mandeville, *The Fable of the Bees or Private Vices, Publick Benefits*, ed. Irwin Primer (New York: Capricorn Books, 1962), p. 710.

122. "A Short Dissuasive from the Sin of Uncleanness" (1701), unpaginated. [Edward Fowler, Lord Bishop of Gloucester], *A Vindication of an Undertaking of Certain Gentlemen, in Order to the Suppressing of Debauchery and Profaneness* (London, 1692). Both of these tracts are connected to the activities of the Society for the Reformation of Manners, the vice society. The first simply declares that by "uncleanness" it means prostitution; the second makes the point implicitly. A sermon from 1727 has not taken on the new uncleanness; see Anthony Holbrook,

Christian Essays upon the Immorality of Uncleanness and dueling delivered in two sermons preached at St. Paul's (London, 1727).

123. On the vigilante societies, see Edward J. Bristow, *Vice and Vigilance: Purity Movements in Britain Since 1700* (Dublin: Gill and Macmillan, 1977), pp. 11–33. Likewise in New England, the battle was over the control of public space and virtue — the early modern culture of carnival and custom versus the new norms of behavior advocated by Puritan divines. On this, see Richard P. Gildrie, *The Profane, the Civil, and the Godly: The Reformation of Manners in Orthodox New England, 1679–1749* (University Park: Pennsylvania State University Press, 1994).

124. *God's Judgments against Whoring, being an Essay towards a General History of it . . . being a Collection of the Most Remarkable Instances of Uncleanness* (London, 1697); for Onan, see pp. 27–28. I have not been able to find the second volume.

125. Josiah Woodward, *A Rebuke to the Sin of Uncleanness. By a minister of the Church of England* (London, 1701). I used the 1704 edition, microfilm, p. 19.

126. John Calvin, for example, wrote *Four Godlye Sermons against the pollution of idolatries* (London, 1561), where the word is used in the sense the *OED* gives from another source: "His purse was verily a puritan for it kept itself from any pollution of crosses." See Edward Reynolds, *The Sinfulness of Sinne*, 4th ed. (London, 1639), pp. 321ff., for the pollution of idolatry, which is part of a whole section on the pollution of sin, considered elsewhere, as a state per se, as the source of guilt, and as an overwhelming and powerful burden on humanity. The prominent Congregational divine Henry Barrows writes about the pollution of false doctrine, "The Pollution of University Learning" (London, 1642). The *OED* gives "he had a pollution of his seed" from 1440. As Chambers's *Cyclopaedia* suggests, "nocturnal pollution" and simply spilling of seed were the usual scientific senses of the word in the early eighteenth century; see above, pp. 35–36. The only use of "self-pollution" I have found is in the entry in Capel, *Tentations: Their Nature, Danger, and Cure* (see n.130 below).

127. See Carol Kazmierczak Manzione, "Sex in Tudor London: Abusing Their Bodies with Each Other," in Murray and Eisenbichler, *Desire and Discipline*, pp. 90–93.

128. For example: W.T., *A godly and profitable treatise, intituled Absalom his fall; or, The ruin of Roysters. VVherein euery Christian may as in a mirrour behold, the vile and abominable abuse of curled long haire, so much now vsed in this our London* (London, 1590); *Cupids tryumph. Though his deity is impeached, by his power he is justified. Against the repraoches [sic] of a coy scornful lady. Being an answer to Cupids courtesie. Whoby experience found that all were stupid, which durst abuse the boundless power of Cupid* (London, 1666 and 1679); John Brinley, *A discourse proving by Scripture & reason and the best authors, ancient and modern, that there are witches: and how far their power extends to the doing of mischief both to man and beast: and likewise the use and abuse of astrology . . .* (London, 1686). To be very precise, "abusers of themselves with mankind" is how Calvin's English translator

renders his French translation of Jerome's Vulgate "neque masculorum concubitores."

129. There is one candidate for a seventeenth-century condemnation of masturbation that would increase my estimate. It is a tract titled *Letters of Advice from Two Reverend Divines to a Young Gentleman, about a Weighty Case of Conscience* supposedly published in 1676. Perhaps such a tract really existed, but it cannot have made much of an impact; there are no contemporary allusions to it, no references from the eighteenth century, and no extant copies. It is not cited in the ESTC. The extant version, if an original ever existed, is as a supplement to some editions of *Eronania* in the 1720s. I suspect the work is a fraud. Of course, other references might be found. But I come to my estimate of three pages after a thorough search of the likely suspects.

130. Richard Capel (1586–1656), *Tentations: Their Nature, Danger, and Cure*, 5th ed. (London, 1655). (There had been four previous editions, in 1633, 1635, 1636, and 1637.) "Epistle to the Reader, n.p.," pp. 2–3, 22–24, 30–40, 205–207, 210–11, 213ff. The book is in four parts; parts 1–3 are 387 pages; part 4, with new pagination but bound with the other three, has 298 pages.

131. Defoe, *The Little Review*, vol. 5, p. 71. Beverland first came to my attention through a brief mention in Michael Stolberg's "Self-Pollution, Moral Reform, and the Venereal Trade: Notes on the Sources and Historical Context of the *Onania* (1716)," *Journal of the History of Sexuality* 9.1–2 (Jan.–April 2000). I am immensely grateful to Theo van der Meer of the University of Amsterdam for sending me the information I have used in these paragraphs. The claim that *De fornicatione* is a satire is made by R. de Smet, *Hadrianus Beverlandus (1650–1716): Non unus e multis peccator. Studie over het leven en werk van Hadriaan Beverland*, Verhandelingen van de Koninklijke Academie voor Wetenschappen, Letteren en Schone Kunsten van België, Klasse der Letteren, vol. 50, 1988, nr. 126, Brussels. It was already regarded as such in G. Peignot, *Dictionnaire critique, littéraire et bibliographique des principaux livres condamnés au feu, supprimés ou censurés* (Paris, 1806), pp. 33–35. Other biographical information comes from P.C. Molhuysen et al., *Nieuw Nederlandsch biografisch woordenboek*, 10 vols. (Leiden, 1911–1937), vol. 7, pp. 126–27, as well as from the bookseller Paul Snijders of The Hague. There is an English-language account of this mad jurist and philologist in E.J. Dingwall, "Hadrian Beverland, Lord of Zealand," in *Very Peculiar People: Portrait Studies in the Queer, the Abnormal, and the Uncanny* (London: Rider, 1950).

132. On these dates, see the discussion in Stolberg, "Self-Pollution, Moral Reform, and the Venereal Trade." If I am right that John Marten wrote *Onania*, then one might be inclined to go for an earlier date. *The Monthly Catalogue, 1714– 1717 [a catalogue of all books, sermons, and pamphlets, published in May 1714, and in every month to this time]* (London, 1714–1717; London: Gregg Press, 1964), 3.6 (Oct. 1716), says that Paul Varenne offers *Onania* for 1 shilling.

133. *The Diary of Samuel Pepys*, ed. Robert Latham and William Matthews

(Berkeley: University of California Press, 1976), vol. 2, p. 204; vol. 2, p. 230; vol. 2, p. 232. References to his giving in to both the playhouse and the pub are everywhere during the first years of the diary. I am grateful to Joseph Roach, who was kind enough to send me his typescript paper "The Practice of Performance: Pepys, Shakespeare, and the Performance of Everyday Life," which he wrote for the 2001 meeting of the Shakespeare Society of America. There he makes the point that both theater and masturbation are forms of vicariousness, both performances that engage fantasy. The index to the Latham and Matthews edition, vol. 10, gives all the instances in which Pepys reports masturbating.

134. *Diary of Samuel Pepys*, vol. 7, p. 365; vol. 8, p. 588; vol. 9, p. 184; vol. 6, p. 331; vol. 2, pp. 230 and 232; vol. 6, p. 191.

135. John Cannon, "Memoirs of the Birth, Education, Life, and Death of Mr. John Cannon. Some time Officer of the Excise and Writing Master at Mere Glastenbury and West Lyford in the County of Somerset, 1684–1742," Somerset Record Office, DD/SAS C/1193/4, pp. 28–29. I am grateful to Tim Hitchcock of the University of North London for sending me his transcription of large parts of this unpublished memoir.

136. Jean Delumeau, *Sin and Fear: The Emergence of a Western Guilt Culture, 13th–18th Centuries*, trans. Eric Nicholson (New York: St. Martins Press, 1900), p. 4.

CHAPTER FOUR: THE PROBLEM WITH MASTURBATION

1. C.F. Lallemand, *Des pertes seminales involontaires* (Paris, 1836–1842), vol. 3, p. 477; Edward Shorter, *The Making of the Modern Family* (New York: Basic Books, 1975).

2. Jean-Louis Flandrin, *Families in Former Times* (Cambridge, UK: Cambridge University Press, 1976), pp. 211 and more generally 189–91 and 209–11.

3. It is still impossible to say what proportion of people masturbate or have masturbated.

4. For a summary of the literature on the collapse of barriers to "sexual-intercourse-so-called" (Henry Abelove's phrase), see Thomas Laqueur, "Sex, Gender, and Desire in the Industrial Revolution," in Patrick O'Brien and Roland Quinault (eds.), *The Industrial Revolution and British Society: Festschrift for R.M. Hartwell* (Cambridge, UK: Cambridge University Press, 1993). Perhaps opportunities to engage in sodomy decreased in the Protestant world and even in some Catholic countries as the monastic life disappeared or was sharply curtailed. Secular authorities cracked down hard in the early eighteenth century on new lay sodomitic male cultures. But there is no evidence that solitary sex in fact led to sodomitic sex, as had so often been claimed, and no reason to believe that it served as a substitute when the real thing was not available. No eighteenth-century commentator linked a putative rise in sodomy to a putative epidemic of masturbation.

5. There would be exceptions in the nineteenth century as masturbation

was mobilized for almost every cause. It was, for example, part of the neo-asceticism of someone like the American health reformer J.H. Kellogg. For him, all sexual activity was potentially enervating, disorderly, and sinful: "Illicit commerce of the sexes is a heinous sin, self-pollution . . . is a crime doubly abominable." Sylvester Graham, an equally fervent foe of masturbation, shared Kellogg's ethos of restraint and sublimation — vegetarianism, temperance. Marriage, he thought, existed not to satisfy but to blunt sexual desire — familiarity breeds disinterest — which was a good thing, since having coition more than twelve times a year was to risk one's health. On Graham, the inventor of the cracker, see Jayme A. Sokolow, *Eros and Modernization: Sylvester Graham, Health Reform, and the Origins of Victorian Sexuality in America* (Rutherford, NJ: Fairleigh Dickinson University Press, 1983), pp. 84–91. Sokolow makes the useful point that sexual restraint, especially with respect to masturbation, was part of a more general reform program meant to cope with the excitement and allure of urban life.

6. See note 35 in ch. 2.

7. There is an excellent summary of Enlightenment views of pleasure in Roy Porter and Lesley Hall, *The Facts of Life: The Creation of Sexual Knowledge in Britain, 1650–1950* (New Haven, CT: Yale University Press, 1995), ch. 3.

8. See Théodore Tarczylo, *Sexe et liberté au siècle des lumières* (Paris: Presses de la Renaissance, 1983), ch. 2. See David Stevenson, *The Beggar's Benison: Sex Clubs of Enlightenment Scotland and Their Rituals* (East Lothian, Scotland: Tuckwell Press, 2001), pp. 69–93 and 98–99. I came upon this book only after mine had already been copyedited.

9. Goss and Co., *The Aegis of Life*, 23rd ed. (London, 1840), p. 59. Roy Porter has argued that, from the eighteenth century on, quacks created and preyed on masturbatory fears by promoting the joys of sexual intercourse under appropriate circumstances. See *Health for Sale: Quackery in England, 1660–1850* (Manchester: Manchester University Press, 1989), pp. 169–79. Goss and Co., *Hygeiana: A Non-medical Analysis of the Complaints Incidental to Females*, 20th ed. (London, 1830), p. 62.

10. John Quincy, *Medicina Statica: Being the Aphorisms of Sanctorius* (London, 1712), aphorisms 34 and 37.

11. The old sin was not entirely dead. In the context of moral theology, it subsisted into the modern period as the long-familiar unnatural vice, as a species of pollution, and as an aspect of the prohibition against birth control, that is, sexual intercourse for its own sake and not for procreation. There were constant casuistic adjustments: in 1665, for example, Pope Alexander VII condemned the view that one had only to confess to pollution if one had also committed sodomy or bestiality because all three were of the same *species infima*. The question of whether a woman can pollute herself in the same sense as a man continued to be debated. In general, the answer is no: no *effusio seminis* takes place, since women have no true semen; therefore, masturbation in women is a species of *tactus*

460

impudici, "indecent touches," whose use was otherwise regulated. But this was not the sort of stuff that drove the new anxiety about solitary sex in modernity. On these points, see Aloysius J. Welsh, *The Scholastic Teaching Concerning the Specific Distinction of Sins in the Light of Moral Theology* (Washington, DC: Catholic University of America Press, 1942), pp. 61–62; Julius Preuss, *Biblical and Talmudic Medicine,* trans. and ed. Fred Rosner (New York: Sanhedrin Press, 1978), pp. 489–90; Cari Capellmann, *Pastoral Medicine,* trans. William Dassel (New York: Pustet, 1879).

12. S.A.D. Tissot, *Onanism; or, A Treatise upon the Disorders Produced by Masturbation; or, The Dangerous Effects of Secret and Excessive Venery,* trans. A. Hume (London, 1761), p. 72.

13. *Ibid.,* p. 32.

14. For the EEG and masturbatory orgasm controversy, see Harvey D. Cohen et al., "Electroencephalographic Laterality Changes During Human Orgasm," *Archives of Sexual Behavior* 5.3 (1976), pp. 188–89, and Benjamin Grabe et al., "EEG During Masturbation and Ejaculation," *Archives of Sexual Behavior* 14.6 (1985); for the forty-one-year-old epileptic, see Daniel E. Jacome, "Absence Status Manifested by Compulsive Masturbation," *Archives of Neurology* 40 (Aug. 1983), pp. 523–24. Apparently, so-called benign non-epileptic paroxysmal events (NEPE) or abdominal pain is commonplace; differentiating those caused by masturbation from those due to an underlying disease is not easy, especially in very young children. One set of pediatricians advises that parents be counseled to recognize masturbation as a normal and commonplace activity that might have certain physical manifestations that mimic something serious and that, once this is clear, many unnecessary diagnostic procedures can be avoided. See David R. Fleisher et al., "Masturbation Mimicking Abdominal Pain or Seizures in Young Girls," *Journal of Pediatrics* 116.5 (May 1990), pp. 810–14; C.H. Wulff et al., "Epileptic Fits or Infantile Masturbation," *Seizure* 1.3 (Sept. 1992), pp. 199–201; S. Livingston, "Masturbation Stimulating Masturbation," *Clinical Pediatrics* 14 (1975), pp. 232–34.

15. "Epilepsy," in Albert H. Buck, ed., *A Reference Handbook of the Medical Sciences,* new rev. ed. (New York: William Wood and Co., 1901), vol. 3, p. 849. There is a fairly large contemporary neurological literature on masturbation and various kinds of seizures, but the old normative questions are both absent and moot.

16. For a powerful version of this view, see G.J. Barker-Benfield, *The Horrors of the Half-Known Life: Male Attitudes Toward Women and Sexuality in Nineteenth-Century America* (1976; New York: Routledge, 2000).

17. Roy Porter, "Sex and the Singular Man: The Seminal Ideas of James Graham," *Studies on Voltaire and the Eighteenth Century* 228 (1984). On Isidore and Harvey, see Thomas Laqueur, *Making Sex: Body and Gender from the Greeks to Freud* (Cambridge, MA: Harvard University Press, 1990), pp. 56, 144.

18. Tissot, *Onanism,* p. 52; "semence," in *Encyclopédie,* vol. 16, p. 939;

Friedrich Hoffmann the Younger, *Opera omnia* (1740), bk. 2, cap. 8, p. 23: "Seminalis liquor delibatissiumus, quai flos sanguinis as liquidi nervorum est, hinc deligenter circumspiciendum, ne immoderate ejus excretio sanitatem offendat." In his day, Hoffmann was considered the greatest of the iatrochemists, those who thought they could understand pathology as a failure of a mechanistically understood physiology. Exactly what he, and indeed other eighteenth-century doctors, understood by semen in these general contexts is difficult to pinpoint. Hoffmann thought that a kind of ether acted through the nervous system on the muscles and kept them, as well as the body's fluids, in motion; it animated life. At times it seems almost as if semen were that ether.

19. Tissot, *Onanism*, p. 2; Winfield Scott Hall, assisted by Jeannette Winter Hall, *Sexual Knowledge* (London: T. Werner, n.d.; first American ed., 1913), pp. 143–44. This appeared in the New Century Series of Physiology. Hall argued that loss from nocturnal emission was not so bad either, because those sperm were dead anyway. He is right that the sperm lost by nocturnal emission are mostly dead; but so would those released in any other way if the subject had not ejaculated for forty-eight hours. Sperm, in short, have a limited life.

20. Tissot's section 6 has nine pages, 48–57, just on "the importance of seminal liquor." Thomas Cogan, *The hauen of health, chiefly made for the comfort of students, and consequently for all those that haue a care of their health, amplified vpon fiue wordes of Hippocrates, written Epid. 6. Labour, meat, drinke, sleepe, Venus: Hereunto is added a preseruation from the pestilence: with a short censure of the late sicknesse at Oxford* (London, 1612), p. 242; Avicenna's *Canon*, from which the *De animalibus* that Cogan cites comes, was available in scores of early modern Latin editions and some vernacular translations.

21. See Albert Müller, *Ueber unwillkürliche Samenverluste und über functionelle Störungen der männlichen Geschlechtsorgane: Eine wissenschaftliche Abhandlung* (Rorschach, 1869). The quotation to this effect is on the title page. In fact, in the text Müller emphasizes the nervous, frictional etiology of masturbatory disease; the problem is that in heterosexual intercourse the degree of friction is determined by the vagina, which after several births becomes slack — hence men tend to be unfaithful to wives who have borne many children. But masturbators have complete control of the amount of force they use and thus overexcite the organs. Seminal loss is not the half of it. See Müller, pp. 23–34.

22. See, for example, the learned and up-to-date discussion "Semen," by the German researchers Wagener and Lueckart, in Robert B. Todd, *The Cyclopaedia of Anatomy and Physiology* (London, 1835–1859), vol. 4, pt. 1, pp. 472–508. There is a lot here on the morphology of sperm, the chemical composition of seminal fluid, and the various stages of spermatogenesis but nothing on life force, vital energy, or highest concoction of blood. In other words, what was new about semen was irrelevant to the masturbation discussion. In fact, this natural philosophy of semen was articulated by a man named Louis de La Caze, whose *Idée de l'homme physique et moral, pour servir d'introduction à un traité de*

médicine (Paris, 1755) greatly influenced the author of the encyclopedia article on masturbation. He was, so thought his research assistant, completely mad, but this seems not to have diminished the appeal of his theories. There is a superb account of this in Anne C. Vila, *Enlightenment and Pathology: Sensibility in the Literature and Medicine of Eighteenth-Century France* (Baltimore: Johns Hopkins University Press, 1998), pp. 48–52. All of these cases are in Tissot, *Onanism*, pp. 36–39.

23. *Onania Examined and detected; or, The ignorance, error, impertinence, and contradiction of a book called Onania discovered and exposed . . . By Philo-Castitatis,* 2nd ed. (London, 1724), pp. 81–82.

24. G. Stanley Hall, *Adolescence: Its Psychology and Its Relationship to Physiology, Anthropology, Sociology, Sex, Crime, Religion, and Education* (1904; New York and London: D. Appleton, 1924), vol. 1, p. 440.

25. Tissot, *Onanisme*, p. 86. Michael Ryan, *Lectures on Population, Marriage, and Divorce* (London, 1831), p. 32.

26. Tissot, *Onanism*, p. 19, for example; "Masturbation," in *Grand Dictionnaire universel du XIXe siècle* (Paris: Administration du Grand Dictionnaire Universel, 1975), vol. 14, pp. 1320–22. The article also provides a useful list of eighteenth- and nineteenth-century medical dissertations on the subject. I am referring to the educator Johann Stuve in his *Über die körperliche Erziehung* (Züllichau, 1781) speaking through the voice of Campe, the leader of the "friends of humanity" and the man who set the prize essay question for the *Berliner Monatsschrift* in 1785. Quoted in Karl Heinz Bloch, *Die Bekämpfung der Jugendmasturbation im 18. Jahrhundert: Ursachen, Verlauf, Nachwirkungen* (Frankfurt am Main, New York: Peter Lang, 1998), pp. 354–55.

27. *Onania*, p. 43; *Dictionnaire portatif de santé*, 4th ed. (Paris, 1771), vol. 2, p. 339; Tissot, *Onanism*, pp. 41 and 41–48 passim. J.G. Zimmermann, "Warnung an Eltern, Erzieher und Kinderfreunde wegen der Selbst-befleckung, zumal bein ganz jungen madchen," *Deutsches Museum* 1 (1778), pp. 453–54; P.J.C. Debreyne, *Essai sur la théologie morale* (Paris, 1844), pp. 111–35, contains some of the goriest tales in this whole sad literature. The works of J.L. Doussin-Dubreuil are also rich on the question of women and masturbation. See his *Des égaremens secrets, ou, De l'onanisme chez les personnes du sexe* (Paris, 1830). This is the source of the illustration and is in the form of letters to mothers to save their daughters from such a fate. His *Nouveau Manuel sur les dangers de l'onanisme*, new ed. (Paris, 1839), letter 8 and esp. p. 125, gives stomach, uterine, and nervous ailments as especially prominent as consequences of the abuse of solitary pleasure.

28. Sigmund Freud, "Some Psychical Consequences of the Anatomical Distinction Between the Sexes," in *The Standard Edition of the Complete Psychological Works of Sigmund Freud*, trans. James Strachey (London: Hogarth, 1953–74), vol. 19, p. 255.

29. J.H. Kellogg, *Natural History and Hygiene of Organic Life*, new rev. ed. (Burlington, IA: I.F. Segner, 1895), p. 231, made a point of remarking on the vice

in girls. One could always blur the lines here. Peter Villaume, writing in the great German pedagogical compendium of the eighteenth century, says that while women and children do not produce semen, they produce something similar which is also, like true semen, a distillation of all the body's parts with especial drain on the brain and spinal fluid; see *Über die Unzuchtsünden in der Jugend* (*About the sins of lasciviousness among youth*) in *Allgemeine Revision*, vol. 7, p. 44.

30. O.S. Fowler, *Amativeness; or, Evils and Remedies of Excessive and Perverted Sexuality* (Wortley, UK, c. 1849), p. 4; in his much longer (more than a thousand pages) and widely selling general textbook on what phrenology had to offer that all-important sphere of human activity — marriage and reproduction — Fowler quotes a leading Philadelphia doctor as the authority for the fact that five-sixths of female complaints are caused, or exacerbated, by masturbation. The claim is accompanied by the sad story of a young dentist's wife who had become a "vacant, staring simpleton" as a result of early self-abuse. O.S. Fowler, *Creative and Sexual Science: or, manhood & womanhood, and their mutual interrelations; love, its laws, power, etc. . . as taught by phrenology and physiology* (Pittsburgh: F.F. Spyer and Co., 1875), see pp. 873–910 for one of the most horrendous accounts on record of the physical ill effects of "personal fornication," "twenty times worse than any other sexual sin" and specifically pp. 877–78, 881, and 886 for the views cited. Thomas Low Nichols, *Esoteric Anthropology (The Mysteries of Man): A comprehensive and confidential treatise on the structure, functions, passional attractions, and perversions . . . and the most intimate relations of men and women* (1853), pp. 280–81. Nichols goes on to say that while some might take the loss of semen to be the primary cause of masturbatory ills, it clearly is not. Nichols's wife, Mary S. Gove Nichols — cited as an authority on masturbation by Fowler — published several oft-reprinted lectures on women's health and anatomy as well as novels and literary studies. Copland does in fact say this in the context of claiming that the "baneful effect of [masturbation] is very much greater in both sexes than is commonly supposed" and is a "growing evil"; see James Copland, "insanity," in *A Dictionary of Practical Medicine* (London, 1858), vol. 2, sec. 303.b. For asylum diagnoses, see Ann Goldberg, *Sex, Religion, and the Making of Modern Madness: The Eberbach Asylum and German Society, 1815–1849* (New York: Oxford University Press, 1999), pp. 88–89. Why this was true is not clear. Goldberg may well be right that German doctors of the period regarded the archetypal male masturbator as stunted, exhausted, listless, and ultimately mad and the female as tending toward the aggressive and nymphomaniacal, but this was not generally the case in nineteenth-century medicine. Harry Oosterhuis, *Stepchildren of Nature: Krafft-Ebing, Psychiatry, and the Making of Sexual Identity* (Chicago: University of Chicago Press, 2001), p. 153. Mary S. Gove [Nichols], *Lectures to Ladies on Anatomy and Physiology* (Boston, 1842), pp. 222–23 and 217–31 generally. Gove surveys the medical literature to produce an impressive list of diseases to which men and women seem equally liable — everything from

464

blindness to St. Vitus's dance and heart palpitations; other diseases, such as menstrual dysfunction and impotence are, of course, sex-specific.

31. Zimmermann, "Warnung an Eltern," p. 455; Christian Gotthilf Salzmann, *Über die heimlichen Sünden der Jugend* (Frankfurt and Leipzig, 1786), pp. 10–11; "manstrupration," in *Encyclopédie*, vol. 10, pp. 51–53; one could multiply these sorts of citations. Dr. Samuel Gottlieb Vogel listed the dangers to each sex separately but argued, in his 1786 *Unterricht fur Eltern*, that they were far greater for girls; he wrote an entire article on the case of a woman who committed suicide as a consequence of the "secret vice." If one could survey the entire eighteenth- and nineteenth-century literature, one would almost certainly find far more cases of boys than of girls masturbating, far more written against the practice in one sex than in the other.

32. Anastasia Verbitskaia, *Moemu chitatelin* (To my readers) (Moscow, 1908), pp. 331–34. I am grateful to Hilda Hoogenbloom for this reference and for the translation. For Verbitskaia's place in the gender politics of late-tsarist Russia, see Laura Engelstein, *The Keys to Happiness: Sex and the Search for Modernity in Fin-de-siècle Russia* (Ithaca, NY: Cornell University Press, 1992), pp. 399–403. Engelstein takes her title from that of Verbitskaia's most famous novel.

33. Tarczylo, *Sexe et Liberté*, ch. 4. See http://jackfilm.8m.com/mp.html. At the time of the correction of the proofs this site is "temporarily unavailable." Since many of the films that feature men are about sperm donation, the comparison as an indicator of erotic interest does not quite work.

34. I rely on Anne Vila's excellent account of the moral physiology of sensibility in *Enlightenment and Pathology*, esp. pp. 43–107.

35. Readers' reactions to reading Rousseau and others were sent to the publisher Panckoucke and are discussed in Robert Darnton, *The Great Cat Massacre* (New York: Vintage, 1985), pp. 243–47; S.A.D. Tissot, "Diseases Incidental to Literary and Sedentary Persons," in *Three essays: First, on the disorders of people of fashion; Second on diseases incidental to literary and sedentary Persons with proper rules for preventing their fatal consequences; Third, on Onanism . . .*, trans. Francis Bacon Lee, M. Danes, and A. Hume (Dublin, 1772), p. 15.

36. Albrecht von Haller, *A dissertation on the sensible and irritable parts of animals. By M.A. Haller, . . . Translated from the Latin. With a preface by M. Tissot, M.D. (De partibus corporis humani sensibilibus et irritabilibus)* (London, 1755), pp. iv and i–xx passim. The English translator is not given; the English preface is reprinted from Tissot's to the Lausanne French edition.

37. On Haller, see *ibid.* and Vila, *Enlightenment and Pathology*, pp. 21–28. Semen, of course, might come back into the picture insofar as it was construed as a kind of spirituous substance that men and women, boys and girls shared as a basic building block of the body. In this sense, it constituted a sort of elementary particle, the quark of life. Nerves and semen had been thought to have a close affinity since Greek Antiquity. But the crucial point is that nerves could be damaged without any loss of what we would recognize as semen.

38. Physician of Bristol, *Tabes dorsalis; or, the cause of consumption in young men and women, with an explication of its symptoms, precautions, and the method of cure ... To which is added, a physical account of the nature and effects of venery, ... By a physician of Bristol. The sixth edition* (London, [1770?]), p. 8. The first three editions, 1753–1758, dealt only with men. The author cites as his authority one of the many English versions of the aphorisms of Sanctorius — Santorio Santorio, professor of medicine at Padua in the late sixteenth and the early seventeenth century and a representative figure in the development of a mechanistic medicine. He is most famous for eating his meals at a chair and table attached to a scale and thereby quantifying "the insensible perspiration" that accounted for the weight loss of metabolism, the difference between input and final weight. The aphorisms, though many are quoted in the eighteenth-century discussion of masturbation as the most dangerous species of venery, do not take up the subject. It was, as noted earlier, a nonsubject before 1714 or so. William Clark, *A medical dissertation concerning the effects of the passions on human bodies; first published in Latin, at Leyden, on the 31st of July, 1727, for acquiring the honour and privilege of doctor in physick ... and now republished in English [Dissertatio medica inauguralis de viribus animi pathematum in corpus humanum]* (London, 1752), p. 38; *A practical essay upon the tabes dorsalis, in the way of aphorism and commentary: In which the history of that distemper is laid down, the rationale of its symptoms given, and the method of cure* (London, 1748), p. 6.

39. Tissot, *Onanism*, pp. 81–83 and 127–28; see on Sanctorius, John Quincy, *Medicina Statica: Being the Aphorisms of Sanctorious* (London, 1712), sec. 6 generally, and pp. 258 and 242–43 specifically.

40. *Précis historique, physiologique et moral, des principaux objets ... qui composent le museum de J-Fois Bertrand-Rival* (Paris, 1805), pp. 344–45.

41. See, for example, the discussion by William Cullen — founder of the Glasgow medical school, one of the most famous clinicians of eighteenth-century nerves, and a great proponent of the view that disease arose from disturbances of nervous energies which were the stuff of life — of *tabes dorsalis*, the disease most associated with masturbation. He did not mention it as a cause and doubted that fluid loss caused the disease at all. William Cullen, *First Lines of the Practice of Physic with Supplementary Notes by Peter Reid* (Brookfield, MA, 1807), pp. 574–79. The book was first published in 1777 and went through more than a score of editions before 1800.

42. Mary Scharlieb and F. Arthur Sibly, *Youth and Sex: Its Dangers and Safeguards for Boys and Girls* (London, c. 1910), p. 44. Scharlieb's contribution on girls in a volume for the distinguished series The People's Books does not worry directly about masturbation; Sibly, who quotes extensively from his contribution to the International Congress on Moral Education in 1908, clearly regards it as the most pressing question imaginable. While in many ways Sibly was typical of those who wrote on masturbation and moral purity, he developed a particularly intrusive and personal system of investigating the solitary sexual lives of each

pupil and treating those in need by hypnosis, a then-novel therapy. Sibly never understood the homoerotic qualities of his preoccupations. On the accusations against Sibly, his firing, and his treatment by Ernest Jones, the translator of Freud and a major figure in the reconceptualization of solitary sex, see Chris Waters's paper "Onanism, Homosexuality, and the Adolescent Boy: The Case of Dr. Arthur Sibly and Dr. Ernest Jones," for which I am grateful to Waters.

43. Sigmund Freud, "On the Universal Tendency to Debasement in Love," in *Complete Works*, vol. 9, p. 182.

44. *The Crime of Onan* (London, c. 1724), p. iii (BL 1173 b.9/11). This is one of the Anodyne-Necklace family of publications; pagination differs from edition to unnumbered edition.

45. *Encyclopédie*, vol. 10, p. 51; Denis Diderot, *D'Alembert's Dream*, in *Rameau's Nephew and Other Works*, trans. Jacques Barzun and Ralph Bowen (Indianapolis: Bobbs-Merrill, 1980), pp. 169–70.

46. *Onania*, p. 90. Of course, children were not meant to have such desire or such pleasures at all, but that is another story, for later.

47. Tissot, *Onanism*, pp. 88 and 155.

48. Christoph Wilhelm Hufeland, *Die Kunst das menschliche Leben*, 3rd ed. (Jena, 1798), pt. 2, pp. 14–16. The English translation, a reworking of an earlier, 1797 version — dedicated to the aphorist, scientist, and general man of letters Georg Christoph Lichtenberg — appeared in London in 1854. Erasmus Wilson, the editor, does not translate this passage and instead remarks that he might "if necessary draw a painful, nay a frightful, picture of the result of these melancholy excesses" but that he refrains. But he warns that "the excesses most to be dread are those … in which the imagination and the feelings play a conspicuous part." The 1797 translation was, in turn, based on a 1794 one. This stuff is clearly centrally located in the Enlightenment world of medicine and letters.

49. D.T. de Bienville, *Nymphomania; or, A dissertation concerning the furor uterinus. Clearly and methodically explaining the beginning, progress, and different causes of that horrible distemper. To which are added, the methods of treating the several stages of it, and the most approved remedies. Written originally in French*, trans. Edward Sloane Wilmot (London, 1775).

50. *Dictionnaire portatif de santé*, vol. 2, p. 340, and the article "Pollution volontaire." "Spermatorrhea" and "onanisme," in *Dictionnaire encyclopédique des sciences medicales*, 3rd ser., vol. 11; "Mary Wood-Allen, *What a Young Woman Ought to Know* (Philadelphia: Vir Publishing Company, 1899, 1905), p. 155. Wood-Allen was head of the purity department of the Women's Christian Temperance Union, but her distinctly American voice, duly translated, seemed to be in much demand all over Europe and in the British Empire.

51. My emphasis. A.P. Buchan, *Venus sine concubitu* (Venus without intercourse) (London, 1818), pp. 50–51 and 43–44. Alexander Peter Buchan was the son and editor of William Buchan, whose *Domestic Medicine* went through scores of eighteenth- and early-nineteenth-century editions and vied with Tissot in

popularity among English-speaking audiences. A.P. not only edited some of his father's works and translated works from French but also published on venereal disease, sea bathing, pediatrics, and classifying diseases; see his notes on his lectures at Westminster Hospital. He says that the ideas in *Venus* were formed fifteen years earlier in the context of his disagreement with John Hunter (see n.53 below). He makes much of the bandied-about fact that hypochondriacal diseases were in the ascendancy. A case in point is an otherwise strong boy who suffered no ill effects from masturbation until he read Tissot and then began thinking he was deadly ill (p. 68). But instead of concluding, as had Hunter and as would some of Freud's colleagues, that guilt about masturbation and not the thing itself caused illness, Buchan takes the view I quote.

52. Thomas Beddoes, *Hygëia; or, Essays Moral and Medical* (Bristol, UK, 1802), p. 48.

53. John Hunter, *A Treatise on the Venereal Disease*, 1st ed. (London, 1786), 2nd ed. (London, 1788), pp. 199–200. See Isabel Hull, *Sexuality, State, and Civil Society in Germany, 1700–1815* (Ithaca, NY: Cornell University Press, 1996), pp. 161–62, for an account of some hostile late-eighteenth-century German reviews of anti-masturbatory literature; like Hunter, one argued that if it were really all that bad "then the whole human race would long since have died out." Because, as I argue, the question is more an ethical than a medical one, such perfectly reasonable views had no impact until the early twentieth century, when the underlying problems of sexuality and self changed.

54. Hunter, *Treatise on the Venereal Disease*, 1st ed., p. 200. The comment is missing in the second edition and by the third edition, in 1810, the whole section has been replaced by a conventional attack on masturbation. See note 57 below.

55. Sándor Ferenczi, "On Onanism," in *Contributions to Psychoanalysis*, trans. Ernest Jones (Boston: Richard G. Badger, c. 1916), pp. 157–63.

56. Duncan Gordon, *A Letter to John Hunter respecting His Treatise on the Venereal Disease... in Favour of Onanism or Masturbation* (London, 1786), pp. 17–18 and passim. Gordon concludes with a sycophantic acknowledgment of Hunter's greatness and the value of his discoveries about venereal disease.

57. John Hunter, *A Treatise on the Venereal Disease enlarged with occasional comments by the editor...*, 3rd ed., ed. Everard Home (London, 1810), pp. 214–15. Home wrote not only on surgical matters — treatment of gunshot wounds, ulcers, constricted urethras, for example — but also on problems in comparative anatomy. Once again, like many of those who wrote against masturbation, he was a leader in his field. He was knighted for his distinction.

58. "Pollution nocturne," in *Encyclopédie*, vol. 10, p. 924, col. 1; Pliny, *Natural History* 36.21–22; Leonard Barkan, "The Beholder's Tale: Ancient Sculpture, Renaissance Narratives," *Representations* 44 (Autumn, 1993), pp. 133–66; "Masturbation," in *Dictionnaire des sciences medicales* (1819). The idea that art produces sexual excitement runs right through the literature on masturbation and deviant sexuality more generally. A late-nineteenth-century American doctor in

an article on nymphomania begins his discussion with the observation that he was "unable to find more than one percent [of those viewing nude statuary in museums or parks] who do not present an increased sexual desire at the sights referred to." L.M. Philips, "Nymphomania — Reply to Questions," *Cincinnati Medical Journal* 10.7 (1895), pp. 467–68.

59. William Farrer, *A short treatise on onanism; or, The detestable vice of self-pollution. Describing the variety of nervous or other disorders, that are occasioned by that shameful practice, or too early and excessive venery, and directing the best method for their cure, By a physician in the country* (London, 1767), p. v. The tract went through at least one more edition the same year.

60. Throughout this book, I have used the terms "fantasy" and "imagination" interchangeably, although there is a long history of the question whether they are the same thing. Coleridge famously distinguished the two. My interest is in our capacity to fantasize, to make something new out of what our senses provide us. This would technically be fantasy. But many of the figures I cite use the term "imagination" — strictly "likeness making" from something less faithful to reality. Just as so many eighteenth- and nineteenth-century figures used the terms promiscuously, so will I. On the intellectual history of the distinction, see the old but excellent survey by Wilma L. Kennedy, *The English Heritage of Coleridge of Bristol, 1798: The Basis in Eighteenth-Century English Thought for His Distinction Between Imagination and Fancy* (New Haven, CT: Yale University Press, 1947). Sigmund Freud, "A Discussion of Masturbation," in *Complete Works*, vol. 12; Anthony Frank Campagna, "The Function of Men's Erotic Fantasies During Masturbation," Ph.D. thesis, Yale University, 1975.

61. This last sense of secrecy is the subject of Frank Kermode's study of the interpretation of the Gospels in *The Genesis of Secrecy: On the Interpretation of Narrative* (Cambridge, MA: Harvard University Press, 1979).

62. *Onania*, p. 11; *Curse of Onan and Eronania* 1173.b.9 (London: Parker, 1724), pt. 2 [separately paginated], pp. 4, vii–viii.

63. Tissot, *Onanism*, p. xi.

64. *Onania*, 17th ed., p. 98.

65. Richard Carlile, *Everywoman's Book*, in M.L. Bush (ed.), *What Is Love? Richard Carlile's Philosophy of Sex* (London: Verso, 1998), pp. 98–99, and commentary, 142–43.

66. I do not mean to imply here that there was not a sense of inner self prior to, or outside, the development of secrecy and privacy. One might read Stephen Greenblatt's account of Spenser, for example, in *Renaissance Self-Fashioning: From More to Shakespeare* (Chicago: University of Chicago Press, 1980).

67. See Richard Rambuss, *Closet Devotions* (Durham, NC: Duke University Press, 1998), pp. 106 and 121, "The Prayer Closet" more generally. Books like *The Puritan Divine* and Oliver Heywood's *Closet-Prayer* were immensely popular, and the whole genre of private devotional literature thrived in seventeenth-century England both among Puritans and among more mainstream Anglicans.

68. G. Giorgi and M. Siccardi, "Ultrasonic Observation of the Female Fetus' Sexual Behavior in Utero," letter in the *American Journal of Obstetrics and Gynecology* 175 (Sept. 1996), p. 753.

69. Zimmermann, "Warnung an Eltern," p. 453. Zimmermann meant here boys; girls, judging by his examples, tend to learn masturbation on their own: itching from worms around the genitals produces pleasure and then self-pollution without irritation. Other doctors had plenty of stories of girls who learned from other girls.

70. Jean-Marc-Gaspard Itard, *The Wild Boy of Aveyron (Rapports et mémoires sur le sauvage de l'Aveyron,* second report 1807), trans. George Humphrey and Muriel Humphrey (New York: Century Co., 1932), pp. 96–99. The bibliographic citation is a bit odd since there is no French text called *The Wild Boy of Aveyron* or even *Rapports et mémoires.* The text is in fact a translation of Itard's *Rapport fait à son excellence le Ministre de l'intérieur sur les nouveaux développements et l'état actuel du sauvage de l'Aveyron* (Paris, 1807).

71. Tissot, *Onanism,* pp. 77 and 44–45; Salzmann, *Uber die heimlichen Sünden,* p. 239.

72. Zimmermann, "Warnung an Eltern," p. 283; Sixt Karl Kapff, *Warnung eines Jugendfreundes vor dem gefährlichsten Jugendfeind; oder, Belehrung über geheime Sünden, ihre Folgen, Heilung und Verhütung, durch Beispiele aus dem Leben erläutert und der Jugend und ihren Erziehern an's Herz gelegt,* 13th ed. (Stuttgart: J.F. Steinkopf, 1880), is the one I looked at. August Strindberg, *The Son of a Servant: The Story of the Evolution of a Human Being, 1849–1867,* trans. and intro. Evert Sprinchorn (Garden City, NY: Anchor Books, 1966), pp. 84–86; Max Hodann, *History of Modern Morals,* trans. Stella Browne (London: Heinemann, 1937), pp. 250–51, says it was Kapff who taught the young Strindberg that he had a secret. Kapff's work, like many of those cited in the first section of this book, was an international phenomenon; it first appeared in German in 1841 and had reached its twenty-second German edition by 1911; the once "secret sin" appeared in most European languages in all manner of places — several German editions printed in the United States, for example, presumably for the large immigrant community; Michael Meyer, *Strindberg: A Biography* (London: Secker and Warburg, 1985), pp. 16–17, citing the quotation from Strindberg's *Samlade skrifter,* vol. 18, pp. 184–85.

73. Many of the eighteenth-century German tracts are explicitly directed to teachers and parents; Tissot clearly has them in mind. I use this example from Mary Ries Melendy, *Perfect Womanhood for Maidens, Wives, Mothers* (K.T. Boland, 1901), a prolific American writer of household medical guides and of a series of books for women on eugenics.

74. *Onania,* 17th ed., p. 18; Sigmund Freud, *Three Essays on Sexuality,* in *Complete Works,* vol. 7, pp. 187 and 187–221 generally.

75. My sense of the civilizing process comes, of course, from Norbert Elias's classic, *The Civilizing Process,* trans. Edmund Jephcott (New York: Urizen Books, 1978).

76. Tissot, *Onanism*, pp. 74, 85, and 152.

77. Tissot, *Onanism*, pp. 44 and 85; Martin Bree, *Observations on the Venereal Diseases, and Certain Disorders Incident to Either Sex, from the Pernicious Habits of Youth* (1780?; London, 1800), pp. 78 and 80; Barkan, "The Beholder's Tale"; Nicholas Francis Cooke, *Satan in Society* (Cincinnati: G.F. Hovey, 1882 [1870], p. 100.

78. Edward O. Laumann, John H. Gagnon, et al., *The Social Organization of Sexuality: Sexual Practices in the United States* (Chicago: University of Chicago Press, 1994), pp. 81 and 564.

79. Jean-Jacques Rousseau, *Confessions*, trans. J.M. Cohen (Baltimore: Penguin, 1963 [1957]), p. 109; Jacques Derrida famously makes the case that masturbation is to sex what writing is to speech, the imagination to reality. It is the correlative in the body of the unboundedness of language. *Of Grammatology*, trans. Gayatri Chakravorty Spivak (Baltimore: Johns Hopkins University Press, 1976), pp. 144–52.

80. *Onania*, 8th ed., pp. 11–12.

81. Jeremy Bentham, "Essay on Pederasty," ed. Louis Compton, repr. in *Journal of Homosexuality* 3.4 (Summer 1978) and 4.1 (Fall 1978), pt. 2, pp. 101–102 and passim.

82. I do not give page numbers because, as I noted earlier, each edition of *Eronania* and the *Curse of Onan* is differently paginated and various editions are not clearly noted on the title pages. These were, after all, mass-produced advertising copy and did not adhere to more elevated literary practices.

83. Sentences like the following are everywhere in Tissot and other eighteenth- and nineteenth-century writers. The secretary of state in Basel writes to Tissot praising his onanism book — "a production of yours" — and saying that doctors must "help youth preserve themselves from the violence of desires which hurry them to *excesses,*" whence "arise these horrid disorders, or such others as disrupt their own and the happiness of society." *Onanism*, p. 149; E. Littré, *Dictionnaire de médecine*, 12th ed. (1865).

84. *Onania*, pp. 60, 149, and 173–74. The Platonic image is in *Gorgias* 493a–d. I used Plato, *Complete Works*, ed. John M. Cooper (Indianapolis, IN: Hackett Pub., 1997), p. 836.

85. Tissot, *Onanism*, pp. 79, 77, 24. Whether we are to credit the claim that the boy in question did it even during his lessons and that he died miserably from his masturbation addiction is another story.

86. Thomas Trotter, *An Essay, Medical, Philosophical, and Chemical, on Drunkenness and Its Effects on the Human Body* (London, 1804), vol. 2, pp. 144 and 170. Trotter (1760–1832) was a much-published naval surgeon. The custom of fashion Trotter is talking about here is the decline of breast-feeding, which resulted in babies' having upset stomachs; these were treated with medicines containing alcohol, which led to the need for more alcohol, and so on.

87. "Manstrupration," in *Encyclopédie*, vol. 10, p. 52; T.M. Caton, *A Practical*

Treatise on the Prevention and Cure of the Venereal Disease (London, 1814), p. 90; Goss and Co., *Aegis of Life*, p. 57. [R.J.] Brodie (Consulting Surgeons), *The Secret Companion: A Medical Work on Onanism or Self-Pollution* (c. 1830). Balm of Zeylanica — whatever that is — at 4 shillings 6 pence a bottle — plus purifying vegetable pills could cure the addiction. Users are warned not to be upset if the medicine does not work right away.

88. V. Sazhin, "The Victor's Hand: Selections from the Correspondence Between V. Belinsky and M. Bakunin," *Erotica in Russian Literature from Barkov to the Present* [*Erotika v russkoi literature ot Barkova do nashikh dnei*], a special issue of *Literary Review* [*Literaturnoe obozrenie*], (Moscow, 1992), p. 39.

89. "Abus," in *Nouveau Dictionnaire de médecine et de chirurgie*, vol. 1; Littré, *Dictionnaire de médecine*.

90. *The Complete Letters of Sigmund Freud to Wilhelm Fliess, 1887–1904*, trans. and ed. Jeffrey Masson (Cambridge, MA: Belknap Press of Harvard University Press, 1985), p. 287 and n.78; André Lorulot, *La Véritable Education sexuelle* (Paris: Les Editions Georges-Anquetil, 1926), p. 241. This is in the context of a book that argues against celibacy — especially clerical celibacy — and offers advice for happy, romantic heterosexual relations.

91. Stopes Papers, Wellcome Library, A 228, 229, 220, 128, 117. Similar expressions are to be found in many other letters.

92. *Reference Handbook of the Medical Sciences* (London, 1923), vol. 6, p. 766.

93. M.N.W. Buet, *Dissertation sur la masturbation et les moyens propres y remédier* (presented to the Faculty of Medicine, Paris, Aug. 24, 1822), pp. 10–11. The "misbehavior" of patients masturbating is an acute source of embarrassment for doctors and the cause of a high proportion of "unnecessary" psychiatric consultations in a major teaching hospital. On this, see A. Kucharski and J.E. Groves, "The So-Called Inappropriate Psychiatric Consultation Request on a Medical or Surgical Ward," *International Journal of Psychiatry in Medicine* 77.3 (1976–1977).

94. For three lurid cases, see Jeffrey Masson, comp., *A Dark Science: Women, Sexuality, and Psychiatry in the Nineteenth Century*, trans. Jeffrey Masson and Marianne Loring (New York: Farrar, Straus and Giroux, 1986).

95. The tics and other involuntary jerking movements of people with Tourette's were said by some doctors in the late nineteenth century to be the result of masturbation. Again, a form of sexuality regarded as essentially excessive was translated into another realm of excess. On Tourette's syndrome and the late-nineteenth-century view that it was a consequence of masturbation, see Howard I. Kushner, "From Gilles de la Tourette's Disease to Tourette Syndrome: A History," *CNS Spectrums* 4.2 (Feb. 1999), and, more generally, Howard I. Kushner, *A Cursing Brain? The Histories of Tourette Syndrome* (Cambridge, MA: Harvard University Press, 1999). Freud's student and colleague Sándor Ferenczi argued more or less the converse, that tics and curses were the result of repressed masturbation in *Contributions to Psychoanalysis*, trans. Ernest Jones

(Boston: Richard G. Badger, 1916), pp. 157–58; Joseph Zohar, Zeev Kaplan, and Jonathan Benjamin, "Compulsive Exhibitionism Successfully Treated with Fluvoxamine: A Controlled Case Study," *Journal of Clinical Psychiatry* 55.3 (March 1994), pp. 86–88; H. Nishimura, M. Suzuki, et al., "Efficacy of Lithium Carbonate on Public and Compulsive Masturbation: A Female Case with Mild Mental Disability," *Psychiatry and Clinical Neurosciences* 51.6 (Dec. 1997), pp. 411–13.

CHAPTER FIVE: WHY MASTURBATION BECAME A PROBLEM

1. I can offer only the classic remark of Simone Weil: "What else are we to think with."

2. The quote is from Michael Mason in *The Making of Victorian Sexuality* (Oxford and New York: Oxford University Press, 1994), p. 194.

3. Jean Stengers and Anne van Neck, *Histoire d'une grande peur, la masturbation* (Institut Synthelabo, 1998), pp. 189–90. The peasant revolts sparked on the eve of the French Revolution were known as the *grande peur*, a term taken as the title for Georges Lefebvre's great history of the subject. The term itself seems somehow timeless but, in fact, seems to have been coined by Lefebvre in the shadow of the Russian Revolution. Robert McDonald, "The Frightful Consequences of Onanism: Notes on the History of a Delusion," *Journal of the History of Ideas* 28.3 (July–Sept. 1967), pp. 431 and 423–31 passim, says that the delusion of masturbatory disease fits well into what he takes to be the history of nineteenth-century repressive sexuality but that an answer to why it happened in the Age of Reason will have to await further work. Michael Mason in *The Making of Victorian Sexuality* regards explaining the coming and going of masturbation as a problem akin to explaining fashion.

4. These are the views of E.H. Hare, "Masturbatory Insanity: The History of an Idea" *Journal of Mental Science* 108.452 (Jan. 1962), pp. 1–25. Robert P. Neuman, "Masturbation, Madness, and the Modern Concepts of Childhood and Adolescence," *Journal of Social History* 8 (Spring 1975), thinks there was an increase in masturbation due to earlier puberty and higher marriage age among the middle classes and that this real social-historical change ran up against a greater anxiety about thrift. All of these particularistic accounts tend to slide into each other. There is an excellent, pointed critique of various explanations in Paula Bennett and Vernon A. Rosario II, "Introduction: The Politics of Solitary Pleasure," in Paula Bennett and Vernon A. Rosario II (eds.), *Solitary Pleasures: The Historical, Literary, and Artistic Discourses of Autoeroticism* (New York: Routledge, 1995), pp. 1–17.

5. The medical-ignorance argument or the allied claim that the newly prominent profession had to offer some sort of explanation for disease can be found in a number of articles. Arthur Gilbert, "Doctor, Patient, and Onanist Diseases in the Nineteenth Century," *Journal of the History of Medicine*, 30 (1975); for the medical-ignorance argument with an emphasis on drastic treatment for men, as opposed to women, see Gail Parsons, "Equal Treatment for

All: American Medical Remedies for Male Sexual Problems, 1850–1900," *Journal of the History of Medicine* 32 (1977).

6. For a powerful argument for isomorphism of the seminal and the sexual economy, see G. J. Barker-Benfield, *The Horrors of the Half-Known Life: Male Attitudes Toward Women and Sexuality in Nineteenth-Century America* (1976; New York: Routledge, 2000). For the limited applicability of this interpretation, see above, pp. 192–209.

7. For an excellent account of masturbation in the context of nineteenth-century constructions of disease, see H. Tristam Engelhardt Jr., "The Disease of Masturbation: Values and the Concept of Disease," *Bulletin of the History of Medicine* 48.2 (Summer 1974). Stengers and van Neck, *Histoire d'une grande peur,* make the case that masturbatory disease is a self-sustaining concept even if the reasons for its rise and fall cannot be assessed.

8. For the Protestant guilt hypothesis, see, for example, Hare, "Masturbatory Insanity," and Rene Spitz, "Authority and Masturbation: Some Remarks on a Bibliographical Investigation," *Yearbook of Psychoanalysis* 9 (1953). Lawrence Stone concludes that "the rise of anxiety about adolescent masturbation in the early and mid-eighteenth century is not easy to account for, since it coincides with the period of greater general adult permissiveness. The late eighteenth and nineteenth-century epidemic of hysteria is more easily explained since it coincided with a rise of Evangelical doctrine and the growing sense of horror and shame about sex..." See *The Family, Sex and Marriage in England, 1500–1800* (New York: Harper and Row, 1977), pp. 515 and 512–17 more generally.

9. The evidence for the Netherlands comes from Theo van der Meer, *Sodoms zaad in Nederland. Het ontstaan van homoseksualiteit in de vroegmoderne tijd* (Nijmegen: SUN, 1995), app. I. I am grateful to him for sending it to me. On the English case, see Tim Hitchcock, *English Sexualities, 1700–1800* (New York: St. Martin's Press, 1997), pp. 60–62, and the references cited there, as well as Arthur N. Gilbert, "Sodomy and the Law in Eighteenth- and Early Nineteenth-Century Britain," *Societas* 8.3 (1978); I am grateful to Eva Österberg of the University of Lund for this information based on her research.

10. This argument has recently been made with some force by Randolph Trumbach, *Sex and the Gender Revolution* (Chicago: University of Chicago Press, 1998), pp. 63–64 and passim.

11. George E. Haggerty, "'What Is This Secret Sin?' Sexuality and Secrecy in the Writings of Horace Walpole," in Maximillian E. Novak and Anne Mellor (eds.), *Passionate Encounters in a Time of Sensibility* (Newark: University of Delaware Press, 2000), pp. 140 and 127–50 passim. For more on the role of secrecy, see pp. 222–35.

12. *Trial of Mr. Foote* bound with *Sodom and Onan: A Satire* (London, 1776); *Onania*, 187.

13. Robert James, "Masturpratio or manustupration," in *A Medicinal Dictionary* (London, 1743–1745), vol. 2; my emphasis. "Manuel Stupration, a Vice not

decent to name, but productive of the most deplorable and generally incurable Disorders."

14. "Onanisme," in *Grand Dictionnaire universel du XIXe siècle* (Paris, 1875); this paragraph refers readers to a major article, five and a half columns long, on masturbation.

15. George H. Napheys, *The Transmission of Life: Counsels on the Nature and Hygiene of the Masculine Function*, new ed. (Philadelphia, 1889), p. 74. Napheys was a well-connected physician who wrote a similar book for women. The book is dedicated to the Reverend John Todd, who thought of masturbation as "the leprosy which fills the whole soul." See his *The student's manual; designed, by specific directions, to aid in forming and strengthening the intellectual and moral character and habits of the student*, 12th ed. (Northampton, 1844).

16. Goss and Co., *Hygeiana: A Non-medical Analysis of the Complaints Incidental to Females*, 20th ed. (London, 1830), p. 62. This was one of the Goss family of books, continuously in print, whose purpose was to make the public aware of a putative disease that the company's medications could supposedly cure.

17. See Harry Oosterhuis, *Stepchildren of Nature: Krafft-Ebing, Psychiatry, and the Making of Sexual Identity* (Chicago: University of Chicago Press, 2000), ch. 4; and Richard von Krafft-Ebbing, *Psychopathia sexualis*, 7th ed., trans. Charles Gilbert Chaddock (Philadelphia: F.A. Davis, 1908), pp. 188–202 and 205–206.

18. L. Thoinot, *Medicolegal Aspects of Moral Offenses*, trans. and enl. by Arthur W. Weysse (Philadelphia: F.A. Davis, 1911), pp. 310–13 and passim.

19. On this point, see Ed Cohen, *Talk on the Wilde Side* (New York: Routledge, 1993). More generally, masturbation was the biggest source of anxiety about sexuality in the same-sex world of the English public school. See J.R. Honey, *Tom Brown's Universe: The Development of the English Public School in the Nineteenth Century* (New York: Quadrangle Books, 1977), p. 169. Symonds is quoted from his memoirs in Oliver Buckton, *Secret Selves: Confession and Same-Sex Desire in Victorian Autobiography* (Chapel Hill: University of North Carolina Press, 1998), p. 73.

20. *The Complete Letters of Sigmund Freud to Wilhelm Fliess, 1887–1904*, trans. and ed. Jeffrey Masson (Cambridge, MA: Belknap Press of Harvard University Press, 1985), p. 41; A.P. Buchan, *Venus sine concubitu* (Venus without intercourse) (London, 1818), pp. 96–98.

21. Charles Baudelaire, "Femmes Damnées" (poem III), in *Les Fleurs du Mal* (Paris: Gallimard, 1972), p. 150. See Vern L. Bullough and Martha Voght, "Homosexuality and Its Confusion with the Secret Sin in Pre-Freudian America," *Journal of the History of Medicine* 28.2 (April 1973), for an excellent survey of the American literature. I have cited more or less at random from different sources because the story everywhere from the eighteenth century on is so similar, however it might be locally inflected.

22. In addition to pp. 148–51 above, see Patricia H. Labalme, "Sodomy and

Venetian Justice in the Renaissance," *Tijdschrift voor Rechtsgeschiedenis* 52.3 (1984). The article is in English.

23. John Marten, *Gonosologium Novum; or, A new system of all the secret infirmities and diseases natural, accidental, and venereal in men and women* (London, 1709), pp. 86 and 89.

24. S.A.D. Tissot, *Onanism; or, A Treatise upon the Disorders Produced by Masturbation; or, The Dangerous Effects of Secret and Excessive Venery*, trans. A. Hume (London, 1761), pp. 80–81 and 149. Cited in Michael Stolberg, "An Unmanly Vice: Self-Pollution, Anxiety, and the Body in the Eighteenth Century," *Social History of Medicine* 13.1 (2000), p. 15, from the manuscript letters in the *Fonds Tissot*.

25. Tissot, *Onanism*, pp. 40–46.

26. Tissot, *Onanism*, p. 46, actually misquotes the line "Ipsa Medullina fluctum cisantis adorat" as "...frictum cirsantis adorat."

27. On this, see the excellent article by Laura Weigert, "Autonomy as Deviance: Sixteenth-Century Images of Witches and Prostitutes," in Bennett and Rosario, *Solitary Pleasures*, pp. 19–47. The connection between perceived religious deviance and sexual deviance is often made in Protestant countries in the context of attacks on Catholicism.

28. Bienville goes through elaborate paeans to his predecessor: he is standing on the shoulders of giants, he cannot possibly approach the master narrator of *L'Onanisme*, and so on. On the nineteenth-century story, see Carol Groneman, *Nymphomania: A History* (New York: W.W. Norton, 2000), pp. 16–17, 29–30, 12, and passim.

29. Auguste Forel, *The Sexual Question: A Scientific, Psychological, Hygienic, and Sociological Study*, trans. C.F. Marshall (New York: Physicians and Surgeons Book Co., 1906), p. 233. Forel does link masturbation to homosexuality in that he thinks inverts give up solo masturbation for mutual masturbation whereas heterosexuals take up vaginal intercourse when the opportunity presents itself. Ellice Hopkins, *The White Cross Army* (London, c. 1880) in a series "Papers for Men Only"; Clement Duke, *The Preservation of Health* (London, n.d., but written for the Howard Medal in Statistical Science, 1884), pp. 145 and 150; Edward Lyttleton, *The Causes and Prevention of Immorality in Schools* (London, 1883), pp. 8 and 15; Elizabeth Blackwell, *The Human Element in Sex: Being a Medical Enquiry into the Relation of Sexual Physiology to Christian Morality* (London, 1885), p. 29; Laura Engelstein finds this sort of thinking in late-nineteenth-century Russia as well. See her *The Keys to Happiness: Sex and the Search for Modernity in Fin-de-siècle Russia* (Ithaca, NY: Cornell University Press, 1992), pp. 221–23.

30. Nicholas Francis Cooke, *Satan in Society* (Cincinnati: G.F. Hovey, 1882 [1870]), pp. 114–15.

31. Johann Peter Frank, *System einer vollständigen medicinischen Polizey*, 11 vols. in 5 (Frankenthal, 1791–1794), vol. 6, pt. 3, sec. 14, pp. 113–16. The "cesspool of masturbation" was also, Frank thought, a cause of suicide and hence a

concern of the state (vol. 12, sec. 8, p. 147). Celibates were far more likely to commit suicide than others, and their "secret vice" is one of the reasons. P.J.C. Debreyne, *Essai sur la théologie morale* (Paris, 1844), pp. 71, and 70–81 more generally; Marc A. Weiner, *Richard Wagner and the Anti-Semitic Imagination* (Lincoln: University of Nebraska Press, 1995), pp. 337–42. Jews fell into the same category as masturbators, and, Weiner argues, so did Jew-like characters in Wagner's operas: Beckmeister in *The Mastersingers of Nuremberg* and Hagan in *The Ring*, for example.

32. Immanuel Kant, "An Answer to the Question: What Is Enlightenment?" in *Perpetual Peace and Other Essays*, trans. Ted Humphrey (Indianapolis: Hackett, 1983), pp. 41–43. The piece was first published in December 1784 in the same *Berliner Monatsschrift* that published four prize essays on how to prevent masturbation. It is not clear, says Kant, that if we looked around we could find a single instance of the disposition to act from pure duty, *Metaphysics of Morals*, trans. with intro. and notes Mary J. Gregor (Philadelphia: University of Pennsylvania, 1971), pt. 1, sec. 2, par. 406.

33. See Isabel Hull, *Sexuality, the State, and Civil Society in Germany, 1700–1815* (Ithaca, NY: Cornell University Press, 1996), ch. 7, for a brilliant account of the view I am discussing here. I am thinking, of course, of *Democracy in America*.

34. Joachim Heinrich Campe, ed., *Allgemeine Revision des gesammten Schul- und Erziehungswesens / von einer Gesellschaft praktischer Erzieher*, 16 vols. (Hamburg, 1785-1792), set the question for the essay contest on the dangers of onanism. I know of no complete bibliography of Campe's *Robinson Crusoe* adaptation, but there are more than 250 separate listings in OCLC. A Swedish version entranced the young Strindberg. Campe's political views are quoted in Nicholas Boyle, *Goethe: The Poet and the Age* (Oxford: Clarendon Press, 2000), pp. 27–28, in what appears to be a correspondence with the young Wilhelm von Humboldt, whom he accompanied to Paris. For this view of Defoe's character, see Isaac Kramnick, *Bolingbroke and His Circle: The Politics of Nostalgia in the Age of Walpole* (Cambridge, MA: Harvard University Press, 1968), pp. 188–204.

35. Foucault discusses the general shift from the power of sovereignty exercised on the body to the more diffuse exercise of power through the discipline of the soul — the inner self — in *Discipline and Punish: The Birth of the Prison*, 2nd ed., trans. Alan Sheridan (New York: Vintage Books, 1995); the making of sexuality as a discursive arena for the creation and the disciplining of desire rather than for its repression and liberation is the theme of *The History of Sexuality, Volume 1*, trans. Robert Hurley (New York: Pantheon Books, 1978); William Hale Hale, the mid-nineteenth-century archdeacon of London, made prescient Foucaultian remarks *avant la lettre* in his *Remarks on the two bills now before Parliament, entitled a Bill for Registering Births, Deaths, and Marriages in England; and a Bill for Marriages in England* (London, 1836), where he argued that once the state held sway over these forms of knowledge, it would have access to the most intimate spaces of our being and would soon be in our bedrooms and living spaces.

36. Jeremy Taylor, "On Chastity," in *The Rule and Exercises of Holy Living* (London, 1651), p. 80; Foucault, *History of Sexuality, Volume 1*, pp. 34–35 and 17–73 generally; *Onania*, p. 23.

37. Tissot, *Onanism*, p. viii; James Hodson, *Medical Facts and Advertisements Submitted to the Consideration of the Afflicted* (London, 1799), p. 8; Brodie (R.J.) and Company, consulting surgeons, *The Secret Companion* (London: published by the author, 1840), p. 35.

38. Frederick Arthur Sibly's paper was first printed in *Papers on moral education, communicated to the first International Moral Education Congress held at the University of London September 25–29, 1908,* ed. Gustav Spiller, published for the Congress Executive Committee (London: D. Nutt, 1908), a prototypical site for the expression of a class of experts who sought to gain dominion over the inner lives of modern citizens. It was reprinted by Lord Baden-Powell in the *Headquarters Gazette* of the Boy Scouts and quoted extensively in Sibly's own *Youth and Sex: Its Dangers and Safeguards for Boys and Girls* (London, c. 1910).

39. Foucault, *History of Sexuality, Volume 1*; Bartholomew Parr, *The London medical dictionary including . . . whatever relates to medicine in natural philosophy, chemistry, and natural history* (Philadelphia, 1819), vol. 1, p. 918. The first edition of the two-volume dictionary appeared in London in 1809.

40. These new arenas of discourse are discussed in Foucault, *History of Sexuality, Volume 1*, pp. 104–105 and 103–31 passim.

41. This formulation is the narrative of the book in which the idea of bio-power was first developed, *Discipline and Punish*, pp. 140 and 102. Isabel Hull argues that by 1800 the German masturbation bubble had burst. This is not the case, as the nineteenth- and twentieth-century German texts I have cited, and many more that could be adduced, prove. The problem of chronology in Foucault's account is not so acute in works after the first volume of the history of sexuality. In the late 1970s, he began to argue that the shift from sovereign power — the power to kill and let live — to governmental power — the power to manage life and let die — had begun in the seventeenth century. Although he never took the explicit argument about medicine and the rise of masturbation, and bio-power more generally, back to an earlier period, he might have. My main critique, however, is as follows: that the process of creating the new anxiety was not one in which governmentality played a crucial role. I am grateful to Michel Feher for straightening me out on this.

42. This is the thesis of John Brewer's rich survey *The Pleasures of the Imagination: English Culture in the Eighteenth Century* (New York: Farrar, Straus and Giroux, 1997), esp. pp. 56–125, although the point is made throughout in different contexts.

43. Montesquieu, *Persian Letters*, trans. C.J. Betts (Harmondsworth, UK: Penguin, 1993), no. 146. By "next" I mean "next in placement." No. 147 is "dated" three years earlier.

44. Sir Richard Steele, *The crisis of property: An argument proving that the*

annuitants for ninety-nine years, as such, are not in the condition of other subjects of Great Britain, but by compact with the legislature are exempt from any new direction relating to the said estates, 2nd ed. (London, 1720). The third quotation is from "Stander-by," *The battle of the bubbles shewing their several constitutions, alliances, policies, and wars, from their first suddain rise to their late speedy decay* (London, 1720), p. 10. The definition and exemplar are from the *OED* entry "bubble."

45. On the problem of reconciling private desire and public good, see J.B. Schneewind, *The Invention of Autonomy: A History of Modern Moral Philosophy* (Cambridge, UK: Cambridge University Press, 1998), esp. ch. 15.

46. For one disease of civilization, gout, in the eighteenth century, see George Cheyne, *The English Malady*, ed. and intro. Roy Porter (1733; London and New York: Tavistock/Routledge, 1991). For a more metaphorical version, see Michael Ignatieff's comments on the Scottish philosopher and political economist John Millar in *Wealth and Virtue: The Shaping of Political Economy in the Scottish Enlightenment*, ed. Istvan Hont and Michael Ignatieff (New York: Cambridge University Press, 1983); *Dictionnaire des sciences medicales* (Paris, 1819); James Copland, *A Dictionary of Practical Medicine* (London, 1858), vol. 3, pt. 2, p. 1010.

47. On this, see below, pp. 284–91.

48. See above, pp. 213ff.

49. Hume's views on this are most succinctly expressed in "Of Commerce" and "Of the Refinement of the Arts" in his *Political Essays*, ed. Knud Haakonssen (1752; Cambridge, UK: Cambridge University Press, 1994), passim and pp. 99 and 105 in particular. For a brilliant introduction to the discussion of the passions and economic thought in the eighteenth century that first formed my thinking on the subject, see Albert O. Hirschman, *The Passions and the Interests* (Princeton, NJ: Princeton University Press, 1997).

50. Jan de Vries, "The Industrial Revolution and the Industrious Revolution," *Journal of Economic History* 54.2 (1994).

51. There had been French imitators of Mandeville whom Hume had cited. Voltaire in his "Défense de Mondain" picked up specifically on Jean-François Melon's *Essai politique sur le commerce* (1734).

52. Bernard Mandeville, *The Fable of the Bees*, ed. and intro. by Irwin Primer (New York: Capricorn Books, 1962). The 1705 poem is printed before the main text: l. 2, p. 27; ll. 156–57 and 166–68, p. 31.

53. This discussion of the meaning of luxury is part of an extensive gloss of verses around l. 200 of the prefatory earlier poem: "Thus vice nurs'd ingenuity / Which join'd with time and industry / Had carry'd life's conveniences, / *Its real pleasures, comforts and ease,* / To such a height, the very poor / Liv'd better than the rich before." *Ibid.*, pp. 32, 104, 77.

54. *Ibid.*, pp. 77, 110, and 110–13 generally.

55. Bernard Mandeville, *A Modest Defense of Public Stews*, Clark Memorial Library Publication 162 (1724; Los Angeles: Augustan Reprint Society, 1973), p.

vi. The piece is in part an attack on the various societies for the reformation of morals, the so-called vice societies; pp. iii–x. See also *Fable*, pp. 106–107.

56. Mandeville, *Fable of the Bees*, pp. 46, 54, 45–46.

57. *Ibid.*, pp. 64–70, passim; ll. 241–408 of "The Grumbling Hive" for the parable of virtue and economic collapse; Mandeville, *In Defense of Public Stews*, p. 74.

58. Mandeville, *In Defense of Public Stews*, pp. vi, 23, 24–27; Mandeville, *Fable of the Bees*, p. 77.

59. Mandeville, *Fable of the Bees*, pp. 90–91 and 94.

60. The old survey of the relationship of the individual to market society by Karl Polanyi, *The Great Transformation*, foreword by Robert M. MacIver (1944; Boston: Beacon Press, 1957), remains as brilliant and thought provoking as it was when it was produced to account for the rise of fascism.

61. Mandeville, *In Defense of Public Stews*, pp. 30–31.

62. Thomas Malthus, *An Essay on the Principle of Population* (London, 1798).

63. Jean-Jacques Rousseau, *The Confessions of Jean-Jacques Rousseau*, trans. J.M. Cohen (Harmondsworth, UK, New York: Penguin Books, [1953] 1989), p. 109.

64. Wilhelm Stekel, *Auto-erotism: A Psychiatric Study of Onanism and Neurosis*, trans. James S. Van Teslaar (New York: Grove Press, 1950), pp. 56–58.

65. The epistemological leap entailed by credit in the late seventeenth and the eighteenth century has been explored most deeply in recent scholarship by J.G.A. Pocock in *Virtue, Commerce, and History: Essays on Political Thought and History, Chiefly in the Eighteenth Century* (Cambridge, UK: Cambridge University Press, 1985) and more generally in *The Machiavellian Moment: Florentine Political Thought and the Atlantic Republican Tradition* (Princeton, NJ: Princeton University Press, 1975). For refinements on Pocock and more specifically on the connection between fiction and credit, see Sandra Sherman, *Finance and Fictionality in the Early Eighteenth Century: Accounting for Defoe* (Cambridge, UK: Cambridge University Press, 1996), pp. 14–54.

66. On the *Spectator*, see Brewer, *Pleasures of the Imagination*, p. 39. Leslie Kurke, *Coins, Bodies, Games, and Gold: The Politics of Meaning in Archaic Greece* (Princeton, NJ: Princeton University Press, 1999).

67. *The Spectator*, no. 3 (March 3, 1711) (London: J.M. Dent, 1951), pp. 1 and 10–13.

68. Archibald Hutcheson as quoted in Sherman, *Finance and Fictionality in the Early Eighteenth Century*, pp. 17 and 187, nn.8 and 9. Sherman's book is one of the most astute and learned critiques in the literature of the credit/fiction homology. Anthony Hammond, *A modest apology, occasion'd by the late unhappy turn of affairs, with relation to publick credit/ by a gentleman* (London, 1724), p. 4.

69. Adam Smith, *An Inquiry into the Causes of the Wealth of Nations* 2.2, pars. 58–59, ed. R.H. Campbell and A.S. Skinner (Indianapolis: Liberty Fund, 1981; repr. of the Glasgow ed.), vol. 1, p. 304; my emphasis. Smith uses a hydraulic

analogy that would not be unfamiliar to doctors: the right kind of credit works like a pond that has a stream running through it; as long as what comes in keeps up with what goes out, all is well irrespective of the total volume that moves through. The second part of the quotation as I give it actually occurs first, par. 58; Maria Edgeworth, "The Dun," in *Works of Maria Edgeworth*, 13 vols. (Boston, 1822–1826), vol. 5, p. 276 (1820). I am grateful to Catherine Gallagher for this reference and for many discussions on the problems of sexuality, credit, and fiction.

70. J.G. Zimmermann, *Solitude: To which are added The Life of the Author, notes...* (London, 1808), vol. 1, pp. 1, 221, and passim. Perhaps in this context we might read David Hume's juxtaposition in his autobiography of the fact that he spent three years in solitude in France with his sad admission that the book he produced during this period — the *Treatise on Human Understanding* — "fell *dead-born from the press*" as a statement about the corporeal dangers of solitary activity. In fact, Hume was in the long run totally wrong about his book, but never mind.

71. John Armstrong, *The Oeconomy of Love: A Poetical Essay* (London, 1736), ll. 94–96, 101–106, 129–30, 139–42. The nineteenth-century author of Armstrong's entry in the *Dictionary of National Biography* thought that "a more nauseous piece of work could not easily be found." Eighteenth-century audiences, perhaps because of the qualities the biographer found so offensive, bought up at least thirty-six editions, not counting its inclusion in complete works. Armstrong's poem *The Art of Preserving Health* went through at least twenty-four editions. "No author of the eighteenth century," writes the *DNB*, "had so masterful a grasp of blank verse" as Armstrong did in this work. Thomas Cooper, the man who brought out the *The Oeconomy of Love*, was a major publisher with a list that includes political works as well as books like *Venetian Tales for the Fair Sex*. T. Cadell and Weyland and Davis published both works in the latter part of the eighteenth century. Armstrong's and Akenside's works traveled in the same circles; they shared publishers for several editions, and *The Pleasures of the Imagination*, like Armstrong's poem, went through more than a score of eighteenth-century editions.

72. D.T. de Bienville, *Nymphomania; or a, A dissertation concerning the furor uterinus. Clearly and methodically explaining the beginning, progress, and different causes of that horrible distemper. To which are added, the methods of treating the several stages of it, and the most approved remedies. Written originally in French*, trans. Edward Sloane Wilmot (London, 1775), p. 158.

73. The doctor is cited in Patricia O'Brien, "The Kleptomania Diagnosis: Bourgeois Women and Theft in Late Nineteenth-Century France," *Journal of Social History* 17.1 (Fall 1983), p. 73. Excessive masturbation was also associated with the far rarer phenomenon of kleptomania in men. See also E.S. Abelson, "The Invention of Kleptomania," *Signs* (Fall 1989). I leave as a question for another occasion the modern notion that the category "compulsive disorders" links kleptomania and masturbation, at least excessive masturbation. Similar

drugs are used to treat both: fluvoxamine, for example. Joseph Zohar, Zeev Kaplan, and Jonathan Benjamin, "Compulsive Exhibitionism Successfully Treated with Fluvoxamine: A Controlled Case Study," *Journal of Clinical Psychiatry* 55.3 (Mar. 1994), pp. 86–88. Several papers report its use to control compulsive shoplifting; Otto Fenichel, *Psychoanalytic Theory of Neurosis* (1946; London: Tavistock/Routledge, 1990), p. 371.

74. Gregory M. Pflugfelder, *Cartographies of Desire: Male-Male Sexuality in Japanese Discourse, 1600–1950* (Berkeley: University of California Press, 1999), pp. 172–73 and 244–45; Timon Screech, *Sex and the Floating World: Erotic Images in Japan, 1700–1820* (Honolulu: University of Hawaii Press, 1999), pp. 31–38; Frühstück, "Debating Sex Education" in *Colonizing Sex: Sexology and Social Control in Modern Japan* (Berkeley: University of California Press, forthcoming 2003).

75. Vinit Sharma and Anuragini Sharma, "The Guilt and Pleasure of Masturbation: A Study of College Girls in Gujarat, India," *Sexual & Marital Therapy* 13.1 (Feb. 1998); Engelstein, *Keys to Happiness*, pp. 227, 234–35. See on the Communist period Eric Naiman, *Sex in Public: The Incarnation of Early Soviet Ideology* (Princeton, NJ: Princeton University Press, 1997), pp. 120–22.

76. Ding Ling, "Miss Sophia's Diary," in *I Myself Am a Woman: Selected Writings of Ding Ling*, ed. and intro. Tani E. Barlow (Boston: Beacon Press, 1989), pp. 50–51.

77. Mary Douglas and Baron Isherwood, *The World of Goods: Towards an Anthropology of Consumption* (London: Allen Lane, 1979), p. 137; Marchmont Nedham, *The Excellencie of a Free-State* (London: 1656), p. 129.

78. Jane Gallop, *Thinking Through the Body* (New York: Columbia University Press, 1988), p. 18.

79. Paul R. Abramson and Steven D. Pinkerton, *With Pleasure: Thoughts on the Nature of Human Sexuality* (New York: Oxford University Press, 1995), pp. 74ff.

80. *Rambler* 89 (Jan. 22, 1751), in *Yale Edition of the Works of Samuel Johnson* (New Haven, CT: Yale University Press, 1958), vol. 3.

81. S.A.D. Tissot, *An Essay on Diseases Incidental to Literary and Sedentary Persons* (London, 1768), pp. 36–37 and 74–76. Anne Vila argues, rightly I think, that Tissot on onanism is but Tissot on the dangers of solitary, intense use of the brain in another register; see her *Enlightenment and Pathology: Sensibility in the Literature and Medicine of Eighteenth-Century France* (Baltimore, Johns Hopkins University Press, 1998), pp. 101–102 and ch. 3 passim. Tissot, *Onanism,* pp. 52 and 48–59 generally. *An essay on the disorders of people of fashion (Essai sur les maladies des gens du monde)* (Edinburgh and London: Alexander Donaldson, 1772) was printed with the book on literary diseases that first appeared in English in 1768. *De la santé des gens de lettres* never had quite the appeal of *Onanism*, but still it found its public; at least 16 French editions, 7 German, 7 English, 4 Italian, plus 1 in Greek, Spanish, and Polish appeared in the eighteenth century. Compiled from Antoinette Suzanne Emch-Dériaz, *Tissot: Physician of the Enlightenment* (New

York: P. Lang, 1992), pp. 331–32. It was printed with his book on onanism in English on occasion, thus linking the two sorts of diseases of civilization.

82. Anthony Comstock, *Traps for the Young*, ed. Robert Bremner (Cambridge, MA: Harvard University Press, 1967), pp. 20–43 and 168–84.

83. Paul Saenger, *Space Between Words: The Origins of Silent Reading* (Stanford, CA: Stanford University Press, 1997), pp. 1–18 and 256–57. See also Saenger's "Silent Reading: Its Impact on Late Medieval Script and Society," *Viator* 13 (1982).

84. I take the general account of the rise of private reading and its relation to privacy from Roger Chartier, ed., *A History of Private Life*, vol. 3, trans. Arthur Goldhammer (Cambridge, MA: Harvard University Press, 1987), in particular the section titled "Literary Practices: Publicizing the Private" by Jean Marie Goulemot, pp. 363–95. Chartier has elaborated in more detail a history of private reading in Roger Chartier, *The Cultural Uses of Print in Early Modern France*, trans. Lydia G. Cochrane (Princeton, NJ: Princeton University Press, 1987). See also the collection *A History of Reading in the West*, eds. Guglielmo Cavallo and Roger Chartier, trans. Lydia G. Cochrane (Amherst: University of Massachusetts Press, 1999) and Saenger, *Space Between Words*, pp. 275–76.

85. The connection between reading and liberty is made explicitly by Jean Starobinski, *The Invention of Liberty, 1700–1789*, trans. Bernard C. Swift (New York: Rizzoli, 1987). Lisa Jardine, *Worldly Goods: A New History of the Renaissance* (London: Macmillan, 1996), pp. 135–80 and 160–61 for these books in particular.

86. Paula Findlen, "Humanism, Politics, and Pornography in Renaissance Italy," in Lynn Hunt (ed.), *The Invention of Pornography* (New York: Zone Books, 1992), p. 63. On Aretino, see the exhaustive study by Bette Talvacchia, *Taking Positions: On the Erotic in Renaissance Culture* (Princeton, NJ: Princeton University Press, 1999), esp. pp. xiii and 19.

87. On these paintings, see Kelly Dennis, "Playing with Herself: Feminine Sexuality and Aesthetic Indifference," in Bennett and Rosario, *Solitary Pleasures*.

88. Max Hodann, *History of Modern Morals,* trans. Stella Browne (London: Heinemann, 1937), front matter; Stopes Papers, A 244, March 9, 1923. The writer's name is known but is not cited to respect the privacy of descendants; A 65, FC, 19/13/19. I have not found this title — *Knowledge a Young Woman Should Have* by Alexander Andrew Philip and H.R. Murray (London: Athletic Publications, [between 1910 and 1920]) must have been a companion piece in a series on sex knowledge. Or, the writer was referring to *Sexual Science* by these same authors and from the same publisher. Tissot, *Onanism*, p. 29.

89. These examples are taken from Alberto Manguel, *A History of Reading* (New York: Viking, 1996), pp. 149–50, 153, 159.

90. *The Inferno of Dante*, trans. Robert Pinsky (New York: Farrar, Straus and Giroux, 1994), canto 5, ll. 107–22 of the English text, p. 53, ll. 121–38 in the facing Italian.

91. *A Practical Treatise upon the Treatment of Tabes Dorsalis*... (1747); Tissot,

Onanism, p. 129; *L'onanismo; ovvero, Dissertazione sopra le malattie cagionate dalle Polluzioni volontarie de Signor Tissot*, 3rd ed. (Venice, 1785), pp. 28–29, n.9.

92. Herbert Maxwell, "The Craving for Fiction," in *The Nineteenth Century* 196 (June 1893); Alfred Austin, "The Vice of Reading," *Temple Bar Magazine* 42 (Sept. 1874). I am grateful to my student Susan Zieger for finding these documents for a set of tutorials we did together. She discusses the problem of reading and addiction in chapter 3 of her Ph.D. thesis, "Addictive Fictions: Medical Knowledge, Novelistic Form, and Habits of Mind in Britain, 1860–1914," University of California, Berkeley, 2002. More generally, see Kelly J. Mays, "The Disease of Reading and Victorian Periodicals," in John O. Jordan (ed.), *Literature in the Marketplace: Nineteenth-Century British Publishing and Reading Practices* (Cambridge, UK: Cambridge University Press, 1995).

93. Isaac Ray, *Mental Hygiene* (1863; New York: Hafner, 1968), pp. 272–73 and 264–75 passim. See also Isabelle Lehuu, *Carnival on the Page: Popular Print Media in Antebellum America* (Chapel Hill: University of North Carolina Press, 2000), p. 131 and passim.

94. Norah March, *Towards Racial Health* (London: Routledge, 1915), p. 85.

95. A.A. Brill, *Psychoanalysis: Its Theories and Practical Application* (Philadelphia: W.B. Saunders, 1922), p. 149.

96. Joseph Addison, "Pleasures of the Imagination or Fancy," *Spectator*, no. 411–12 (June 21–23, 1712); Wilma L. Kennedy, *The English Heritage of Coleridge of Bristol, 1798: The Basis in Eighteenth-Century English Thought for His Distinction Between Imagination and Fancy* (New Haven, CT: Yale University Press, 1947), pp. 1–19. On Augustine and the history of the imagination more generally before the eighteenth century, see J.M. Cockering, *Imagination: A History of Ideas*, ed. and intro. Penelope Murray (London: Routledge, 1991), p. xiii and the first four chapters of the book, which are the most learned and reasonable account of the subject I have encountered.

97. *Spectator*, vol. 3, pp. 277ff. in the Everyman Library ed.

98. Shelley is quoted in Cockering, *Imagination*, p. vii; Charles Darwin, *The Descent of Man, and Selection in Relation to Sex* (Princeton, NJ: Princeton University Press, 1981), pt. 1, ch. 2, p. 45.

99. For the story up to roughly the late seventeenth century, see Cockering, *Imagination*, pp. 1–101 and 141–95. For the story beginning with Locke, see the remarkable book by Ernest Lee Tuveson, *The Imagination as a Means of Grace* (Berkeley: University of California Press, 1960), pp. 72–91 and throughout; the imagination is everywhere in Hume but especially in the *Treatise of Human Nature*. For an excellent reading, see Annette C. Baier, *A Progress of Sentiments: Reflections on Hume's "Treatise"* (Cambridge, MA: Harvard University Press, 1991), pp. 7–15 and 257–58; there is a succinct summary of Kant on the subject in Eva T.H. Brann's enormous and learned compendium on the imagination in the thought of almost everyone, *The World of the Imagination: Sum and Substance* (Savage, MD: Rowman and Littlefield, 1991), p. 505 and throughout. For Kant on the imagination as "an

active faculty" that "represents appearances in association" and "plays a part in the transcendental unity of apperception," see *Critique of Pure Reason* A115ff.

100. I base this list on the excellent survey of the question in Wolfgang Iser, *The Fictive and the Imaginary: Charting Literary Anthropology* (Baltimore: Johns Hopkins University Press, 1993), pp. 171ff.

101. I take this characterization of the novel from Catherine Gallagher's *Nobody's Story: The Vanishing Acts of Women Writers in the Marketplace, 1670–1820* (Berkeley: University of California Press, 1994), whose influence on my thinking about markets, fiction, and the imagination goes well beyond this short quotation.

102. See Albert Ward, *Book Production, Fiction, and the German Reading Public, 1740–1800* (Oxford: Clarendon Press, 1974), esp. ch. 3 on the growth of the novel-reading public in Germany, pp. 59–91, for a case study. The point holds true throughout western and, later, the rest of Europe.

103. *Critical Review* 33 (London: 1772), p. 327, as well as the other quotations are cited in James Raven, "From Promotion to Prescription: Arrangements for Reading and Eighteenth-Century Libraries," in James Raven, Helen Small, and Naomi Tadmor (eds.), in *The Practice and Representation of Reading in England* (Cambridge, UK: Cambridge University Press, 1996), p. 179 and passim. On female novel writing and harlotry, see Gallagher, *Nobody's Story*. Colman is cited in G. J. Barker-Benfield, *The Culture of Sensibility: Sex and Society in Eighteenth-Century Britain* (Chicago: University of Chicago Press, 1992), p. 327. I came upon this book late in my writing and find in it a wealth of material and interpretation of the sexual dangers of novel reading and consumerism, especially for women. Barker-Benfield suggests briefly that "to previous speculations explaining masturbatory phobia one may add the notion that masturbation became a sexual expression of consumer psychology, whatever cultural meanings it had previously" (p. 330).

104. Jan Goldstein, *Console and Classify: the French Psychiatric Profession in the Nineteenth Century* (Cambridge, UK: Cambridge University Press, 1987). Etienne Bonnot de Condillac, *An Essay on the Origin of Human Knowledge*, trans. Thomas Nugent (1756; Gainesville, FL: Scholars' Facsimiles and Reprints, 1971), pt. 1, sec. 2.

105. That reading novels had somatic effects is, of course, the basis of the sensational fiction of Wilkie Collins and his successors. On this, see David Miller, "'Cage aux folles': Sensation and Gender in Wilkie Collins's *The Woman in White*," in Catherine Gallagher and Thomas Laqueur (eds.), *The Making of the Modern Body: Sexuality and Society in the Nineteenth Century* (Berkeley: University of California Press, 1987), pp. 107–36. The quotations from Beddoes, Coleridge, and the *Methodist Magazine* are from the extensive collection of anti-novel sentiments in James Tinnon Taylor, *Early Opposition to the English Novel* (New York: Columbia University Press, 1943), pp. 102–103 and 105–106. Beddoes is cited only indirectly, pp. 107–108. Thomas Clarkson in his *Portrait of*

Quakerism makes the claim that "a physician of the first eminence" told him about the dire effects of novel reading. That physician, we know, is Beddoes in his *Hygeia: or, Essays, Moral and Medical, on the Causes Affecting the Personal State of our Middling and Affluent Classes* (Bristol, 1802–1803), essay 3, pp. 77 and 76–80 passim. Sheridan quoted in Raven, *Practice and Representation of Reading*, p. 190; on Rousseau's readers, see Robert Darnton, *The Great Cat Massacre* (New York: Vintage, 1985), pp. 243–47.

106. This example — many more could be cited — is from the *Ladies Mercury* (Feb. 28, 1693), pp. 2–3.

107. *Onania . . . also the Sixth Supplement*, 15th ed. (1730), p. 125 of the *Supplement*. The story from Dr. Carr follows p. 128. The source for this is in n. 7, ch. 2 above. The *Supplement* goes on to cite other medical literature that purports to correlate the size of the clitoris with salaciousness, especially one often reprinted and pirated text by "Dr. Drake," which must be James Drake, *Anthropologia nova; or, A new system of anatomy: describing the animal oeconomy, and a short rationale of many distempers incident to human bodies: in which are inserted divers anatomical discoveries, and medicinal observations, with the history of the parts: illustrated with above fourscore figures, drawn after the life: and to every chapter a syllabus of the parts describ'd, for the instruction of young anatomists* (London, 1707), which does in fact make this point. The nun's story was, of course, a standard Protestant and Enlightenment anti-clerical trope. On "Aristotle," see Roy Porter, "'The Secrets of Generation Display'd': *Aristotle's Master-Piece* in Eighteenth-Century England," in Robert Maccubbin (ed.), *Unauthorized Sexual Behavior During the Enlightenment* (Williamsburg, VA: College of William and Mary, 1985). The line between pornography and acceptable literature was a fine one. We know that medical or quasi-medical books served a dual purpose. On this bridging of worlds, see Peter Wagner, "The Discourse on Sex — or Sex as Discourse: Eighteenth-Century Medical and Paramedical Erotica," in Roy Porter and George Rousseau (eds.), *Sexual Underworlds of the Enlightenment* (Manchester, UK: University of Manchester Press, 1987), and Peter Wagner, "The Veil of Science and Morality: Some Pornographic Aspects of the *Onania*," *British Journal for Eighteenth-Century Studies* 6 (1983).

108. Ludmilla Jordanova shares de Lignac's high regard for Tissot's literary skills. She offers her judgment in "The Popularization of Medicine: Tissot on Onanism," *Textual Practice* 1.1 (1987). Louis-François de Lignac, *De l'homme et de la femme considérés physiquement dans l'état du mariage* (1772); S.A.D. Tissot, *Three essays: First, on the disorders of people of fashion. . . ,* trans. Francis Bacon Lee (Dublin, 1772), p. iii. The second is on the diseases incidental to literary and sedentary persons translated by Danes, and the third is a reprinting of Hume's *Onanism*.

109. Bienville, *Nymphomania*, pp. 76 and 161.

110. *Ibid.*, p. 32. This is Mary D. Sheriff's formulation in "Enthusiasm, Nymphomania, and the Imagined Tableau," in Lawrence Klein and Anthony J.

La Vopa (eds.), *Enthusiasm and Enlightenment in Europe, 1650–1850* (San Marino, CA: Huntington Library, 1998).

111. Anthony J. La Vopa, "The Philosopher and the Schwärmer," in Klein and La Vopa, *Enthusiasm and Enlightenment in Europe.*

112. *The Confessions of St. Augustine*, trans. and intro. John K. Ryan (Garden City, NY: Image Books/Doubleday, 1960), bk. 1, ch. 13, p. 56; bk. 3, ch. 2, p. 78. The long history of anti-theatricality of which Augustine and Rousseau, not to speak of Plato, are all parts, is exhaustively told in Jonas A. Barish, *The Antitheatrical Prejudice* (Berkeley: University of California Press, 1981).

113. Johann Georg Heinzmann quoted in Reinhard Wittmann, *Geschichte des deutschen Buchhandels* (Munich: C.H. Beck, 1991), pp. 186–87.

114. On sexuality and the anti-philosophe tradition, see Darrin M. McMahon, *Enemies of the Enlightenment: The French Counter-Enlightenment and the Making of Modernity* (New York: Oxford University Press, 2001), p. 38. The would-be masturbation involves a scene where Mlle de L'Espinasse is puzzled that she can't find the hand of the sleeping D'Alembert, who represents in this dialogue the voice of Diderot. In the persona of a dreamer, Diderot can be as radical as he wants. The real Mlle de L'Espinasse was so outraged by the manuscript that she made her friend D'Alembert insist that Diderot destroy it in her presence. He threw what he thought was the only copy in the fire, and what we have is printed from a fair copy that had been made by a German journalist's clerk without the author's permission. Denis Diderot, *Rameau's Nephew and Other Works*, trans. Jacques Barzun and Ralph Bowen (Indianapolis: Bobbs-Merrill, 1980), pp. 168–69. On the connection between pornography and modernity more generally, see Margaret Jacobs, "The Materialist World of Pornography," in Hunt, *Invention of Pornography*, pp. 159 and 157–202 passim.

115. *The Gladstone Diaries*, vol. 4, 1848–54, edited by M.R.D. Foot and H.C.G. Mathew (Oxford: Clarendon Press, 1974), entry for 19 July 1848, p. 55.

116. For the connection between the world of pornography and radicalism in England, see Iain McCalman, *Radical Underworld: Prophets, Revolutionaries, and Pornographers in London, 1795–1840* (Cambridge, UK: Cambridge University Press, 1988). For the pornography-Enlightenment-materialism link in France, see in particular Robert Darnton, *The Forbidden Best-Sellers of Pre-revolutionary France* (New York: W.W. Norton, 1995), although my views on this subject are clearly influenced by his other books and his teaching. On Diderot and on this subject more generally, see Angelica Goodden, *The Complete Lover: Eros, Nature, and Artifice in the Eighteenth-Century French Novel* (Oxford: Clarendon Press, 1989), p. 211 and passim.

117. Material in this and the following paragraph is from John Cannon, "Memoirs of the Birth, Education, Life, and Death of Mr. John Cannon. Some time Officer of the Excise and Writing Master at Mere Glastenbury and West Lyford in the County of Somerset, 1684–1742," Somerset Record Office, DD/ SAS C/1193/4, p. 41 (1700). My thanks again to my former student Tim Hitchcock

for sending me his transcript. On the popularity of *Aristotle's Master-Piece* and a general introduction to this guide to the business of reproduction, see Porter, "'Secrets of Generation Display'd'," pp. 5–7. There were at least twenty eighteenth-century English editions.

118. *Onania*, 8th. ed. (1723), pp. 17, vii, and throughout.

119. Tissot, *Three essays:... Second on Diseases Incidental to Literary and Sedentary Persons with proper Rules for preventing their full consequences...*, trans. M. Danes, pp. 31–35.

120. Bienville, *Nymphomania*, pp. 30 and 44.

121. That pornography is a prototypical form of the novel and not sharply differentiated from it in the eighteenth century is the central claim of Jean Marie Goulemot's *Forbidden Texts: Erotic Literature and Its Readers in Eighteenth-Century France*, trans. James Simpson (Philadelphia: University of Pennsylvania Press, 1994). The book was first published in France in 1991 with a title taken from Rousseau: *Ces livres qu'on ne lit que d'une main* (Those books which one only reads with one hand). Lynn Hunt in her introduction to *The Invention of Pornography* suggests that this is a distinctly gendered view. Bernadette Fort, "Accessories of Desire: On Indecency in a Few Paintings by Jean-Baptiste Greuze," *Yale French Studies* (special issue on libertinage and modernity) 94 (1998), allies herself solidly with those who argue that images like Greuze's *Lady Reading* and, by extension, even more explicit images of women erotically self-absorbed in literature are "timeless emblem[s] of femininity," "seductive icons" that "put men in the position of both interpreting and mastering her charms." See also Dennis, "Playing with Herself."

122. Darnton in a lecture said that he had seen evidence, to wit, stains, which he took to be semen, on the pages of books. These suggest, if not prove, that pornography was read with one hand by men in the eighteenth century. Women would leave no such traces, so their absence is not evidence that they did not read such works. Their use of pornography as an incitement to masturbation is a big theme in the pornography itself. See, for example, Darnton's discussion of *Thérèse philosophe* in Robert Darnton, *Forbidden Best-Sellers of Prerevolutionary France* (New York: W.W. Norton, 1993), pp. 96 and 222. There is textual evidence that, at the very least, women were represented not as passive sexual objects in pornography but as active agents who might have appealed to female readers. See Dorelies Kraakman, "Reading Pornography Anew: A Critical History of Sexual Knowledge for Girls in French Erotic Fiction, 1750–1840," *Journal of the History of Sexuality* 4.4 (1994). On the importance of the imagination in looking at images in Rousseau and Diderot, see Goodden, *Complete Lover*, p. 155.

123. The quotation is from Brewer, *Pleasures of the Imagination*, p. 103. The proportion of female to male readers of novels and of married to single — especially vulnerable — female readers is impossible to discover. A recent survey cautiously concludes that although there was a sizable female audience for fiction,

"eighteenth century women were not as early and widely addicted to novels as contemporary moralists asserted." See Jan Fergus, "Women Readers: A Case Study," in Vivien Jones (ed.), *Women and Literature in Britain, 1700–1800* (Cambridge, UK: Cambridge University Press, 2000), pp. 171–72.

124. Bernard Mandeville, *The Virgin Unmask'd; or, Female Dialogues Betwixt an Elderly Maiden Lady and Her Niece* (1709; London, 1724), cited in Barker-Benfield, *Culture of Sensibility*, p. 327. Barker-Benfield makes the connection to Marshall and says that Mandeville had wanted to support a fellow author prosecuted for spreading such female masturbation techniques. I have not followed up this claim.

125. I take these images, the quotation, and my view of absorbed reading in Dutch art from Svetlana Alpers, *The Art of Describing: Dutch Art in the Seventeenth Century* (Chicago: University of Chicago Press, 1983), pp. 192–94. The quotation is on p. 194.

126. See Peter Wagner, *Eros Revived: Erotica of the Enlightenment in England and America* (London: Martin and Secker, 1988), pp. 247 and 219.

127. For Dorat and an excellent discussion of the relationship between erotic text and image, see Philip Stewart, *Engraven Desire: Eros, Image, and Text in the French Eighteenth Century* (Durham, NC: Duke University Press, 1992), fig. 3.18, p. 100; fig. 6.4, 180; 8.12, 286; 3.17-98-99. Translation from Dorat as quoted in Stewart. For the place of Nerciat in the corpus of erotic literature, see Patrick Kearney, *A History of Erotic Literature* (n.p.: Dorset Press, 1993), pp. 83–86.

128. I am grateful to Michel Feher for this reformulation of my argument in response to an earlier draft of this chapter.

CHAPTER SIX: SOLITARY SEX IN THE TWENTIETH CENTURY

1. Habuto Eiji in *Tôkyô Nichinichi Shinbun*, 12 November 1913, cited in Frühstück, *Colonizing Sex: Sexology and Social Control in Modern Japan* (Berkeley: University of California Press, forthcoming 2003), p. 95.

2. Jean Laplanche and J.B. Pontalis, *The Language of Psycho-analysis* (1967; London: Karnac Books, 1988), p. 446. The full claim is this: "The origin of autoeroticism is thus considered to be that moment — recurring constantly rather than fixed at a certain time — when sexuality draws away from its natural object, finds itself delivered over to phantasy and in this very process is constituted qua sexuality." On narcissism, see Sigmund Freud, "Instincts" (1916–1917), in *Introductory Lectures*, vol. 10 of *The Standard Edition of the Complete Psychological Works of Sigmund Freud*, trans. James Strachey (London: Hogarth, 1953–74), p. 227.

3. See Ed Cohen, "(R)evolutionary Scenes: The Body Politic and the Political Body in Henry Maudsley's Nosology of "Masturbatory Insanity." *Nineteenth-Century Contexts* 11.2 (1987), p. 184; Arthur N. Gilbert, "Masturbation and Insanity: Henry Maudsley and the Ideology of Sexual Repression," *Albion* 12.3 (1980).

4. Hugh Northcote, *Christianity and Sex Problems*, 2nd rev. ed. (Philadelphia: F.A. Davis, 1916), pp. 35–36. F.A. Davis also published Havelock Ellis in the United States.

5. A.A. Brill, *Psychoanalysis: Its Theories and Practical Application* (Philadelphia: W.B. Saunders, 1922), pp. 146–47.

6. See Harry Oosterhuis, *Stepchildren of Nature: Krafft-Ebing, Psychiatry, and the Making of Sexual Identity* (Chicago: University of Chicago Press, 2000), for this benign and, I think, perceptive interpretation of a development that is usually interpreted far more negatively.

7. Schreber's world is well described in William G. Niederland, *The Schreber Case: Psychoanalytic Profile of a Paranoid Personality* (New York: Quadrangle Books, 1974); Thomas Smith Clouston's *Clinical Lectures on Mental Diseases* was not exceptional and still found an audience for its sixth edition (Philadelphia and New York: Lea Bros., 1904).

8. Cyril Bibby, *Sex Education: A Guide for Parents, Teachers, and Youth Leaders* (New York: Emerson Books, 1946). The latest edition of the book he mentions that I have seen is John Thompson, *Man and His Sexual Relations, including childhood, youth, manhood & married life, with the physiology and pathology of his reproductive organs*, 2 vols., new enl. ed. (South Cliff, Scarborough, UK, [1892?]). It is indeed retrograde, but I assume that Bibby is referring to some later popular rip-off.

9. Sigmund Freud, "On the Grounds for Detaching a Particular Syndrome from Neurasthenia Under the Description 'Anxiety Neurosis'" (1895), in *Complete Works*, vol. 3. Freud's views on this point were based on the interviews that a student, Felix Gattel, conducted with one hundred consecutive cases, among whom he found masturbation to be a common experience at the Vienna Psychiatric Hospital. See Makari, "Between Seduction and Libido," p. 643.

10. Sigmund Freud, "A Discussion of Masturbation: Concluding Remarks" (1911–1913), in *Complete Works*, vol. 12. The Hugo novel has not been traced, says the English editor James Strachey.

11. Dr. Pouillet, *Essai medico-philosophique sur les formes, les causes, les signes, les conséquences et le traitement de l'onanisme chez la femme* (Paris: Adrien Delahaye, 1876). I do not know who Pouillet was, but he was cited often during the next thirty years.

12. Bernard S. Talmey, *Woman: A Treatise on the Normal and Pathological Emotions of Feminine Love* (1904; New York: Practitioners' Publishing Company, 1908), pp. 1127–35. The author, a pathologist at Mothers and Babies Hospital in New York, regards masturbation in both sexes as a form of hyperesthesia; Iwan Bloch, *Das Sexualleben unserer Zeit in seinen Beziehungen zur modernen Kultur* (Berlin, 1908), published in English under the title *The Sexual Life of Our Time in Its Relations to Modern Civilization* (New York: Falstaff Press, 1937), p. 422.

13. G. Stanley Hall, *Life and Confessions of a Psychologist* (New York: D. Appleton and Co., 1924), pp. 132–34. Hall says that as a psychologist of adoles-

cent sexuality he owed readers an account of his own sexual coming of age. Tarnovski is presumably Veniamin Mikailovich Tarnovski, the author of *La Famille syphilitique et sa descendance; étude biologique* (Clermont: Diax, 1904). Hall, in short, thought of masturbation in the same context as hereditary syphilis.

14. G. Stanley Hall, *Adolescence: Its Psychology and Its Relations to Physiology, Anthropology, Sociology, Sex, Crime, Religion, and Education* (1904; New York: D. Appleton, 1924), vol. 1, pp. 432–53.

15. John F.W. Meagher, *A Study of Masturbation and the Psychosexual Life*, 3rd ed., reed. and rev. Smith Ely Jelliffe (Baltimore: W. Wood, 1936). Jelliffe was an internationally known biologist and the author of major university and high-school textbooks; Charles William Malchow, *The Sexual Life: Embracing the Natural Sexual Impulse* (Mosby: St. Louis, 1923), pp. 90–91; Charles William Malchow, *The sexual life embracing the natural sexual impulse, normal sexual habits and propagation; together with sexual physiology and hygiene*, 7th ed. (St. Louis: Mosby, 1931).

16. For the debate, see note 17 below. See Elizabeth Blackwell, *The Human Element in Sex: Being a Medical Enquiry into the Relation of Sexual Physiology to Christian Morality* (London: J.A. Churchill, 1885), pp. 26–27.

17. I am grateful to Leslie Hall of the Wellcome Library, who is working on a biography of Stella Browne, for suggesting that I look at this debate and telling me about its context. See Hall's "'I Have Never Met the Normal Woman': Stella Browne and the Politics of Womanhood," *Women's History Review* 6.2 (1996). See generally, Margaret Jackson, *The Real Facts of Life: Feminism and the Politics of Sexuality, c. 1850–1940* (Bristol, PA: Taylor and Francis, 1994). This debate goes on in almost every issue of the *Freewoman* for the first half of 1912; but especially on the question of insanity, see letters section for July 11 and July 18.

18. Stopes Collection, Wellcome Library, A 126, A 239, A 168.

19. Bloch, *Sexual Life of Our Time*, p. 411; Alan R. Mootnick and Elaine Baker, "Masturbation in Captive Hylobates (Gibbons)," *Zoo Biology* 13.4 (1994); F.B.M. de Waal, cited in Paul Abramson and Steven Pinkerton, *With Pleasure: Thoughts on the Nature of Human Sexuality* (New York: Oxford University Press, 1995), p. 25.

20. Elie Metchnikoff, *The Nature of Man: Studies in Optimistic Philosophy*, ed. P. Chalmers Mitchell (London: William Heinemann; New York: G.P. Putnam's Sons, 1903), pp. 95–99.

21. The anti-tight-clothes view was popularized by Bernhard Christoph Faust, *Wie der Geschlechtstrieb der Menschen in Ordnung zu bringen* (Braunschweig, 1791), intro. J.H. Campe, whom we have encountered before. Faust's views were everywhere in western Europe and the United States through his more popular *Health Catechism*, which went through scores of editions. For a general contemporary account of this new view, see Havelock Ellis, *Studies in the Psychology of Sex*, 3rd ed. (Philadelphia: F.A. Davis, 1920), vol. 1, pp. 161–277 in particular, although the whole section on autoeroticism is on point.

22. Ellis, *Studies in the Psychology of Sex*, vol. 1, pp. 261, 265–66, 274, 160–286 passim. Ellis's six-volume study began to appear in 1897.

23. Jones, *Free Associations*, pp. 57 and 219.

24. Auguste Forel, *The Sexual Question: A Scientific, Psychological, Hygienic, and Sociological Study*, trans. C.F. Marshall (New York: Physicians and Surgeons Book Co., 1906), pp. 228–34.

25. Hermann Rohleder, *Die Masturbation: Eine Monographie für Ärzte und Pädagogen* (Berlin, 1899).

26. See Oosterhuis, *Stepchildren of Nature*, pp. 70–71, 131–33, and passim. Masturbation figures as a repulsive and dangerous practice in many of Krafft-Ebing's case reports; see *Psychopathia Sexualis*, 7th ed., trans. Charles Gilbert Chaddock (Philadelphia: F.A. Davis, 1908), pp. 188–89.

27. I quote from Johannes Rutgers, *How to Attain and Practice the Ideal Sex Life*, trans. Norman Haire (New York: Cadillac Publishing Co. [1940]). Margaret Sanger very much admired Rutgers, a physician and editor of the Netherlands Medical Yearbook as well as the author of birth-control books and pamphlets translated into all European languages, as well as Esperanto.

28. This reading of the picture as an expression specifically of Schiele's castration anxiety and his masturbatory guilt as elements in his process of self-discovery is Danielle Knafo's, discussed in Magdalena Dabrowski and Rudolf Leopold, *Egon Schiele: The Leopold Collection, Vienna* (New York: Museum of Modern Art, 1997), p. 17; see figure 9 in this catalog. It is not the only image of masturbation in this artist's works, and I do not take it as characteristic of his views on the subject, if indeed he had any. This image is pretty clearly about female power and self-possession through autoeroticism although there is no title to that effect. What otherwise is she doing with her finger; what otherwise are we to make of her look?

29. *Ibid.*, plate 148, p. 334, as being about autoerotic power, but the image seems fairly straightforward about that. What, otherwise, is she doing with her finger?

30. The phrase is Joyce McDougall's, *Theatres of the Mind: Illusion and Truth on the Psychoanalytic Stage* (London: Free Association Books, 1986), p. 250.

31. This original, and, I think, correct, claim about how masturbation bridges seduction and libido theory is made by Makari, "Between Seduction and Libido."

32. This point is Richard Wollheim's in *Sigmund Freud* (New York: Viking, 1971), p. 20.

33. Sigmund Freud, *Studies on Hysteria*, in *Complete Works*, vol. 2, III, p. 3.

34. *The Complete Letters of Sigmund Freud to Wilhelm Fliess, 1887–1904*, trans. and ed. Jeffrey Masson (Cambridge, MA: Belknap Press of Harvard University Press, 1985), pp. 338 and 390 as discussed in Makari, "Between Seduction and Libido," p. 654.

35. Makari, "Between Seduction and Libido," p. 661; all of this comes from the Dora case, *Fragments of an Analysis of a Case of Hysteria*, in *Complete Works*, vol. 7.

36. Sigmund Freud, *General Theory of Neurosis*, in *Complete Works*, vol. 16, p. 309.

37. Sigmund Freud, "'Civilized' Sexual Morality and Modern Nervous Illness" (1908), in *Complete Works*, vol. 9, p. 187. Here he still thinks that the pressures come largely from outside. Later he will place more emphasis on the superego. In either case masturbation is a critical site of sublimation.

38. *Ibid.*, pp. 187–89 and 198–99; Sigmund Freud, "On the Universal Tendency to Debasement in Love," in *Complete Works*, vol. 11, p. 182 and "The Psychology of Love I: A Special Type of Object Choice Made by Men," in *Complete Works*, vol. 9, p. 172.

39. Sigmund Freud, *Three Essays on Sexuality* (1905), in *Complete Works*, vol. 7, pp. 180–82, 189–90, 219–21, and 234.

40. *Ibid.*; *New Introductory Lectures* (1932), in *Complete Works*, vol. 22, pp. 118 and 128. I have omitted a discussion of Freud's account of the amnesia of infantile masturbation, which is the paradigmatic form of infantile amnesia and explains why guilt in neurotics is attached to memories of some masturbatory activities, as well as the role of masturbation in hysteria, obsession, and other neuroses, because it is not crucial to the metapsychological story Freud is telling when he describes the clitoris-to-vagina transfer. For a more general account of this, see my "Amor Veneris, vel Dulcedo Appeletur," in Michel Feher with Ramona Naddaff and Nadia Tazi (eds.), *Zone 5: Fragments for a History of the Human Body* (New York: Zone Books, 1989).

41. Laura Hutton, *The Single Woman and Her Emotional Problems* (London: Baillière, Tindall and Cox, 1937), pp. 84–85.

42. André Green, *On Private Madness* (London: Karnac Books, 1997), p. 132.

43. D.M. Dunlop et al., *Textbook of Medical Treatment*, 2nd ed. (Edinburgh: E. and S. Livingston, 1943). I have looked at a number of English and German textbooks that follow this model, but one would have to do a more thorough survey to track the acceptance of Freudian views. It is probably an uneven development. For example, in Frederick W. Price, ed., *A Textbook of the Practice of Medicine* (London: Henry Frowde and Hodder, 1926), pp. 1609–10, published in the prestigious Oxford Medical Publications series, there is a combination of what strikes us as old-fashioned, if in new language — "autointoxication from the genital glands" — and contemporary: "Psychoanalysis may sometimes prove of use in revealing the cause of" epochal disorders, although other causes should be considered before one turns to sexual ones. Other books in the same series have more in common with Dunlop. See, for example, Henry A. Christian, *Psychiatry for Practitioners* (New York: Oxford University Press, 1927), pp. 140–41.

44. For the older view, which harks back to late-nineteenth-century texts and forward into the late 1920s, see Arthur Preuss, *A Handbook of Moral Theology*, 3rd ed. (1918; St. Louis and London: Herder, 1928), pp. 73–77. This book is based on Anton Koch, *Lehrbuch der Moraltheologie*, the earliest edition of which I could find was 1905. For a history of the subject and the "contemporary view,"

see Charles E. Curran, *Contemporary Problems in Moral Theology* (Notre Dame, IN: Fides Publishers, 1970), pp. 161–76; the part on integration of the personality is on p. 176; On "conjugal onanism," that is, birth control, see John C. Ford and Gerald Kelly, *Marriage Questions* (Westminster, MD: Newman Press, 1964), pp. 259–61 and 270–71ff.; John C. Ford and Gerald Kelly, *Contemporary Moral Theology* (Westminster, MD: Newman Press, 1958), pp. 230 and 233–39. There follows a fascinating discussion of the role of psychology in pastoral practice on questions of sexuality. On moral pedagogy, see Bernard Häring, *The Law of Christ*, trans. Edwin G. Kaiser (Westminster, MD: Newman Press, 1966), p. 304; Ernie Zimbelman, *Human Sexuality and Evangelical Christians* (Lanham, MD: University Press of America, 1985), p. 306.

45. See José Pierre, ed., *Investigating Sex: Surrealist Research, 1928–1932*, trans. Malcolm Imrie (London: Verso, 1994), pp. 6–7, 22–23, 29, 33, 103, and passim. On Duchamp, see Amelia Jones, *Postmodernism and the En-gendering of Marcel Duchamp* (Cambridge, UK: Cambridge University Press, 1994), pp. 196–98.

46. These are the famous words of hope from the last paragraph of Foucault's introduction to the history of sexuality.

47. Joyce McDougall, *Theatres of the Mind: Illusion and Truth on the Psychoanalytic Stage* (London: Free Association Books, 1986), p. 250, see also 101; R.D. Hinselwood, *A Dictionary of Klinean Thought* (London: Free Association Press, 1991), entry: "masturbation phantasies"; Helen Deutsch, *The Psychology of Women* (New York: Gruen and Stratton, 1944), vol. 1, p. 87. Deutsch also thought that the guilt associated with masturbation could inhibit reproduction and make conception more difficult. See *ibid.*, vol. 2, p. 140.

48. Martha Shelley, "Lesbianism and the Women's Liberation Movement," in Barbara A. Crow (ed.), *Radical Feminism: A Documentary Reader* (New York: New York University Press, 2000), p. 307, originally published in 1970. Morton Hunt, *Sexual Behavior in the 1970s* (New York: Playboy Press, 1974), pp. 100 and 72.

49. On "J." and the publishing history of her books, see Terry Garrity and John Garrity, *Story of "J"* (New York: William Morrow, 1984). The first and most important by far is *The Sensuous Woman; The First How-to Book for the Female Who Yearns to Be All Woman* (New York: L. Stuart, 1969).

50. Naomi McCormick, *Sexual Salvation: Affirming Women's Sexual Rights and Pleasures* (Westport, CT: Praeger, 1994), for example, makes this explicit.

51. Anne Koedt, *The Myth of the Vaginal Orgasm*, in Crow, *Radical Feminism*, pp. 372 and 377; originally published in 1970.

52. Lonnie Barbach, *For Each Other: Sharing Sexual Intimacy* (Garden City, NY: Anchor Books, 1983), pp. 184–85. Betty Dodson, *Liberating Masturbation: A Meditation on Self Love* (New York: Bodysex Designs, 1974). "I had visions of the redemption of masturbation in a fashionable Madison Avenue Gallery," writes Dodson having finally persuaded her models to pose while "jerking off" — far more difficult than getting anyone to pose having intercourse — and the gallery owner to show the resulting four pictures. See p. 11 on this adventure.

494

53. Seneca, *Letters to Lucilius* 23.4, quoted in Michel Foucault, *History of Sexuality: The Care of the Self* (New York: Pantheon, 1986), pp. 66–67. I am grateful to Michel Feher for pointing out this link.

54. Federation of Feminist Women's Health Centers, *A New View of a Woman's Body: A Fully Illustrated Guide*, illustrations by Suzann Gage, photographs by Sylvia Morales (West Hollywood, CA: Feminist Health Press, 1991).

55. Rebecca Chalker, *The Clitoral Truth: The Secret World at Your Fingertips* (New York: Seven Stories Press, 2000).

56. On this moment in lesbian sexual politics, see Lillian Faderman, "The Return of Butch and Femme: A Phenomenon in Lesbian Sexuality of the 1980s and 1990s," *Journal of the History of Sexuality* 2.4 (April 1992), especially the interview with Susie Bright, formerly sex-advice columnist in *On Our Backs*, p. 582. An odd little 1960s book that claims to have been written by a psychotherapist says that based on her patients it is a "ridiculous idea" that women are not aroused by pornography: "I have yet to meet a woman who is not." Although she says she sees mostly lesbians, the pornography she speaks of is heterosexual. See Yvonne Johanet, *I, Lesbian* (North Hollywood, CA: Brandon House, 1964), p. 34. This book is part of a large collection of lesbian fiction in the Duke University Library Sexuality Collection; it presents itself as being a first-person, true-to-life account.

57. This clearly only scratches the surface of the subject. There are lots of collections of porn intended for women in any bookshop. I surveyed all the issues of *On Our Backs* available in the Duke Sexuality Collection, but my examples are drawn from the following: Summer 1984, p. 23; Summer 1987, p. 12; the masturbation scene as part of S/M fiction is in Spring 1988, p. 35.

58. So says the label in the Tate Modern, which discussed Acconci's work in the context of the New York art world of the 1970s.

59. I want to thank my daughter Hannah Laqueur for first alerting me to Acconci. See Lucy Soutter, "Community vs. Context in the Reception of Eleanor Antin's Retrospective," presented at the Eighty-ninth College Art Association conference in Chicago, Feb. 28 – March 3, 2001, at http://web.ukonline. co.uk/n.paradoxa/2001panel4.htm. Interview on Feb. 21, 2001, at http:// kunst.no/kit2001/Kate_Fowle/kate_fowle.html.

60. Her home page is at http://gatesofheck.com/annie. She may be moving in a more spiritual direction if her recent collaboration with the "erospiritualist" and teacher of male masturbation Joseph Kramer is any indication. For an account of her remarkable career, follow the links on her home page, or see Annie Sprinkle, *Post-Porn Modernist: My 25 Years as a Multimedia Whore*, rev. ed. (San Francisco: Cleis Press, 1998).

61. Amelia Jones, "Sexual Politics: Feminist Strategies, Feminist Conflicts, Feminist Histories," p. 32, and Susan Kandel, "Beneath the Green Veil: The Body in/of New Feminist Art," pp. 191–92, in Amelia Jones (ed.), *Sexual Politics: Judy Chicago's "Dinner Party" in Feminist Art History* (Berkeley: University of

California Press, 1996). I am grateful to Elizabeth Dungan for allowing me to use, and quote from, an unpublished interview she conducted with Zoe Leonard on January 13, 2002. Readers can get a sense of how Leonard's series of photographs of female genitals installed between eighteenth-century portraits look at http://www.icca.ro/artelier/nr5/roxana_marcocia.html.

62. See Jean-Jacques Lebel, "Picasso's (Erotic) Gaze," in Jean Clair (ed.), *Picasso Erotique* (New York: Prestel, 2001), p. 67 and passim. I have not seen the video. A number of the images in the enormous Tate exhibit *Surrealism: Desire Unbound* support the claim. See the catalog *Surrealism: Desire Unbound*, ed. Jennifer Mundy (London: Tate Publishing Company, 2001). Unfortunately, the catalogue does not have an image of Dalí's guilt-stricken illustration for the frontispiece to Georges Hugnet's *Onan*.

63. On Benglis, the best thing I have read is an unpublished paper by Cherie Caswell, Dec. 8, 1993, written for Professor Anne Wagner's graduate seminar. Caswell makes the point about double masturbation, which she then gives a Lacanian explanation.

64. John R. Burger, *One-Handed Histories: The Eroto-Politics of Gay Male Video Pornography* (New York: Haworth Press, 1995), pp. x, 30, and passim.

65. Joanie Blank (ed.), *First Person Sexual* (San Francisco: Down There Press, 1996).

66. Amy Scholder (ed.), *Fever: The Art of David Wojnarowicz* (New York: Rizzoli, 1999), pp. 7 and 116–17 and passim. Richard Marshall, *Robert Mapplethorpe* (New York: Whitney Museum, 1990), p. 66.

67. In fact, Elder was concerned about the ignorance and prejudice that surrounded discussion of masturbation although this was not part of the public discussion at the time of her firing. In an on-line magazine interview/article called "Mword" she is quoted as saying that a friend, a senior citizen, had written her asking that she tell children about masturbation. This friend had spent her youth in the agonies of fear that she would go blind from her secret practices but after consideration decided that this would be a better option than stopping. Elders responded that her mandate had been to tell "children the truth about their bodies and sex," a truth that many were afraid of. http://www.nerve.com/Elder/mword. See *Washington Post*, Dec. 12, 1994, p. A20; *Wall Street Journal*, Dec. 12, 1994; *New York Times*, Dec. 18, 1994, p. 15.

68. See for a summary the site "Masturbation in Film" and the linked site "The Internet Movie Database." Barbarella does enjoy — burns up — the orgasm machine run by the mad scientist; Nadia, the Czech exchange student in *American Pie*, masturbates looking at the main character's porn magazines and suffers no humiliation. But in general masturbation is that rare thing in modern talk about sexuality: something best left unspoken and so discomforting that it can only be broached under the protection of a joke. If there is a taboo topic in our culture, this may be it.

69. http://www.jackinworld.com.

Index

499

Marshall, John, 341.
Marten, John, 29–30, 32, 44, 85, 173, 207, 261, 336–37. *See also Onania.*
Martial, 99, 106, 109–10.
Masters, William, and Virginia Johnson, 74–75, 77, 402.
Mather, Cotton, 34.
Maudsley, Henry, 363–64.
Maxwell, Herbert, 316.
McAllister, Dawson, 417.
McDougall, Joyce, 72, 397–98.
Meagher, John, 371–72.
Medicine, and masturbation, 40–41, 83–95, 186, 192ff., 271–73; to "cure" masturbation, 15–16, 25–26, 33, 34, 44–47.
Melendy, Mary Ries, 230.
Menuret de Chambaud, Jean Jacques, 37, 212–13.
Metchnikoff, Elie, 67.
Millett, Kate, 81.
Montaigne, Michel de, 168.
Montesquieu, Baron de, 279.
Moravia, Alberto, 68.
Musonius Rufus, 104.

NACHMANIDES, 123.
Nauman, Bruce, 414.
Nearkos, 96, 97.
Nerciat, Andréa de, 355, *356.*
Nerves, and masturbation, 204–207.
Nietzsche, Friedrich, 67.
Nothnagel, Hermann, 364.
Nougaret, P.J.B., *353.*
Novels, 269, 303, 306, 316, 320–30. *See also* Reading.
Nymphomania, 215, 262, 263.

ONAN, story of, 15, 20, 35, 42, 47, 112–17, 119, 125–35.
Onania: 13–16, 25–37; authorities cited in, 84–85; date of, 179, 249; epistolary style of, 272, 324–26; on excess, 261–62; on homosexuality, 256–57; on imagination, 211; on secrecy, 224, 232.

Onania Examined, 30–32, 261.
Onanism (L'Onanisme). See Tissot, Samuel Auguste David.
Onanism, coinage of term, 35.
Ostervald, J.F., 170.
Our Bodies, Ourselves, 75–77, 400.
d'Outremont, Phillippe, 167.
Ovid, 107.

PAGET, SIR JAMES, 17.
Parker, Henry, 33, 170.
Paul of Hungary, 151–52.
Penitentials, 141–42, 145–47.
Pepys, Samuel, 180–82, 334.
Péret, Benjamin, 396.
Peter Damian, 148–51.
Peter Lombard, 151.
Philo of Alexandria, 126.
Picasso, Pablo, 411.
Pleasure, sexual, 138–40, 154, 189–92.
Pliny, 86–87, 220–21.
Pollution, 35, 117–18, 169–70, 171–74.
Pontalis, J.B., 360.
Pope, Alexander, 108.
Pornography, 309, 330–57.
Porter, Roy, 8.
Print culture, 25ff., 303, 308–11.
Privacy, 225–26. *See also* Secrecy.
Progrès du Libertinage, Le, 347, *353.*
Protestantism, and masturbation, 126–30, 253–54.
Proudhon, Pierre-Joseph, 257.

QUENEAU, RAYMOND, 396.

RARE VERITIES, 30.
Ray, Isaac, 316–17.
Raymond of Peñafort, 139.
Reading, 302–17, 320–58. *See also* Novels.
Reubens, Paul, 63.
Rohleder, Hermann, 379–80.
Roman culture, masturbation in, 96, 99, 104–107.
Romano, Giulio, 308.
Roth, Philip, 361.

Designed by Bruce Mau with Julie Fry
Typeset by Archetype
Printed by Bowne of Toronto on Sebago acid-free paper
Bound by Acme Bookbinding

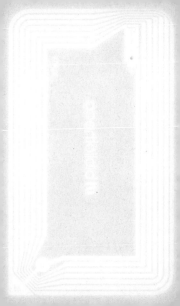